Assessing Children's Vision: A Handbook

Assessing Children's Vision

A Handbook

Susan J. Leat PhD
Assistant Professor, School of Optometry, University of Waterloo, Ontario, Canada

Rosalyn H. Shute PhD
Senior Lecturer, School of Psychology, The Flinders University of South Australia; Visiting Psychologist, Women's and Children's Hospital, Adelaide, South Australia

Carol A. Westall PhD
Director of Visual Electrophysiology Unit, Department of Ophthalmology, Hospital for Sick Children; Associate Professor, University of Toronto, Toronto, Ontario, Canada

Order of authorship is alphabetical

With a chapter on Visual Acuity by Kathryn Saunders PhD
School of Biomedical Sciences, University of Ulster, Coleraine, Northern Ireland

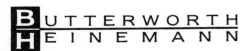

OXFORD   AUCKLAND   BOSTON   JOHANNESBURG   MELBOURNE   NEW DELHI

Butterworth-Heinemann
Linacre House, Jordan Hill, Oxford OX2 8DP
225 Wildwood Avenue, Woburn, MA 01801-2041
A division of Reed Educational and Professional Publishing Ltd

A member of the Reed Elsevier plc group

First published 1999

British Library Cataloguing in Publication Data

Leat, Susan
    Assessing children's vision: a handbook
    1. Pediatric opthalmology   2. Pediatric optometry   3. Vision –
    Testing
    I. Title   II. Shute, Rosalyn H.   III. Westall, Carol A.
    618.9′2′09775

Library of Congress Cataloguing in Publication Data

Leat Susan J.
    Assessing children's vision: a handbook/Susan J. Leat, Rosalyn
    H. Shute, Carol A. Westall; with a chapter on Visual acuity by
    Kathryn Saunders.
    p.   cm.
    Includes bibliographical references and index.
    ISBN 0 7506 0584 7
    1. Vision disorders in children – Diagnosis – Handbooks, manuals,
    etc.   2. Vision – Testing – Handbooks, manuals, etc.   I. Shute,
    Rosalyn H.   II. Westall, Carol A.   III. Title.
    [DNLM: 1. Vision Disorders – in infancy & childhood.   2. Vision
    Disorders – diagnosis.   3. Vision Tests – in infancy & childhood.
    4. Vision Tests – methods.   WW 600 L438a]
    RE48.2.C5L413
    618.92′0977075–dc21   98–10424
                                                            CIP

ISBN 0 7506 0584 7

Printed and bound in Great Britain by Martins the Printers, Berwick on Tweed

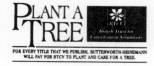

Contents

Foreword

The current interest in the measurement and management of vision in children is relatively new amongst optometrists. To an outsider, it may seem surprising that the science of optometry, arguably several hundreds of years old, has for so long neglected the youngest and most vulnerable members of our population. The explanation is simple: we had to wait until the revolutionary development of techniques (most notably Preferential Looking) which allow us to assess vision in non-communicating subjects. Once the techniques became feasible, researchers and practitioners could begin to understand the ways in which vision develops in children. And it is only when we know the rate and manner in which the system progresses in the normal case that we can begin to identify and then to manage the defects which can arise.

When the authors and I began to work in this field, we had to learn the techniques as we went along, by trial and, I'm sure often, by error. The present and future generations of optometrists are much luckier; they now have the present volume, among others, to guide them in their pursuit of this vital knowledge. The student and the established practitioner will find in this book not only the experimental data so important in clinical science but also the step-by-step instructions on how to carry out the new procedures. Furthermore, we have to avoid treating the child as simply 'a pair of young eyes': this book deals with the whole child, including their feelings and fears. Children with all forms of disabilities are much more at risk of eye disorders than are the general paediatric population; these children need our skills all the more. This book puts great emphasis on our understanding of multiple disabilities and the complex needs of children with visual and other problems.

Our learning is by no means over. There is so much more we have yet to discover about visual development, and how we, as clinical researchers and practitioners, can ameliorate the effects of abnormal development. There will always be children who need our skills and we, the professionals, have a duty to continue the learning process. I hope this book will encourage as many as possible to join us in this exciting journey.

J. Margaret Woodhouse
Cardiff, UK

Preface

The idea of writing this handbook of child visual assessment originated several years ago, when we were all working in the School of Optometry, University of Wales, College of Cardiff. We came to realize that we had a very fruitful combination of expertise in the field of children's vision. Dr Susan Leat is an optometrist with particular interests in low vision and special needs populations, Dr Carol Westall an optometrist specializing in eye movements, strabismus and electrophysiology and Dr Rosalyn Shute a psychologist with expertise in children, health issues and vision care. In Cardiff, we were all involved in research, clinical practice and teaching, and these domains of activity were mutually influential. For example, our undergraduate and postgraduate students would undertake research on issues suggested by our clinical practice, and findings would feed back into that practice and into future teaching. One of our former students, Dr Kathryn Saunders, has contributed a chapter to this book as well as the delightful illustrations; we hope that these will not only be informative, but serve to humanize the material.

In Cardiff, we worked together in the Visual Assessment Unit, which included a children's clinic known colloquially as the 'infant clinic' because the majority of the children were at the lower end of the age range. This book similarly gives great emphasis to the early months and years of life as being crucial in terms of future visual functioning. We also devoted a weekly clinic to less routine cases, where we saw many infants, children and adults with special needs, who so often seem to fall through the net in terms of vision care services. We must thank our former Cardiff colleague, Dr Margaret Woodhouse, for her enthusiastic work in this area. Providing quality vision care for children with disabilities is a central concern of ours, and this is reflected by the fact that special needs issues are fully integrated into the various chapters of this book, rather than being given a single, separate section.

In some respects it was sad when our team became dispersed around the world in 1991, Susan and Carol taking up new posts in Canada and Rosalyn in Australia. However, several years of work in new countries and new clinical, teaching and research settings have undoubtedly been of great benefit in terms of further broadening the experience we have been able to bring to this book. Furthermore, we have not assumed that our readers are based in any particular country, but have discussed issues of practice in a way that is applicable to a range of industrialized nations, making the book international in its scope and approach.

Although this handbook has been basically written for the optometry profession we have gone to some trouble to make it accessible to a wider readership. We anticipate that the core readership will consist of students of optometry and experienced optometrists who are new to working with young children. Students should be able to make use of the handbook right from the beginning of their professional training as we have included some basic material about the visual system and provided brief definitions and explanations of various technical terms, especially early in the book. In addition, each of the chapters begins with a brief introduction to the topic in hand. In this way, we hope that the book will also be accessible to others who might find the material (or parts of it) of interest, such as special needs teachers and parents of children with low vision or other disabilities. Much of the book will also be of value to non-optometrist eye professionals, such as ophthalmologists and orthoptists (or students working in these fields). Physicians seeking further information about children's vision care should also find the book of value. We have indicated a few places where we believe the material could be skipped over by knowledgeable eye professionals or where the non-specialist reader may wish to turn to other sources for further information.

The opening chapters provide a background for those that follow. We begin with a brief description of early child development and the development of the eye and visual system. We also consider the development of children with disabilities and the effect on development when a child has low or absent vision, whether this occurs in isolation or in association with other impairments. We stress the importance of early visual assessment for all children and summarize some of the main risk factors for oculovisual problems. We have also emphasized the importance of effective communication with children and their parents: all the technical skill in the world will be ineffective if we cannot take an adequate history and gain a child's confidence, and we have presented practical (but research-based) ideas for achieving this. Various aspects of the oculovisual examination are then detailed, including assessing signs and symptoms, ocular health and refractive status. A brief chapter on general principles of psychophysical testing of children paves the way for subsequent chapters on the measurement of visual functions, including visual acuity, contrast sensitivity, binocularity, visual fields, colour vision and eye movements. We have also included a chapter on electrophysiological testing.

The final chapter focuses upon implementing management plans on the basis of the information gained from assessment. The importance of collaborating with other workers involved with the child is emphasized. We believe it is a strength of our book that the information and advice we have presented are solidly research-based, although we have blended this with our clinical experience and, above all, have aimed to produce a *practical* book. We have also introduced some topics which are increasingly impinging upon children's eye care, including child abuse and ethical and legal issues. Overall, we would describe our view of child vision care as a holistic one.

There are some issues which we have not covered extensively. These include children's learning and reading disabilities and the broad area of vision training (although broadly accepted principles of orthoptic training are mentioned in Chapter 14). Our reasons for excluding these are that we have concerned ourselves with topics which we consider clearly within the scope of optometry and which can be substantiated by good research. We have also focused upon topics in which we have personal expertise. For the latter reason, we have not covered contact lens prescription in any depth.

We decided upon alphabetical order of authorship to reflect the fact that we have contributed equally to the book. We shared authorship of the three introductory chapters and the last one. Carol and Susan jointly wrote the chapters on ocular health and contrast sensitivity. Carol wrote the chapters on binocular vision, eye movements and electrophysiology, Susan wrote those on refraction and visual fields and Rosalyn wrote those on psychophysical testing and colour vision. However, we offered extensive suggestions on each others' work and Rosalyn was primarily responsible for integrating and editing the various contributions. Kathryn Saunders wrote the acuity chapter. It is no easy matter to co-ordinate a project of this scale with the contributors and publisher spread across three continents. Electronic mail proved invaluable, and we are deeply grateful to Caroline Makepeace and her colleagues at Butterworth-Heinemann for their encouragement and patience.

We would also like to acknowledge a number of people who read and made suggestions about portions of the text. These include: Anthony Cullen (Department of Optometry, University of Waterloo); Jeff Hovis (Department of Optometry, University of Waterloo), who also provided Fig. 7:1; Steve Kraft (Hospital for Sick Children, Toronto); Alex Levin (Hospital for Sick Children, Toronto), Carole Panton OC (C) (Hospital for Sick Children, Toronto), Steffan Shute, LLB (Hons); Marlee Spafford, OD, FAAO (Department of Optometry, University of Waterloo); Kathryn Saunders (School of Biomedical Sciences, University of Ulster); Elen Shute (for editorial assistance); the editorial services of the Hospital for Sick Children, Toronto; Bill and Eileen Westall (for proofreading assistance). Any errors remain, of course, our responsibility. Finally, we would like to thank Margaret Woodhouse most warmly for her enthusiastic involvement in the conception of this book.

Susan Leat, Waterloo, Canada
Rosalyn Shute, Adelaide, Australia
Carol Westall, Toronto, Canada

The developing child and visual system

INTRODUCTION

In this introductory chapter we provide a broad overview of children's general development and the development of the visual system. We also consider how general development is affected when a child has a visual impairment.

We begin by providing an outline of children's early development, establishing the central role that vision normally plays. The anatomy of the eye and visual system are then described. Knowledgeable eye practitioners may pass over the material on definitions of ocular components and basic eye anatomy and function; these sections have been included with the aim of making the book accessible to interested non-specialist readers. The sections on the anatomy and function of the visual pathway may, however, be of value to practitioners who are unfamiliar with the recent research evidence to which we have referred. The remainder of the chapter addresses issues of atypical development, and describes how children's development is affected by poor or absent vision, whether this occurs in isolation or in association with other sensory, motor or intellectual impairments.

THE DEVELOPING CHILD

The relevance of child development to vision care

Traditionally, eye professionals have not been expected to know a great deal about general child development. Such knowledge is becoming of increasing clinical value, however, as specially designed children's tests enable the assessment of various visual functions at ever earlier ages. Those who are accustomed to clinical work with adults may at first be puzzled and frustrated by children's unusual and sometimes uncooperative reactions. The vision care of children can, however, become deeply satisfying when our clinical practice is underpinned by a broad understanding of child development.

A knowledge of how children at various stages of development are likely to respond, what it is reasonable to expect of them and how best to communicate with them and their parents all contribute to effective vision care. An awareness of developmental milestones enables the practitioner to organize the testing situation in a way which takes account of an infant's capabilities and to appreciate when a child's development is delayed. It is also invaluable to have some understanding of the integral part that vision plays in a child's general development, especially in the formative early months. A recognition of how the 'developmental tasks' facing a child change over time gives context to visual assessment, so that the meaning of vision (and visual impairment) for the child's present and future functioning is apparent. This is important both for the child who is developing in a typical way and for the child whose development is atypical, for example, as a result of hearing impairment or low birth weight.

Typical development

What is development?

It is not a straightforward matter to conceptualize the myriad changes that occur during childhood, and many different developmental theories have been proposed. One way of looking at development is to conceive of people at various stages of life as facing certain developmental tasks which are determined by a combination of biological and environmental (including cultural) forces. These forces shape the emerging self, which in turn becomes an additional impetus for change (Havighurst, 1972). The tasks of infants (as outlined below) are probably universal, whereas those listed here for older children are particularly influenced by Western industrialized societies.

The infant's tasks include acquiring motor skills (such as walking) and forming concepts and learning language to describe social and physical reality; close relationships with caregiving figures such as parents are needed at this time when the child is immature both physically and in terms of understanding 'how the world works'. The older child's tasks include learning more advanced physical skills for games, building a positive self-concept and good peer relationships, developing basic literacy and numeracy skills and concepts necessary for everyday living, achieving independence in performing personal tasks and developing attitudes towards social groups and institutions. During adolescence, tasks include developing an ideology and more mature peer relationships, accepting one's physique, preparing for a career and achieving socially responsible behaviour and emotional independence from parents. Tasks for later stages of life have also been outlined, but the only ones that need concern us here are the parental tasks of rearing children and guiding them towards becoming happy and responsible adults. Although Havighurst's approach to development is descriptive rather than explanatory (Sugarman, 1986), it is useful in several ways.

First, it provides a brief guide to the kinds of developmental issues likely to be relevant for a child of a particular age. Secondly, it enables us to see the child, even in infancy, not as a passive, randomly-behaving entity, but as striving towards particular goals (and, as we shall see later, vision normally plays a central role in achieving many of these). This view of the child also means that he or she is not a passive recipient of our vision-testing procedures, but actively interprets what happens and responds in ways which influence test outcomes. A third advantage of Havighurst's view is that it involves the notion that tasks build upon one another in a hierarchical fashion: developmental tasks need to be successfully accomplished to lead to happiness and success with later tasks, while failure leads to unhappiness, social disapproval and difficulty with later tasks. For example, an infant whose early language development is impeded for some reason will face problems later in learning to read, which may in turn lead to poor general academic achievement, low self-esteem and lack of career opportunities later in life. This notion of the hierarchical organization of developmental tasks gives a sense of the importance of early visual or more general developmental problems for the later life of the child.

Now that a broad framework for understanding development has been established, some specific aspects will be outlined. Emphasis is given to the early months of rapid change, a time when visual problems can fundamentally affect general development as well as later visual functioning. Throughout this section, some implications of stage of development for vision testing are also mentioned, a theme which will be carried further in Chapter 3. The amount of detail given here is necessarily limited, but those interested in further reading will find many introductory texts on child development to choose from (e.g. Berk, 1997).

Infants' sleeping patterns, personality and mood

Although it often seems to weary new parents that their offspring do not sleep enough, the phrase 'sleeping like a baby' is well justified considering that the average newborn sleeps 18 to 20 hours a day. It may therefore be difficult to catch a very young infant awake for vision testing, although Buncic (1983) reports that it is sometimes possible to carry out certain important examination procedures on a sleeping infant: these are retinoscopy (which determines any need for a spectacle correction) and fundoscopy (examination of the back of the eye). Gradually, infants spend more time in a state of alert inactivity, when a good response to testing of any kind is likely (Helms and Turner, 1981). By a month old, the baby will be spending about 20 hours a week in this alert but inactive state.

Infants have individual patterns of wakefulness, and also seem to differ in personality right from birth, some being more 'fussy' than others and therefore harder to examine (Kagan, Rosnik and Snidman, 1988). Most babies will not be very happy when a meal is due and some object to wet and dirty nappies. When making an appointment for vision testing, parents will be able to say when the child is likely to be at his or her best. A really infant-friendly practice or clinic would have somewhere for babies to be fed and changed. A child who is under the weather will not respond well and a rescheduled appointment is advisable for the sake of all concerned.

Motor development

Infants reach motor milestones during the first year or so in a sequence which is almost invariable, although there is considerable variability in timing, especially for the later milestones, such as walking, which can occur several months earlier or later than average (Bayley, 1969). For the gross motor skills described below, we have indicated both average age and and the age by which 90% of infants have reached each milestone. It is important to remember that there is a great degree of individual variation, but serious delay in several motor skills would be a cause for concern.

When a newborn baby (neonate) is held upright, the head is floppy, but by an average of 6 weeks it is held erect and steady (90% of infants achieve this skill by 4 months, Figure 1.1). Sitting alone is achieved at an average of 7 months, with 90% able to do so by 9 months (Figure 1.2). Crawling also first occurs at an average of 7 months, with 90% doing so by 11 months (Figure 1.3), although some infants omit the crawling stage. Infants are able to pull themselves up into a standing position (by grasping furniture) by an average of 8 months, with 90% able to do so by a year (Figure 1.4). Standing alone is achieved at an average of 11 months, with 90% able to do so by 16 months (Figure 1.5). Walking alone generally occurs shortly before the first birthday, with 90% doing so by 17 months. During the second year further motor skills develop, such as stooping, running, jumping and being able to kick a ball (Figure 1.6).

Vision testing during these months is best carried out with the child sitting on an adult's lap (Figure 1.1) although some toddlers will like to sit on a chair alone as long as a parent is nearby. The infant's head will have to be supported (under the chin) in the early weeks to direct

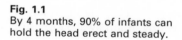

Fig. 1.1
By 4 months, 90% of infants can hold the head erect and steady.

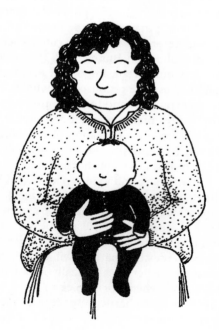

Fig. 1.2
By 9 months, 90% of infants can sit
without support.

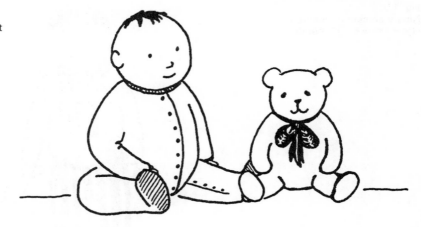

Fig. 1.3
By 11 months, 90% of infants
are able to crawl.

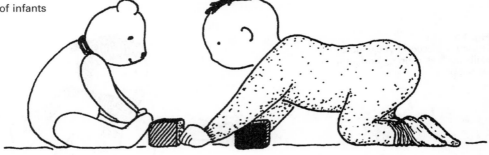

Fig. 1.4
By the first birthday, most infants
can pull themselves into a
standing position.

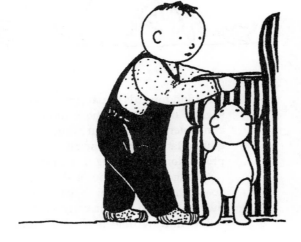

Fig. 1.5
Ninety percent of children can stand alone by 16 months.

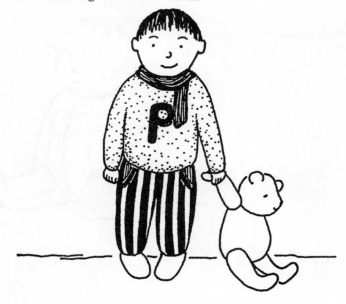

Fig. 1.6
During the second year, motor skills such as running and jumping develop.

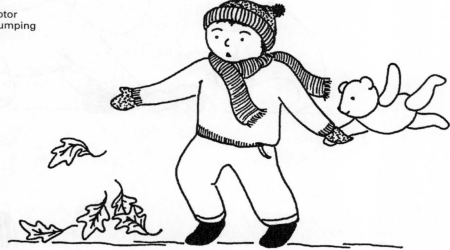

attention towards visual targets. Occasionally, with a young infant or a slightly older child whose motor development is delayed, it is most convenient to carry out some procedures with the child lying on an adult's lap or on a mat on the floor or table (taking suitable safety precautions) or sitting in a pushchair/stroller or wheelchair.

Changes in gross motor skills are paralleled by developing hand-eye co-ordination. Visual behaviour is initially independent of arm movements, and in the early weeks the infant will look at patterns and follow moving objects visually. Such behaviours offer ways of assessing infants' vision long before they can give verbal or pointing responses. Around 4 months, the infant will reach for objects but miss, but will grasp an object placed in the hand. These behaviours become co-ordinated at about 5 months, when the child will reach towards and grasp nearby objects. Around 9 months finer control of thumb and forefinger is developing, and pointing occurs around 11 months; it is possible to obtain pointing responses to vision tests from some infants around this time (Shute et al., 1990).

By the second birthday the child can throw a ball, build a tower of bricks, scribble, open a door and help in dressing and undressing. Toys in the waiting room can keep the active toddler amused, and are also useful for maintaining the child's attention to vision testing procedures in preference to other interesting aspects of the room.

Social and communicative development

The infant has the important task of learning to recognize and form attachments with a small number of caretaking figures and of laying the foundations for later communicative competence. Babies recognize their own parents from a young age; for example, the mother's voice is discriminated from that of a stranger within only 12 hours of birth (DeCaspar and Fifer, 1980).

Babies look at faces with interest from birth, although this attractiveness must result from patterns of contrast rather than detail given the immaturity of the newborn's visual system. Around 2 months the baby smiles at faces and this is very rewarding for parents, as is making eye contact with their baby.

The baby vocalizes when talked to at about 3 months, and 'pseudo-conversations' between parent and child occur long before the baby uses actual words. The child therefore learns at a very early age the important concept of turn-taking in interactions (Schaffer, 1989).

In these early months, although the baby can distinguish familiar from new people, all are responded to in a friendly manner. Later, around 8 months, crying occurs in the absence of an attachment figure and wariness of strangers develops (Sroufe and Waters, 1977); these self-protective behaviours continue for many months and have implications for health care workers in interacting with older infants and toddlers.

By around 9 months the average baby can say one clear word, increasing to three by a year. By 21 months word combinations appear and the child tries to tell others about experiences. However, it may be difficult for those unfamiliar with the child to decipher his or her speech for some time. In addition, young children have difficulty in taking another person's perspective, and so do not realize that a stranger will not know about certain facts which are familiar to the child. Parents are often good interpreters, repeating indistinct speech and explaining the situation to which the child is referring. Errors of grammar, such as referring to sheep as 'sheeps' are common in the early years (Berko, 1958) and, rather than suggesting incompetence, show that the child is acquiring linguistic rules (normally, we do add an 's' to indicate a plural).

During the early years the child continues to learn rules about interactions, rules which are not always obvious even to the adults involved. For example, adults often use questions as a way of controlling children's behaviour rather than as a way of trying to elicit information, as when a parent holds out a hand and says, 'Are you coming with me?' – a positive answer is certainly expected, even if not always received! Such hidden rules have implications for communicating successfully with children (Chapter 3).

Most children from middle childhood onwards accept parental separation and may prefer the independence of vision testing without the presence of a parent. Peer relationships are becoming increasingly important, and occasionally a child presents for vision testing because he or she is hoping for spectacles like those of a friend. Increasing participation in organized physical activities by older children and adolescents raises sports vision issues, such as eye safety and which correctives are suitable for swimming or ball games.

Cognitive development

The great developmental psychologist Piaget (cited in Donaldson, 1978) maintained that children's understanding of the world develops through modifications of mental representations of the world, or schemas. New information which does not fit within existing schemas results in readjustment and the formation of more highly developed schemas. These are initially based on physical actions, such as sucking and grasping objects, but become increasingly abstract. An important message of Piaget's theory is that although children's thinking can seem strange to adults, it in fact has its own logic.

One aspect of understanding the physical world to which Piaget gave particular attention was the notion that objects still exist when out of sight (object permanence) – babies will search for hidden objects late in their first year whereas previously they acted as if out of sight meant out of mind. More recent research suggests that children acquire this understanding earlier than Piaget thought (around 4 months) but that they can only demonstrate this under special laboratory conditions (e.g., Baillargeon, Spelke and Wasserman, 1985). In general, recent research indicates that infants are more cognitively capable than previously thought.

The same is true of older children. Piaget maintained that children did not develop certain thinking skills until around 7 years old. Other researchers, however, notably Donaldson (1978), have shown that young children are more capable than Piaget imagined. The problem is that adults ask questions in a way that fools children into giving wrong answers. If children are asked questions in ways that make sense to them and without pressure to give an expected answer to an adult authority figure, they display more sophisticated thinking. This has implications for the eye professional who is communicating with children and trying to get the best out of them (Chapter 3).

The work of Donaldson and other psychologists has demonstrated how closely social interaction and cognition are linked. A

further example of this, in which vision is central, is mutual attention. By the end of the first year, babies can co-ordinate their direction of gaze with that of other people, which means that the
attention of infant and adult is directed at the same object, which
the adult will point towards, name and otherwise bring into
the interaction (Collis and Schaffer, 1975), thus helping the
child to learn about it.

Emotional development
In terms of emotional expression, also, it has been found that infants
are more capable than was previously thought. For example, even
when newly born the infant can express certain emotions, such as
disgust (Izard, 1982). That newborns can show distress may seem
obvious, but until recently there was a belief that newborns do not feel
pain; this has been proved wrong by both behavioural and physiological measures (Field, 1992). As already mentioned, social smiling
appears at a few weeks, and at 3–4 months expressions of anger,
surprise and sadness appear. A little later comes fear, followed by
shyness, while guilt and contempt are first expressed around the
second birthday.

Through emotional expression, infants can communicate their
feelings and needs, enabling parents and other carers to adjust the
physical or social environment to ensure the child's well-being.

One aspect of children's emotional development which has been
studied in some depth is the nature of their fears at various ages (e.g.
Ollendick and Francis, 1988). Infants are fearful of loss of support,
loud noises, strangers (in the second half of the first year, as discussed
above) and sudden, unexpected looming objects. Between 1 and 2
years, fear of loud noises continues, fear of the dark is common and
fear of separation from parents continues and may persist into the fifth
year. In middle childhood, children's fears are more concerned with
bodily injury and in connection with achievement, while the 10 or 11
year old becomes increasingly concerned about school tests and
examinations, physical appearance and social comparison. These
changing fears are closely associated with the nature of developmental
tasks at various stages of childhood, with an emphasis on maintaining
physical safety and proximity to caregivers in the early years of
dependence, while shifting towards fears based more on social
judgement as the child grows older. Such fears can be considered
quite normal unless they are expressed strongly at later ages than
normal and interfere with the child's functioning.

In terms of vision testing, the youngster who displays positive
emotions is rewarding and relatively easy to test, but one who hides,
struggles or cries creates a difficult situation and may be labelled as
uncooperative. It is important that we do not take such behaviour as a
personal insult, nor blame the parents for being unable to control
their child; rather, we need to take account of the child's stage of
development and recognize that he or she has a point of view on the
situation which may be quite appropriate, if inconvenient.

VISION IN DEVELOPMENT

Many aspects of development depend upon, or are guided by, vision. Indeed, it is clear that right from birth, despite having limited visual capabilities in comparison with adults, the infant is essentially a visual creature. Vision is used for exploring the environment before infants are mobile or even able to reach out and grasp objects. They can scan the environment, looking for edges and contours, track moving objects, and bring the source of a sound into view. Haith (1980) proposed that the scanning occurs in the early weeks in a way that enables the child to attain a certain level of visual stimulation.

The visual scanning and tracking behaviour of infants has been investigated in some depth. Saccades, small amplitude low frequency eye movements which bring visual targets from the periphery to the centre of the field of vision, are present in newborns, although they are rather slower and less accurate than those of adults. This represents a basic mechanism for responding to visual information which is usually assumed to be unlearned and which improves rapidly over the first few months of life (Aslin, 1987). Once the newborn has the target in the centre of the visual field, it is scanned, but the nature of the scanning changes. At 1 month, there is a tendency to fixate the external boundaries of objects, where there is high contrast, such as the chin or hairline of a face, but a month later internal, finer-detailed features are scanned. When the object of regard moves, fixation is sustained by smooth pursuit eye movements – infants display this behaviour at about 1 month, and it improves over several months (Hainline, 1985) (eye movements are discussed in detail in Chapter 12).

Right from birth, therefore, the infant is gathering information visually, and soon begins to integrate visual input with that from the other senses. As well as playing an important part in social, cognitive and communicative development, vision guides motor development – for example, the baby learns to reach and to crawl towards visible objects, expanding spatial knowledge and developing muscular strength and co-ordination in the process. Later, after outlining the anatomy and development of the eye and visual system, we will discuss the profound effects of lack of vision on a child's development.

ANATOMY OF THE EYE AND VISUAL SYSTEM

A detailed description of the anatomy of the eye and visual system is beyond the scope of this handbook; interested readers are referred to Snell and Lemp (1989) for more information. Here we will simply provide an outline of the structures and their function, sufficient for the reader without any prior knowledge of the topic.

Ocular components and related terminology

Please note that the following definitions are not given in alphabetical order. The outer parts of the eye are described first, followed by the inner components, moving from front to back, in the same way that light travels through the eye (See also Figures 1.7–1.9).

Extraocular muscles – A group of six muscles for each eye which control the direction of gaze of the eye. These include the superior and inferior recti, the medial and lateral recti and the superior and inferior obliques.

Cornea – The clear anterior (front) portion of the fibrous coat of the eye, continuous structurally with the sclera (see below). It is responsible for the greater part of the refractive power of the eye (its ability to bend light rays).

Sclera – The tough white protective part of the eye which gives the eye its rigidity.

Conjunctiva – The thin layer of fine, transparent membrane filled with blood vessels over the sclera at the front of the eye and the inside of the lids.

Iris – The diaphragm which is in front of the lens and which is continuous with the choroid (see below). The iris imparts the eye with its colour. It is circular with a central hole (the pupil) which is the 'window' controlling the amount of light which enters the eye.

Anterior chamber – The fluid-filled space between the iris and the cornea.

Lens – The crystalline structure behind the pupil, which helps focus the image on the retina. The lens gives the eye its ability to change focus (accommodate). The outer coat of the lens is like a bag and is called the capsule. The lens is suspended by fibres attached to the cilary body.

Ciliary body – The muscles of the eye that are responsible for changing the shape of the lens when the eye accommodates.

Aqueous humour – Watery substance in front of the lens of the eye.

Vitreous humour – Jelly-like substance behind the lens of the eye.

Retina – The light-sensitive layer at the back of the eye that converts light into electrical signals and performs some initial analysis of the retinal image.

Choroid – The vascular layer between the retina and the sclera which provides some layers of the retina with nutrients.

Ganglion cells – The last level of nerve cells in the retina, the axons of which project to the lateral geniculate nucleus (LGN) in the midbrain (see below).

Cones – The receptor cells in the retina which are sensitive to light and which are responsible for colour vision, vision in normal day illumination and detailed vision.

Rods – The receptor cells in the retina which are responsible for vision in dim lighting conditions. They are not sensitive to colour, nor do they see fine detail.

Fovea (fovea centralis) – The depression in the centre of the retina, 1.5 mm in diameter, which is responsible for fine visual discrimination.

Foveola – A small area of 0.4 mm diameter at the centre of the fovea which contains only cones (rod-free area). This area of the retina is responsible for the finest detail vision.

Macula – The area around and including the fovea which contains yellow pigment and which is 3–5 mm in diameter.

Retinal image – The optical image on the retina. This is inverted (upside down) and laterally reversed.

Optic nerve – The nerve which takes neural signals from the retina to the brain.

Optic disc – The point at which the optic nerve exits from the eye. This is seen as a light pinkish-yellow disc when the retina is viewed. The retinal artery and retinal vein can be seen entering the eye at the optic disc.

Fundus – The view of the retina, retinal vessels and sometimes the choroidal blood vessels as seen with an ophthalmoscope. Examination of the eye in this way is known as ophthalmoscopy or fundoscopy.

Axial length – Length of the eye from the apex of the cornea to the retina.

Chiasm – The junction of the right and left optic nerves where the optic nerve fibres which have arisen from the nasal half of each retina cross over to the opposite hemisphere.

Optic tract – The nerve fibres that take the visual signal from the optic chiasm to the lateral geniculate nucleus.

Lateral geniculate nucleus (LGN) also known as the lateral geniculate body – The structure in the midbrain where the axons from the ganglion cells of the retina terminate, synapse and from where the neural signal is then transmitted via the optic radiations to the visual cortex.

Optic radiations – The fibres which transmit the visual signal through the brain from the LGN to the visual cortex.

Visual cortex, striate cortex or visual area 1 – The first visual area of the brain. The incoming fibres from the optic radiations make their first synapse here (see below).

Synapse – Electrical junction between two nerve cells (see Figure 1.9).

Dioptre – A unit of measurement to describe the refraction (bending) of light at a surface. The dioptre is the inverse of the focal length of the refracting surface when measured in metres. Abbreviated to D.

Visual acuity (VA) – The smallest detail that an eye is capable of discerning (see section later in this chapter on 'Development of Visual Functions').

Visual field – The widest extent in space in which objects can be detected by a stationary eye (monocular) or eyes (binocular).

Refractive error – The spectacle lenses needed to focus a relaxed eye for distance objects. Spectacle lenses are graded in terms of dioptric power.

Anatomy and function of the eye

The cornea is the main refracting component of the eye. Approximately 66% of the bending or refracting of the incoming light takes place at the anterior corneal surface, the rest being accomplished by the lens. The lens also changes in shape, the surfaces becoming steeper, causing an increase in dioptric power in order for the eye to

Fig. 1.7
The eye cut in horizontal section.
(From Stein, H.A., Slatt, B.J. and
Stein, R.M., 1994. *The Ophthalmic
Assistant: A Guide for Ophthalmic
Medical Personnel*, 6th edn. St
Louis, Baltimore, Mosby, p. 5.
Reproduced by kind permission of
Mosby-Year Book Inc.)

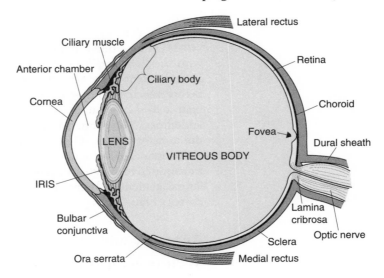

focus for objects closer than infinity, a process known as accommodation. During accommodation the anterior lens surface changes more than the posterior surface. The converging light rays form an inverted image on the retina, the light sensitive surface lining the back of the eye.

The refractive error of an eye is determined by the combination of all the ocular components and the axial length of the eye. If the total dioptric power of an eye is greater than that required by its axial length, the result is myopia, otherwise known as short-sight or near-sight. If the dioptric power is less than that required for its axial length, the result is hypermetropia or hyperopia (long-sight or far-sight). In both cases the result is a blurred image (Chapter 5).

The position and curvature of each refracting surface will influence the total dioptric power of the eye, thus influencing its refractive error. The 'refractive index' of various ocular components also needs to be considered (this index describes the degree to which light is bent when it travels from one substance to another, e.g. from air into water, and is dependent upon the speed of light through each substance). The refractive index of the lens has a considerable influence on the refractive error of an eye. On the other hand, the refractive indices of the aqueous and vitreous vary little between individuals and therefore play little part in explaining why one eye becomes myopic while another remains hyperopic. Similarly, the refractive index of the cornea plays little part in determining the refractive error outcome. This is because the anterior and posterior surfaces of the cornea are virtually parallel and therefore practically 'cancel each other out'. The corneal curvature, on the other hand, plays a large part, because of the large change in refractive index between the air and the aqueous.

The optical components of the eye cause an upside-down image to be formed (hopefully in focus) on the 'image plane' of the eye – the receptive cells of the retina.

The retina is the first sensory relay of the visual system. The cornea and lens of the eye focus the light onto the retina (see Figure 5.1(a), p. 124). The retina is made up of several layers of neural (nerve) cells, with the light sensitive receptors being in the more posterior layer. First the light has to pass through the other (inner) layers of the retina before reaching the light-sensitive receptors. The small particles of light, called quanta, are 'captured' by the outer segments of the rods and cones. The captured quanta cause chemical changes resulting in the transformation of light energy to electrical signals. This process is called phototransduction. Once initiated the electrical signals are transmitted through the retina to the optic nerve, optic tracts and lateral geniculate body or nucleus (LGN) in the brain to the visual cortex (Figure 1.8).

Anatomy and function of the visual pathway

As shown in Figure 1.8, afferent (eye-to-brain) fibres (axons, Figure 1.9) from the ganglion cells of the retina pass through the optic nerve towards the chiasm and from there to the LGNs. At the chiasm, the fibres which originate from the temporal (outer) retinae of each eye, stay on the same side (right or left) and continue to the LGN located

Fig. 1.8
The visual pathway. One half of the visual field from each eye is projected to one side of the brain. Thus visual impulses from the right visual field of each eye will be transmitted to the left occipital lobe. (From Stein, H.A., Slatt, B.J. and Stein, R.M. (1994) *The Ophthalmic Assistant: A Guide for Ophthalmic Medical Personnel*, 6th edn. St Louis, Baltimore, Mosby. Reproduced with permission of Mosby-Year Book Inc.)

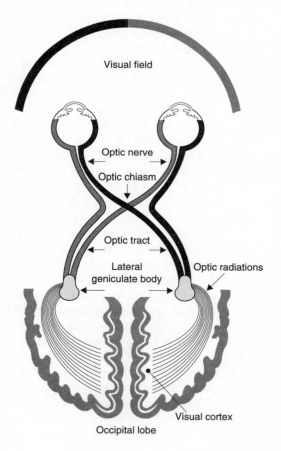

Fig. 1.9
Schematic representation of three
nerve cells, showing nerve cell
bodies, axons, and dendrites. Not
all nerve cells have axons with
myelin sheaths. Those with myelin
sheaths are called medullated
nerve fibres. The dendrites are
branches of the cell which meet
with other cells forming synapses
(electrical junctions).

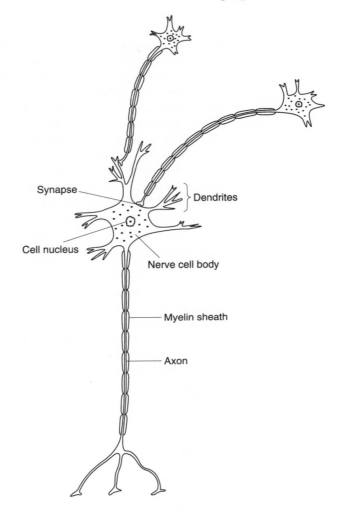

in the brain hemisphere on the same side. Conversely, fibres from the
nasal portion of each retina cross (decussate) at the chiasm and pass
to the LGN in the opposite hemisphere. Normally, 53–60% of the
retinal fibres cross at the chiasm (Townsend, Selvin and Griffin,
1991). Thus fibres from both right retinae are brought together at the
LGN. This is a 'relay station', i.e. there is a synapse (junction) of two
nerve cells. One interesting anomaly of decussation is found in
albinism, in which a greater percentage of fibres (75%) cross at the
chiasm (Holdeman, 1994) (Chapter 13).

Further initial analysis of the neural signal takes place in the LGN.
Here the visual pathways are separated into 'fine' and 'coarse' systems. The parvocellular layers contain the cell bodies of the smaller
axons responsible for fine, detailed vision and colour vision. The
magnocellular layers contain the cell bodies of larger axons responsible for visual functions such as motion detection and the ability to
see coarse information/shapes of low contrast.

From the synapse at the LGN, the fibres pass on to the visual cortex (visual area 1) of the same side. This is the first point where neural signals resulting from similar images from the two eyes are brought together. Thus the neural image from the right retina of each eye proceeds to the right visual cortex. Because of the lateral inversion due to the optics of the eye, this corresponds with objects seen in the left visual field. The left visual field is thus analysed by the right visual cortex. Correspondingly, both sensory and motor control of the left side of the body are dealt with in the right side of the brain. Thus in cases of stroke (cerebral vascular accident or CVA) giving rise to one-sided visual field loss (hemianopia) and motor deficits, both the field loss and motor problems occur on the side of the body opposite to the site of the stroke in the brain (right hemisphere stroke causing left-sided deficits and vice versa).

DEVELOPMENT OF THE EYE AND VISUAL PATHWAY

During fetal and postnatal development the cells of the body multiply and form new connections, resulting in tissue growth and increased neural communication. Certain developmental stages are easy to appreciate: we are aware that the infant is growing, that motor co-ordination is improving and that communication is developing. What is not so obvious is that the eye is growing and developing, neural connections are being made and the visual pathways and visual cortex are also developing. The maturation of the eye, visual pathways and their neural connections are associated with the development of visual functions.

Development of ocular components

The eye of the preterm neonate is smaller in all its dimensions than that of the full-term neonate. The axial length is of the order of 12 mm at 26 weeks gestational age (26 weeks after conception), 15 mm at 34 weeks and 16 mm at 36 weeks (Isenberg, 1994; O'Brien and Clark, 1994), compared with an average of 16.5–17.3 mm in the full-term neonate. From full-term birth the axial length continues to increase to an average of 23 mm at adulthood (Larsen, 1971; Tucker et al., 1992; Isenberg, 1994). Most of this change occurs in the first 2 years of life when there is a total increase of 3.8 mm. Between the ages of 2 to 3 years there is a further 1 mm increase. The period up to the age of 3 years is called the infantile period. There is a second, slower growth period for the axial length, which is from age 3 to 14 years and is termed the juvenile period. Most of this axial length increase, particularly that which happens after 3 years of age, is due to changes in the depth of the vitreous chamber. Similar changes take place in the other overall diameters of the eye, i.e. the transverse (side-to-side) and vertical diameters. All these overall diameters are consistently greater and grow more rapidly in boys than girls, except for corneal diameter (Isenberg, 1994; O'Brien and Clark, 1994).

Corneal diameter is 8.2 ± 0.5 mm at 34 weeks (Musarella and Morin, 1982) and 9 mm at 37 weeks gestational age (Tucker et al., 1992). At full-term birth it measures 9.8 mm with a range of 9–11 mm and then continues to increase up to the age of 2 years at which time it has reached its adult size of 12 mm. At full-term birth, the corneal diameter is slightly (0.3 mm) larger in girls than boys. This is one dimension of the eye for which we need accurate statistics, to enable us to detect those that are larger or smaller than the normal; a large diameter cornea may indicate glaucoma, when there is damaging increased pressure within the eye, while a small one may indicate that either the cornea itself or the whole eye is abnormally small (micro-cornea or microphthalmos).

The cornea is steeper in premature than full-term infants, being about 9 D steeper (60 D) at 28 weeks gestation and 4 D steeper (54 D) at 30–35 weeks. The corneal surface continues to flatten in the first few months of life. As a result of this, the corneal power decreases from a mean of 51–48.4 D at birth to 44 D at one year (Gordon and Donzis, 1985). There is another period of corneal flattening in the late teens.

The anterior chamber depth averages 2.6 mm at birth and deepens by about 1.4 mm from birth to adolescence. Most of this change happens in the first 18 months, but there is a steady increase until the mid-teens (Larsen, 1971).

The lens of pre-term neonates has 9 D greater power than that found in full-term neonates. At full-term birth, the lens is almost spherical and has a dioptric power of 34.4 (Gordon and Donzis, 1985). There is some uncertainty about whether, during the first years of life, the anterior–posterior length of the lens decreases or remains constant (O'Brien and Clark, 1994). However, it is generally agreed that there is an increase in the transverse diameter and a flattening of the lens surfaces. Thus the lens becomes less spherical and its dioptric power decreases. This, together with the flattening cornea, compensates for the increasing axial length. These changes result in an increase in the total lens mass (Weale, 1982).

Changes in the lens continue up to the middle teenage years (Garner et al., 1995; Zadnik et al., 1995). There is co-ordinated growth between the lens and the axial length, which allows the eye to maintain near-emmetropia, that is, for the relaxed eye to focus distant objects clearly on the retina. If this co-ordinated growth process (emmetropization) did not occur, and the changes in the optical components of the eye happened independently, there would be large fluctuations in the refractive error. The process of emmetropization is discussed further in Chapter 5.

Adhesions between the lens and the vitreous are strong in infants and, for this reason, if an infant has a cataract (opaque lens) the extra-capsular method of cataract surgery is used, in which the lens capsule is left in place. The sclera of newborns is much more pliable and half the thickness of the sclera of adults. This means that there is more danger of collapse during surgery in infant eyes (Isenberg, 1994).

Iris pigmentation is lighter in infants, the adult colour of the iris developing fully by 9–12 months. In general, the darker the iris at birth, the more darkly pigmented it will become later.

Pupil diameters from birth to 6 months postnatal age are smaller than in adults, when measured in the light. It is thought that this smaller pupil is due to the earlier development in strength of the sphincter (constrictor) muscle compared to the dilator (which opens the pupil). The reflex constriction of the pupil to direct light (pupil light reflex) starts to be evident at 31 weeks gestational age, and increases in magnitude over the next few weeks. However, even at term and until 6 months postnatal age the response is smaller and slower than in the adult. Pupil diameters in low lighting (mesopic levels) are larger in premature neonates, being 4.7 mm at 26 weeks gestational age and decreasing to 3.5 mm at 30 weeks gestational age. This decrease in mesopic pupil diameter happens at about the same time as the emergence of the pupillary light reflex (Isenberg et al., 1990; Robinson and Fielder, 1990).

It is very common to observe in preterm babies the remnants of a structure called the hyaloid canal. This is a system of blood that extends from the optic disc to the posterior lens surface, supplying nutrients to the lens during embryological development. This structure regresses from 34 weeks to 41 weeks gestation and is not usually present in full-term infants. However, when the gestational age is less than 34 weeks the hyaloid vasculature is usually present. Rarely, the partial remains of this structure extend from the disc and remain into adulthood. This is called a Bergmeister's papilla and has little functional relevance.

Retinal development

There are two main aspects of postnatal retinal development: the expansion of the retina and the development of the fovea. The area of the retina at birth is only about half that of the adult, yet the whole complement of retinal cells is already present; this means that mitosis (cell division) has finished, so retinal expansion takes place by the spreading out of the cells and by individual cell development. The development of the retina, such as cell development and differentiation of the layers occurs in a centripetal direction, i.e., from the centre to the periphery, and continues after full-term birth up to the second year (for a more detailed description see Chapter 10).

In the adult, the foveal area is much thinner than the rest of the retina. The ganglion cells are moved to each side so that the incident (incoming) light does not have to pass through several layers of retinal cells to reach the cones. This area, called the foveal pit, starts to appear at 24–26 weeks gestational age. At birth, this foveal depression is still forming. The ganglion cell layer has started the process of thinning, but the fovea is still overlaid with 1 or 2 layers of ganglion cells, and is undeveloped and relatively undifferentiated. The rod-free foveola is much larger at birth than in the adult and the cones are more widely spaced within it. The cone outer segments are much fatter and shorter than in the adult, which means that less light is captured, therefore visual signals have to be much stronger to cause the light-initiated changes in electrical activity in the retina.

Two main changes take place in the fovea postnatally. First, there is thinning of the cone outer segments: the cones move centripetally (inwards), becoming thinner and more tightly packed, and the area of the fovea decreases. Secondly, there is centrifugal (outward) movement of the inner retinal layers away from the foveola. Thus there is a shearing action taking place at the edges of the fovea and the net effect is an amazing increase in cone density. From birth to 45 months there is a 2.5 × increase in cone density and a further 35% increase to adulthood (Yuodelis and Hendrickson, 1986). By 15 months the cone outer segments are 7 × longer than at birth, but still shorter than in the adult. At 45 months they are longer again but still 30–50% shorter than adult outer segments (Hendrickson, 1993). The foveola reaches the size of that found in the adult between 15 and 45 months.

It has been suggested that the mid-periphery develops before the fovea. By 13 months rod outer segments in the mid periphery are of a similar length to those found in adults (Hendrickson, 1993). Rod and cone receptors in the mid-periphery are more mature than foveal receptors (Hendrickson, 1993). Hendrickson suggests that newborn infants may use their peripheral retina for visual functions which are later performed by the central retina.

Development of the visual pathway

Conduction of impulses along nerve fibres is enhanced by a covering called the myelin sheath (Figure 1.9). The myelin sheath of the optic nerve and optic tract fibres increases in thickness over the first two years after birth (Reagan, 1989). Cells of the LGN parvocellular layers mature more quickly than cells of the magnocellular layers. Parvocellular and magnocellular cells mature by 12 and 24 months respectively (Reagan, 1989). The visual cortex is still developing after birth. The number of synapses in the visual cortex remains constant for the first 2 months after birth, then increases rapidly to more than double by 8 months of age. Synaptic density then reduces to adult levels over about the next 11 years.

Measurement and development of visual functions

Measurement of visual functions

In young infants, who cannot respond verbally, we can measure visual functions by using either behavioural or electrophysiological techniques, both of which give valuable information. An example of a behavioural technique is forced choice preferential looking (FPL), where the infant's direction of gaze is observed in response to a real stimulus and a null or control stimulus presented simultaneously. Electrophysiological techniques (such as visual evoked potentials or VEPs) measure electrical responses of the nervous system as a result of visual stimulation. It is important to note that visual development as measured with FPL appears slower than with VEPs since behavioural methods are also dependent upon the maturation of higher cortical processes.

The best-known visual function is acuity, which in adults is the lowest line that can be read on an eye care practitioner's letter chart when wearing an appropriate spectacle correction. Clinically, distance (4 metres or more) visual acuity is often described as a Snellen fraction such as 6/6 (metric) or 20/20 (imperial). The Snellen fraction represents distances – the numerator is the distance at which the letter is viewed and the denominator is the distance at which the elements of that letter subtend 1 minute of arc (1/60 degree) visual angle at the eye. Thus a 6/6 (or 20/20) letter is one which is viewed at 6 metres (20 feet) and whose elements subtend 1 minute of arc at that distance. A letter twice that size has elements that subtend 1 minute of arc at 12 metres (40 feet). It is therefore described as a 6/12 or 20/40 letter (Figure 1.10 a, b). This means that the minimum size of detail that an eye with 6/12 acuity can see is twice the size that an eye with 6/6 acuity can see.

Visual acuity may also be measured using a series of lines or checks as the target instead of a letter. A series of equal width equi-distance bars is called a grating, and a series of equal width equi-spaced squares is a checkerboard. The object of measurement using a grating or checkerboard is to determine the smallest bar/square width that can

Fig. 1.10
Angular subtense and visual acuity. (a) A 6/6 letter. Each limb of the letter subtends 1 minute of arc (1/60th of a degree) at the eye when at a distance of 6 m. Therefore the whole letter subtends 5 minutes of arc. In order to recognize the letter, the observer must be able to 'resolve' or see the separate limbs of the letter, i.e. to resolve detail of 1 minute of arc. (b) Each limb of a 6/12 letter subtends 2 minutes of arc and the whole letter subtends 10 minutes of arc. It is twice the size of a 6/6 letter. (c) A 30 cycle per degree square-wave grating. Each black bar and each white bar subtends 1 minute of arc. One cycle is represented by one black and one white bar and subtends 2 minutes of arc. Therefore there are 30 cycles in each degree.

(a)   6/6 (20/20) letter at 6 m

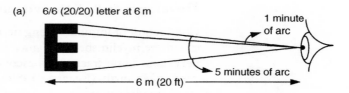

(b)   6/12 (20/40) letter at 6 m

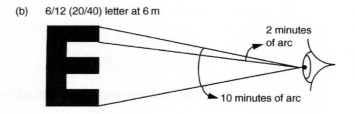

(c)   30 cycle per degree grating

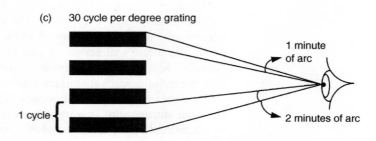

be detected. The visual acuity, or grating acuity, is described in terms of minutes of arc subtended by each bar/square.

Another way of describing visual acuity recorded with a grating/ checkerboard is in terms of spatial frequency (Figure 1.10 c). Spatial frequency is defined in terms of cycles in 1 degree. One cycle equals 2 bars (1 white and 1 black) or 2 checks (1 white and 1 black). For example, if a child's resolution limit is found to be a grating where each bar subtends 1 minute of arc then the grating acuity is 1 minute of arc. When each bar subtends 1 minute of arc, then 1 cycle (of 1 black and 1 white bar) will subtend 2 minutes of arc. Within 60 minutes of arc (1 degree) there will be 30 cycles, therefore it is a 30 cycle per degree grating (Figure 1.10 c). A halving or doubling of spatial frequency is known as an octave.

In subsequent chapters we will refer to target size in minutes of arc and spatial frequency in terms of cycles per degree.

Vision is always documented in terms of acuity (Chapter 7), therefore it is not surprising that good acuity is often thought to be synonymous with good vision. The way we see is, however, determined by much more than the ability to resolve fine details. While visual acuity is the smallest letter or stripe width visible using high-contrast targets (usually black on white), contrast sensitivity is measured using targets in various shades of grey and is the lowest contrast letter or stripe visible to an observer; Chapter 8 describes the development and measurement of the contrast sensitivity function. The development and measurement of binocular visual functions such as stereopsis (the ability to perceive small differences in depth) are discussed in Chapter 9. Chapter 10 describes the development and measurement of vision in the peripheral visual fields and Chapter 11 describes the development and measurement of colour vision.

Development of visual functions

Monocular grating acuity measured by VEPs increases from 5 cycles per degree at 1 month to about 16.3 cycles per degree at 8 months (Norcia, Tyler and Hamer, 1990). There is little change in visual acuity between 8 and 13 months of age, although there is still a small improvement after this age with adult grating acuity reaching 30 cycles per degree. Contrast sensitivity measured using VEPs increases by a factor of 4–5 across all spatial frequencies between 4 and 9 weeks of age. Contrast sensitivity to low spatial frequencies (wide stripes or large checks) shows little improvement after that time, whereas contrast sensitivity to high spatial frequencies continues until at least 30 weeks of age (Norcia et al., 1990). There is a much slower improvement in contrast sensitivity to both high and low spatial frequencies over the next few years. These developments can be explained by the following factors (Norcia et al., 1990).

1. Increased length of cone outer segments results in increased quantal catch and therefore increased sensitivity.
2. Reduced cone spacing would be expected to result in the detection of finer detail.

3. Development of the fovea might help explain the increase in contrast sensitivity to high spatial frequencies.
4. Increased myelination and cortical development may explain some of the changes beyond 8 months.

The development of the various visual functions is discussed further in the relevant chapters.

ATYPICAL DEVELOPMENT

So far in this chapter we have overviewed general child development and the development of the visual system. We now turn to another important foundation area upon which later chapters will build: the child who is not developing typically. Some such children have visual impairments occurring in isolation, while others have a combination of difficulties. Early visual assessment of all these children is essential to maximize their developmental opportunities.

The language of atypical development

Confusion often surrounds the use of words such as disability and handicap, but the World Health Organization's terminology has gained widespread usage (WHO, 1980). A distinction is made between disorder, impairment, disability and handicap, which separates out the physical aspects from social effects which can accrue. A *disorder* is any deviation from the normal structure due to development, physiology or pathology, such as the presence of a cataract. An *impairment* is a limitation of basic functioning as compared with age norms, such as impaired motor co-ordination or low visual acuity. A *disability* results when an impairment prevents a person from carrying out a specific task, such as being unable to read because of low vision. *Handicap* refers to the disadvantage which results from the existence of disability, such as being denied access to public buildings because of using a wheelchair.

These distinctions help to draw attention to the fact that some typical features of people with impairments are not inevitably part of their physical condition, but result from social forces which it may be possible to change. Despite this advantage of the WHO terminology, objections may be made to its negative tone, and the more positive-sounding term 'challenge' is often used these days to refer to a problem faced by those with impairments or their carers (as in 'physically challenged' and 'challenging behaviour'). Both types of terminology are used in this book.

We may note in passing at this point that issues of terminology are important for the clinician's everyday communications also. For example, the use of a phrase such as 'a normal child' may distress the parent of a child with an impairment who, by implication, has an 'abnormal child'. As a general rule, we should avoid labelling a child. The worst kind of labelling occurs when people are referred to by their condition (as in 'I had a cataract in here this morning'), but more subtle labelling also needs attention. For example, it is preferable to refer to a child 'with a visual impairment' rather than 'a visually impaired child', so that the child is a child first and foremost and not totally defined by the condition. (We have generally followed this usage in this book, although there is occasional departure for the sake of clarity of written expression.)

In the next section we will briefly examine some circumstances which can lead to atypical development, including preterm birth, and the presence of intellectual, hearing, motor and multiple impairments (note that these are not mutually exclusive categories). An understanding of the ways in which impairments can interfere with developmental tasks will alert the vision care worker to developmental patterns which differ from usual and thus necessitate different approaches to vision testing. Furthermore, children with impairments such as cerebral palsy and reduced hearing frequently have visual problems which compound their disability and handicap, and although their visual assessment may prove challenging, it is vital for the promotion of the child's total development.

Infants born preterm

Until recently, the term 'premature' was used to apply generally to infants of low birth weight (less than 5.5 lb or 2500 g). Today, a distinction is made between those who are small but full-term and those who are preterm (born before 37 weeks from conception), the latter being at greater risk of medical problems (Kopp, 1987). With modern care, babies born as much as 3 months early, weighing less than 2 lb ('kilogram kids'), can survive, but the incidence of permanent problems is greater the less mature the infant was at birth. Further information about the incidence of preterm births is given in Chapter 3.

Neurological problems may arise, which seem to result from general circulatory problems: there is rupture of the fragile capillaries around the spaces in the brain (ventricles), resulting in intraventricular haemorrhage. If this is mild, there is no permanent damage, and the infant may eventually be indistinguishable from a baby born at full term, but if it is severe the infant may die, or survive with cerebral palsy and intellectual impairment. The condition of an infant at birth is indicated by an Apgar score, which can range from 0 to 10, calculated by adding scores from 0–2 on each of five aspects of condition (heart rate, respiration, muscle tone, body colour and reflexes). A score of 3 or less indicates a life-threatening emergency, around 5 is suggestive of later developmental difficulty, while 7–10 indicates a healthy baby. Two scores may be given, one immediately after birth and a second several minutes later. Parents often remember their child's Apgar score, and this can be useful in history-taking.

Children who are born preterm, even if they have no neurological abnormalities, generally lag behind in development in the early years (even when a correction is made for degree of prematurity). They tend to be smaller and lighter until 5 or 6 years of age. In general, they tend to obtain lower scores on cognitive and motor development tests during the first 5 years (e.g. Holwerda-Kuipers, 1987), those from economically-deprived backgrounds having the lowest scores of all. Most catch up, however, and there are generally significant impairments in IQ only in some babies of very low birth weight who have had additional problems.

Infants born preterm may behave differently from those born at full-term in being less socially responsive and more restless, with cries which are particularly distressing and hard to terminate (Friedman, Jacobs and Wertmann, 1982). Later, there is an increased incidence of distractibility, hyperactivity, autism and accident-proneness.

Some developmental problems do seem to be due to immaturity at birth *per se*, but there may be other reasons, such as birth complications, multiple births and the abnormal early environment of the hospital incubator. Parental behaviour and attitudes may be affected as a result of the unusual social circumstances, and sometimes there are feelings of guilt ('What did we do wrong?') and disappointment; the mother may hold the baby at a distance instead of cuddling it, and some feel less attached to their baby even months later. Preterm infants are also at increased risk of neglect and abuse (Leifer et al., 1972).

Preterm babies seem more content when surrounded by fur-like material or when well wrapped. They may prefer the stimulation of softness against the skin and the feeling of security from being well wrapped, even when this is not necessary for warmth. Stimulation of infants born too early, for example, playing heart beat recordings and rocking them, has resulted in more advanced sensory and motor skills and exploratory behaviour in the short term (e.g. Burns et al., 1983), although care must be taken not to overstimulate very immature infants (Lester and Tronick, 1990). Programmes to help parents adapt to the special needs of their baby have resulted in cognitive advantages at 7 years of age (Achenbach et al., 1990).

Intellectual impairment

Intellectual impairment can result from chromosomal abnormality (such as Down syndrome), trauma, hypoxia (shortage of oxygen), prenatal infection, prematurity, metabolic disease, toxins and neurological disease. However, in about half of cases the cause is unknown. The learning problems may stem from a short attention span or poor short-term memory, but the extent of the difficulty varies enormously. It was usual, at one time, to categorize people with intellectual impairments on the basis of IQ scores; in comparison with the population average of 100, those with an IQ of 70 or less were considered to have an intellectual impairment. Although in some parts of the world such categorization is still used as a basis for service provision, there has been a move towards considering the special needs of each child, based not simply on an IQ score but on the total circumstances of the child, naturalistic observations supplementing formal tests (Smith and Cowie, 1988). Manuals for IQ tests sometimes warn against diagnosing intellectual impairment on the basis of IQ alone, advising that functional assessment should also be made. Visual assessment should be an integral part of defining a child's needs.

Down syndrome is the commonest cause of intellectual impairment, affecting around one baby in 500. Such a child may not be noticeably different in development from other children at first, but is likely to begin to fall behind by the end of the first year (Lewis, 1987). It has been suggested that Down syndrome decreases the intellectual ability by a constant subtractive factor compared to what might have been if the child had not had Down. However, environment and the amount of stimulation have a large effect, and there is evidence that early intervention, before 6 months, promotes good development. At this stage, the parents may still be struggling to come to terms with their child's condition (indeed, this is likely in all cases where a child has been born with some kind of impairment). The vision care specialist needs to be aware of this, and to be able to provide accurate information sensitively to parents about the child's vision. If vision is in the normal range for the child's age, it may be particularly reassuring for parents to be told this.

The baby and young child with Down syndrome seems to take longer to process information than other children: they may need to look and listen to stimuli for longer in order to recognize them, and are slower to smile or laugh. It is important, therefore, during testing, to give them enough time to respond. They may also forget skills they have demonstrated previously, and so may be erratic during assessment. It may be worthwhile, therefore, to see the child more frequently than usual, particularly if his or her visual performance seems low. Further information about the incidence of Down syndrome and associated ocular abnormalities is given in Chapter 3.

Hearing impairment

Just as many 'blind' children have some usable vision, so many children characterized as 'deaf' have some hearing, which they can be assisted to use with the help of amplification and auditory training.

For the child with profound, congenital deafness, the task of acquiring language is seriously undermined. Unable to hear the speech of others or to monitor their own vocalizations, their speech often remains unintelligible even to their specialist teachers (Conrad, 1981). Communicating with others is therefore a major problem for children with congenital deafness, and can create problems of loneliness and isolation.

Nor is the difficulty simply a communicative one. The child misses out on language-based opportunities for conceptual development, and is therefore likely to achieve low scores on intelligence tests which tap into such abilities, although he or she may perform on a comparable level with hearing children if the tests used are not language-dependent (Wiley, 1971).

What is fundamentally a sensory impairment can therefore result in secondary disabilities and handicaps related to social, cognitive and emotional development. Early intervention, including the supply of alternative or supplementary communication systems, such as sign language, is thus essential.

Some suggestions for working with children with hearing impairments are listed below, based on those made by Patton et al. (1987). They include:

- eliminate background noise
- use writing when necessary to communicate with older children
- talk to the child directly, not to the interpreting carer
- use gestures and facial expressions
- attract attention by waving hand or touching shoulder
- speak naturally and clearly, not over-dramatically
- if working regularly with children with hearing impairments, understand how hearing aids function; men should trim facial hair to permit lipreading.

For further details on the visual assessment of children with hearing impairments, see Shute (1993).

Motor impairments

The following descriptions of some common causes of motor impairment are based partially on Halliday (1989).

Cerebral palsy (CP) describes a group of non-progressive conditions in which motor control is impaired due to damage to areas of the brain which control motion. There are three main types of cerebral palsy, depending upon the area of the brain damaged early in life. Damage to the motor cortex (66–78% cases of CP) results in spasticity (stiffness, jerkiness and lack of muscular control) of some or all limbs. Athetosis, or dyskinesia (20% of cases), results from damage in the basal ganglia of the brain and is characterized by lack of motor control, writhing movements and often grimacing and dribbling; these children generally have unimpaired intelligence, but are more likely to have impaired hearing. In ataxia (10%) damage to the cerebellum results in unsteadiness and difficulty in balance and co-ordination. Some children with cerebral palsy are subject to epilepsy and intelligence may or may not be impaired. There is often speech/language impairment, and communication aids may be used. More information about causes and ocular complications of CP are given in Chapter 3.

Muscular dystrophies are degenerative conditions, with increased wasting and weakness of muscles eventually leading to early death. Cognitive abilities are preserved.

Spina bifida is a developmental abnormality of the spinal cord. In its more severe forms it involves permanent damage to the spinal cord, resulting in paralysis and lack of sensation below the lesion. If there is also hydrocephalus (water on the brain) which is not treated intelligence can be impaired (see Chapter 3 for more information about spina bifida and hydrocephalus).

Vision care facilities need to be able to meet the needs of children with motor impairments. Wheelchair facilities are required, and procedures may have to be adapted to cope with problems such as lack of gross and fine motor control and the use of alternative communication methods such as symbol boards.

Multiple impairments

It is a difficult task to try and understand the development of children with multiple impairments (some combination of visual/hearing/ neurological/motor difficulties, with or without intellectual impairment and other health problems). Given the extent to which an isolated impairment can impact on development, it is not surprising that children with multiple impairments have even greater difficulty in fulfilling their developmental tasks. However, unravelling the interacting mechanisms leading to delayed development is a challenging task, and few studies have been directed at this (Hogg and Sebba, 1986).

Their abilities (visual, cognitive or whatever) may be untestable using standard techniques which rely on sensory and motor capacities they do not have, so there may be uncertainty about their true abilities. As they do not reach the usual developmental milestones even those with average or high intellectual ability may seem intellectually impaired. Disability may be compounded by handicap if people have low expectations of the child and do not provide an appropriately stimulating physical and social environment.

Rogow, Hass and Humphries (1984) have observed that many such children demonstrate language and symbolic capabilities much later than usual, perhaps at 5 years old, and some then prove capable of academic learning. What can be achieved in some cases has been demonstrated by work in the former Soviet Union: children with profound impairments of both vision and hearing have proved able, with intensive and appropriate intervention within a residential setting, to develop language and cognitive skills that have taken them through university. The lesson from this appears to be that, although it is a very difficult task to determine the developmental limits of a child with multiple impairments, 'writing off' a child too soon will create a self-fulfilling prophecy.

VISUAL IMPAIRMENT AND DEVELOPMENT

Visual impairment in children with atypical development

We have already seen that children with a range of non-visual impairments are at risk of being unable to fulfil their developmental tasks. As we shall see shortly, children with very low vision are similarly at risk in terms of their general development and indeed, given the co-ordinating role which vision normally plays, those whose impairment is of a visual nature are at particular risk of broader developmental problems. Children with multiple impairments involving low vision in addition to some other sensory, motor or neurological limitation are especially vulnerable. This is an important issue given that visual problems are frequently associated with other difficulties.

In the case of low birth weight infants, relatively little is known about the relationship between neurological problems and visual development, but it seems that severe visual deficits are likely if the brain ventricles are dilated with associated haemorrhaging. When saving the lives of preterm babies first became possible in the 1950s and 1960s, there was a high incidence of retinal abnormality, due at least in part to high oxygen levels. The incidence of this 'retinopathy of prematurity' (ROP) dropped as oxygen levels became subject to more careful monitoring, but a resurgence has been noted in recent years, possibly because younger and younger babies are surviving with improved care (see Chapters 3 and 4 for further discussion of ROP). Other possible consequences of prematurity are strabismus (eye turn) and myopia and astigmatism (errors of focus causing blurred vision, see Chapter 5).

Children with intellectual impairment are at high risk of ocular anomaly, those with the severest intellectual impairment also being most likely to have a high degree of visual difficulty (Warburg, 1970, 1982). Woodruff (1977) found visual anomalies in two-thirds of a sample of Canadian children with intellectual impairment living in the community. In a Danish study, 5% of children with intellectual impairment had a visual acuity of less than 6/60, compared with less than 1% in the general child population (Warburg, 1982). Ocular problems in children with intellectual impairments often remain undetected into adulthood, and high incidences of optic atrophy, high myopia, cataract, retinal disease and keratoconus (abnormal cornea) have been found (Jacobson, 1988). Reduced accommodative capacity has been demonstrated in children with Down syndrome (Meades, Woodhouse and Leat, 1990) and CP (Leat, 1996).

Children with hearing impairments are also at higher than usual risk of visual problems (e.g., Suchman, 1968), with the type of visual problem being related to the cause of the hearing problem (Woodruff, 1986). Inherited deafness appears to have the lowest rate of associated visual difficulty, while congenital rubella is associated mainly with refractive errors. In cases of neonatal sepsis and rhesus incompatibility, higher rates of strabismus and amblyopia (poor acuity uncorrectable with spectacles) have been reported, as well as hyperopia and myopia. Loss of hearing resulting from meningitis has been reported to be associated with hyperopia.

Strabismus and nystagmus (involuntary eye jerks) are common in children with CP, while untreated hydrocephalus can result in blindness (Halliday, 1989).

Children with profound multiple impairments are at high risk of visual problems. Orel-Bixler, Haegerstrom-Portnoy and Hall (1989) examined 59 people with multiple impairments between the ages of 3 and 33 years: they found significant refractive error in 73%, strabismus in 71%, and nystagmus in 36%. Groenendaal and van Hof-van Duin (1992) found, by measuring a wide range of visual functions, that 100% of children who had suffered perinatal hypoxia (oxygen deprivation) had visual defects (ranging from total blindness to motility defects and slight loss of VA). Jackson et al. (1991) found that 11% of a population with multiple physical impairments had acuity lower than 6/18 and that 8.3% would benefit from some kind of optical low vision aid. Girls with Rett syndrome, which causes severe physical as well as intellectual impairment, often have high refractive errors but are more likely than other children with multiple impairments to have intact visual pathways (Saunders, McCulloch and Kerr, 1995). Children with profound multiple impairments present perhaps the greatest challenge in terms of visual assessment. It is important that assessment is attempted, however, given the high incidence of visual problems in this population.

Further details are given in Chapter 3 about visual problems resulting from a range of genetic, prenatal, perinatal and postnatal factors.

Effects of visual impairment on development

The effects of severe visual impairment on development have come to be understood by studying children who are blind or have low vision in the absence of other impairments, and it has been found that they are at a distinct developmental disadvantage (Fraiberg, 1977; Lewis, 1987).

Motor development

The lack of visual incentive means that they reach for objects later than other babies, may not crawl at all (resulting in lack of development in strength of shoulder, arm and leg muscles) and tend to walk later. When walking does start, children with severe visual loss are likely to be apprehensive since they cannot see what lies ahead, and there is a resultant tendency to lean backwards and to develop a strange gait. Lack of vision, then, reduces the child's opportunities for exploration, even through non-visual means. Indeed, in comparison with the busy hands of children with sight, their hands may be 'floppy' and underused, which may be exacerbated by carers who have a tendency to do more than usual for the child (Jan, Freeman and Scott, 1977).

A child who does not see distance detail or objects will also have less incentive to hold the head up to view the environment, retarding development of the neck and shoulder muscles. This can be observed in some children and adults without sight who have never learned to hold their head erect, letting it flop forward or sometimes backwards in an abnormal posture. Posture and gait and activities such as feeding independently are further affected by the child's lack of opportunity to learn by observing others.

These problems with motor development can be prevented through deliberate effort and training, possibly involving input from a physiotherapist.

Social and communicative development

The child may also experience problems related to social development and communication. Since the normal patterns of eye contact and smiling between parent and infant are disrupted, parents may inadvertently decrease contact and interaction with the child, reducing his or her opportunity to learn through such social interactions.

Some aspects of language development may be delayed, as in learning to reverse the use of the words 'I' and 'you' in conversation (Andersen, Dunlea and Kekelis, 1984). Furthermore, they cannot observe facial expressions, and often lack expressiveness themselves, making it difficult for them to learn about emotional expressiveness and for others to 'read' their emotions. As they miss subtle visual feedback from other people they may also be prevented from modifying socially unacceptable mannerisms.

Lack of eye contact may interfere with both the early attachment process and with later social interactions, when subtle changes in eye contact control the flow of conversation – a later manifestation of the turn-taking normally observed in infant–parent interactions. This early turn-taking is often absent, with the adult monopolizing the conversation. Facial signals can be replaced by touch signals (for example, fingering the face and then stopping fingering being equivalent to gazing and looking away; Fraiberg, 1977). The eye professional can likewise use touch in situations where he or she would be chatting with a fully-sighted youngster to establish rapport.

At school, mainstreamed children with visual impairments may have social difficulties. They have difficulty integrating into the play of other children, which is frequently very visually based. An example known to us is a child whose high myopia was not recognized for several years and who did not understand what was happening in skipping games. Children with visual impairments may also be separated from their peers through being taken out of the usual curriculum for orientation and mobility training or special education sessions. They may be called names by other children or regarded as mentally impaired.

Despite such social difficulties, youngsters with visual impairments are generally well adjusted, with a dislike of being patronized (Tobin and Hill, 1987, 1988, 1989).

Cognitive development

A child with visual impairment may be cognitively delayed. He or she is not only deprived of a sensory mode, but has difficulty in integrating information coming in from the other senses, since vision normally fulfils this function. It is often thought that children without vision develop 'supersenses' such as very acute hearing. This is not true, although they may ultimately learn to make good use of their remaining senses.

The child will lose out on an enormous number of incidental learning opportunities with regard to the environment which sighted children enjoy. This has a negative effect on the development of spatial concepts and the end result can be a very patchy under-standing of the world. For example, when a toy rolls out of reach, the child may imagine that it has disappeared and not seek it, so that the concept of object permanence will take longer to develop. Mother may suddenly appear and disappear without any explanation, unless she knows that she must communicate verbally what she is doing and when she is coming and going. This sudden appearance of objects can also be frightening as when, for example, a parent suddenly starts brushing the child's hair or picks her or him up without any prior warning.

Knowledge and understanding about things which cannot be touched will not develop naturally. Large distant objects such as cars, trees, clouds and mountains may not be appreciated at all or not appreciated in their entirety. For example, a child may think of a tree as a large rough round thing (the trunk which they can feel) without developing a concept of the leaves and branches at all, while the quarter moon might be imagined to be shaped like a slice of cake. Rooms may look round, rather than square, since the contrast which defines the corners cannot be seen, and concepts of distances of objects may be lacking.

It has been suggested that children with severe visual impairments do not learn stages or levels of visual perceptual skills as quickly as normal or cannot progress through certain stages. These stages or levels include such tasks as learning to see things in three dimensions, ability to copy/draw shapes, discrimination and matching tasks and figure–ground relationships (Faubert, Overbury and Goodrich, 1987). It has been further suggested that these sorts of skills are necessary to begin learning to recognize letters and words and therefore to read (Quillman, Mehr and Goodrich, 1981; Faubert, Overbury and Goodrich, 1987; Rosner and Rosner, 1990) so that the child who lacks them may face educational problems.

Emotional development

Babies with severe visual impairments show a fear of strangers at the same age as other infants, and may initially be very wary of a stranger's voice, and object strongly to being held by someone new but, as with sighted infants, they will probably be happy to interact with a stranger if they can remain on the lap of a parent or other familiar person. 'Separation anxiety' in response to parental absence develops at a later age than usual, perhaps because of a delay in learning about object permanence, but it persists longer than usual, and the child may become exceptionally distressed if he or she suddenly realizes that a parent has left the room. Because of separation anxiety, one would not normally expect to test any small child's vision without the parent being present, and in the case of a child with severe visual impairment parental reassurance may be required at an older age than usual. A 'clingy' child with a visual impairment does not necessarily have overprotective parents, therefore – it is simply harder for him or her to come to understand matters related to parental disappearances and reappearances.

Children also go through an adjustment period as they come to terms with the fact that they are 'different' from other children, that they may never see as others do and that they may never be able to drive or take up certain kinds of employment. There may also be fears that they will never be able to have intimate personal relationships. Children, as well as adults, can experience depression.

Behavioural problems

Problems with parenting and the child's behaviour may arise for a number of reasons. As discussed above, the initial relationship between parent and child may be detrimentally affected, parents may feel guilty about their child's condition although they are not to blame and they may behave in ways that others regard as overprotective or which are viewed as 'spoiling' the child, and which may result in behavioural problems.

Conversely, children with severe visual impairment are often labelled as 'good', but we should recognize that a passivity which makes them easily manageable may well reflect the negative effects of visual loss in terms of difficulty in interacting with the world.

There may be difficulty with developing a normal diurnal cycle of sleep and wakefulness since day and night appear the same to them. It may therefore be difficult for parents to teach their child to adopt a routine which fits in with the rest of the family.

Eye poking and other self-stimulation behaviour such as rocking and head nodding are common, and these behaviours ('blindisms') are even more common in children who are also developmentally delayed (van Dijk, 1982). Although some of these behaviours are observed in sighted children, they normally disappear with age. Eye poking is by far the most common stereotyped behaviour in pre-schoolers without vision, occurring in four main circumstances, which may vary in different children: under conditions of boredom; when high cognitive demands are placed on the child; when the child is highly aroused; and during eating (Troster, Brambring and Beelman, 1991). Continuation of eye poking is harmful to the eyes and to the child's appearance, and blindisms are also a social problem (Hyvarinen, 1994). Psychologists are able to devise methods for reducing the occurrence of such undesirable kinds of behaviour.

Intervention

Children with severe visual impairments should be considered as 'developmental emergencies' (Hyvarinen, 1994), and intervention should start immediately. Although severe visual impairment has the potential to retard a child's development in a pervasive way, with motor, social, cognitive and emotional spheres all being affected, the situation is far from hopeless and, as noted earlier, most children with severe visual impairments develop into well-adjusted teenagers. Habilitation consists of attempting to minimize these impacts of visual impairment by deliberate intervention, which should begin as soon as a visual impairment has been recognized (see Chapters 2 and 14).

CONCLUSION

This chapter has laid some foundations for those that follow. We have presented an outline of the basic structure and development of the eye and visual system; this will be further elaborated in later chapters. We have briefly described some central features of early childhood development, emphasizing the important role that vision normally plays. We have drawn attention to some important ways in which early development can be affected by sensory, motor and neurological impairments and, in particular, by low or absent vision. As will be discussed in the following chapter, early visual assessment and intervention have a vital part to play in promoting the successful fulfilment of a child's developmental tasks, regardless of whether he or she is found to have a mild or profound visual deficit, and whether that deficit occurs in isolation or in association with other impairments.

REFERENCES

Achenbach, T.M., Phares, V., Howell, V.A. and Nurcombe, B. (1990). Seven-year outcome of the Vermont Intervention Program for Low-Birthweight Infants. *Child Development*, **61**, 1672–1681.

Andersen, E.S., Dunlea, A. and Kekelis, L.S. (1984). Blind children's language: resolving some differences. *Journal of Child Language*, **11**, 645–664.

Aslin, R.N. (1987). Visual and auditory development in infancy. In J. Osofsky (ed.), *Handbook of Infant Development*, pp. 5–97, New York; Wiley.

Baillargeon, R., Spelke, E.S. and Wasserman, S. (1985). Object permanence in five-month-old infants. *Cognition*, **20**, 191–208.

Bayley, N. (1969). Bayley Scales of Infant Development. New York: Psychological Corporation.

Berk, L.E. (1997). *Child Development*. 4th edn. Boston, Allyn and Bacon.

Berko, J. (1958). The child's learning of English morphology. *Word*, **14**, 150–177.

Buncic, J.R. (1983). Ocular examination in infants and children. In J.S. Crawford and D.J. Morin (eds), *The Eye in Childhood*, New York, Grune & Stratton.

Burns, K.A., Deddish, R.B., Burns, K. and Hatcher, R.P. (1983). Use of oscillating waterbeds and rhythmic sounds for premature infant stimulation. *Developmental Psychology*, **19**, 746–751.

Collis, G.M. and Schaffer, H.R. (1975). Synchronization of visual attention in mother-infant pairs. *Journal of Child Psychology and Psychiatry*, **16**, 315–320.

Conrad, R. (1981). Sign language in education: some consequent problems. In B. Woll, J.G. Kyle and M. Deuchar (eds), *Perspectives on BSL and Deafness*. London, Croom Helm.

DeCaspar, A. and Fifer, W. (1980). Of human bonding: newborns prefer their mothers' voices. *Science*, **208**, 1174–1176.

Donaldson, M. (1978). *Children's Minds*. London, Fontana.

Faubert, J., Overbury, O. and Goodrich, G.L. (1987). A hierarchy of perceptual training in low vision. *Canadian Journal of Optometry*, **49**, 68–73.

Field, T. (1992). Infants' and children's responses to invasive procedures. In A.M. LaGreca, L.J. Siegel, J.L. Wallender and C.E. Walker (eds), *Stress and Coping in Child Health*. New York, Guilford.

Fraiberg, S. (1977). *Insights from the Blind. Comparative Studies of Blind and Sighted Infants*. New York, Basic Books.

Friedman, S., Jacobs, B. and Wertmann, M. (1982). Preterms of low medical risk: spontaneous behaviors and soothability at expected date of birth. *Infant Behavior and Development*, **5**, 3–10.

Garner, L.F., Maurice, K.H., Kinnear, R.F. and Frith, M.J. (1995). Ocular dimensions and refraction in Tibetan children. *Optometry and Vision Science*, **72**, 266–271.

Gordon, R.A. and Donzis, P.B. (1985). Refractive components of the human eye. *Archives of Ophthalmology*, **103**, 785–789.

Groenendaal, F. and van Hof-van Duin, J. (1992). Visual deficits and improvements in children after perinatal hypoxia. *Journal of Visual Impairment and Blindness*, **86** (5), 215–218.

Hainline, L. (1985). Oculomotor control in human infants. In R. Groner, G.W. McConkie and C. Menz (eds), *Eye Movements and Human Information Processing*, pp. 71–84. Amsterdam, Elsevier.

Haith, M.M. (1980). *Rules that Babies Look By*. Hillsdale, N.J., Lawrence Erlbaum.

Halliday, P. (1989). *Special Needs in Ordinary Schools: Children with Physical Disabilities*. London, Cassell.

Havighurst, R.J. (1972). *Developmental Tasks and Education*, 3rd edn (1st edn, 1948). New York, David McKay.

Helms, D.B. and Turner, J.S. (1981). *Exploring Child Behavior*. New York, Holt, Rinehart and Winston.

Hendrickson, A. (1993). Morphological development of the primate retina. In K. Simons (ed.), *Early Visual Development, Normal and Abnormal*, pp. 287–295. Oxford, Oxford University Press.

Hogg, J. and Sebba, J. (1986). *Profound Retardation and Multiple Impairment. Vol. 1, Development and Learning*. London, Croom Helm.

Holdeman, N.R. (1994). Metabolic disease. In B.H. Blaustein (ed.), *Ocular Manifestations of Systemic Disease*. New York, Churchill Livingstone.

Holwerda-Kuipers, J. (1987). The cognitive development of low-birthweight children. *Journal of Child Psychology and Psychiatry and Allied Disciplines*, March, **28**, 2, 321–328.

Hyvarinen, L. (1994). Assessment of visually impaired infants. *Low Vision and Vision Rehabilitation*, 7, 219–225.

Isenberg, S.J. (1994). Physical and refractive characteristics of the eye at birth and during infancy. In S.J. Isenberg (ed.), *The Eye in Infancy*. St. Louis, Mosby.

Isenberg, S.J., Molarte, A. and Vazquez, M. (1990). The fixed and dilated pupils of premature babies. *American Journal of Ophthalmology*, **110**, 168.

Izard, C.E. (1982). *Measuring Emotions in Infants and Young Children*. New York; Cambridge University Press.

Jackson, A.J., Morrison, E., O'Donoghue, E. E. et al. (1991). The provision of ophthalmic services for a rehabilitation day centre population with multiple physical handicaps. *Ophthalmic and Physiological Optics*, **11**, 314–318.

Jacobson, L. (1988). Ophthalmology in mentally retarded adults. *Acta Ophthalmologica*, **66**, 457–462.

Jan, J., Freeman, R. and Scott, E. (1977). *Visual Impairments in Children and Adolescents*. London, Grune and Stratton.

Kagan, J., Rosnik, J.S. and Snidman, N. (1988). Biological bases of childhood shyness. *Science*, **240**, 167–171.

Kopp, C. (1987). Developmental risk: Historical reflections. In J. Osofsky (ed.), *Handbook of Infant Development*, pp. 881–912. New York, Wiley.

Larsen, J.S. (1971). The sagittal growth of the eye, IV: Ultrasonic measurement of the axial length of the eye from birth to puberty. *Acta Ophthalmologica*, **49**, 872.

Leat, S.J. (1996). Reduced accommodation in children with cerebral palsy. *Ophthalmic and Physiological Optics*, **16**, 385–390.

Leifer, A., Leiderman, P., Barnett, C. and Williams, J. (1972). Effects of mother-infant separation on maternal attachment behaviour. *Child Development*, **43**, 1203–1218.

Lester, B.M. and Tronick, E.Z. (1990). Introduction. In B.M. Lester and E.Z. Tronick (eds), *Stimulation and the Preterm infant: the Limits of Plasticity*. Philadelphia, W.B. Saunders.

Lewis, V. (1987). *Development and Handicap*. Oxford, Blackwell.

Meades, J., Woodhouse, J.M. and Leat, S.J. (1990). Assessment of accommodation in children. *Ophthalmic and Physiological Optics*, **10**, 413.

Musarella, M.A. and Morin, J.D. (1982). Anterior segment and intraocular pressure measurements of the anaesthetized premature infant. *Metab Ped Sys Ophthalmol* **8**, 53.

Norcia, A.M., Tyler, C.W. and Hamer, R.D. (1990). Development of contrast sensitivity in the human infant. *Vision Research*, **30**, 1475–1486.

O'Brien, C. and Clark, D. (1994). Ocular biometry in pre-term infants without retinopathy of prematurity. *Eye*, **8**, 662–665.

Ollendick, T.H. and Francis, G. (1988). Behavioral assessment and treatment of childhood phobias. *Behavior Modification*, **12** (2), 165–204.

Orel-Bixler, D., Haegerstrom-Portnoy, G. and Hall, A. (1989). Visual assessment of the multi-handicapped patient. *Optometry and Vision Science*, **66**, 530–536.

Patton, J.R., Payne, J.S., Kaufman, J.M. et al. (1987). *Exceptional Children in Focus.* Columbus, Merrill Publishing.

Quillman, R.D, Mehr, E.B. and Goodrich, G.L. (1981). Use of Frostig Figure Ground in evaluation of adults with low vision. *American Journal of Optometry and Physiological Optics*, **58**, 910–918.

Reagan, D. (1989). *Human Brain Electrophysiology.* New York, Elsevier.

Robinson, J. and Fielder, A.R. (1990). Pupillary reaction and response to light in preterm neonates. *Archives of Disease in Childhood*, **65**, 35.

Rogow, S.M. Hass, J. and Humphries, C. (1984). Learning to look: cognitive aspects of visual attention. *Canadian Journal of Optometry*, **46**, 31–34.

Rosner, J. and Rosner, J. (1990). *Pediatric Optometry*, 2nd edn. Boston, Butterworths.

Saunders, K.J., McCulloch, D.L. and Kerr, A.M. (1995). Visual function in Rett syndrome. *Developmental Medicine and Child Neurology*, **37**, 496–504.

Schaffer, R. (1989). Early social development. In A. Slater and G. Bremner (eds), *Infant Development*. Hove, Lawrence Erlbaum.

Shute, R.H. (1993). A silent examination. *Optician*, October 8, No. 5422, Vol. 206, pp. 18–20.

Shute, R., Candy, R., Westall, C and Woodhouse, J.M. (1990). Success rates in testing monocular acuity and stereopsis in infants and young children. *Ophthalmic and Physiological Optics*, **10**, 133–136.

Smith, P.K. and Cowie, H. (1988). *Understanding Children's Development.* Oxford, Blackwell.

Snell, R.S. and Lemp, M.A. (1989). *Clinical Anatomy of the Eye.* Boston, Blackwell Scientific.

Sroufe, L.A. and Waters, E. (1977). Attachment as an organisational construct. *Child Development*, **48**, 1184–1189.

Suchman, R.G. (1968). Visual impairment among deaf children. *Volta Review*, **70**, 31–37.

Sugarman, L. (1986). *Life-span Development: Concepts Theories and Interventions.* London, Routledge.

Tobin, M.J. and Hill, E.W. (1987). Special and mainstream schooling. Some teenagers' views. *New Beacon*, **LXXI**, 3–6.

Tobin, M.J. and Hill, E.W. (1988). Visually impaired teenagers: Ambitions, attitudes and interests. *Journal of Visual Impairment & Blindness*, **82**, 414–416.

Tobin, M.J. and Hill, E.W. (1989). The present and future: concerns of visually impaired teenagers. *British Journal of Visual Impairment*, **VII**, 55–57.

Townsend, J.C., Selvin, G.J. and Griffin, J.R. (1991). *Visual Fields, Clinical Case Presentations.* Boston, Butterworth-Heineman.

Troster, H., Brambring, M. and Beelman, A. (1991). Prevalence and situational causes of stereotyped behaviours in blind infants and preschoolers. *Journal of Abnormal Child Psychology*, **19**(5), 569–590.

Tucker, S.M., Enzenauer, R.W., Levin, A.V. et al. (1992). Corneal diameter, axial length, and the intraocular pressure in premature infants. *Ophthalmology*, **99**, 1296–1300.

van Dijk (1982). Effect of vision on development of multi-handicapped children. Symposium on Early Visual Development. *Acta Ophthalmologica*, **157** (suppl.), 91–97.

Warburg, M. (1970). Tracing and training of blind and partially sighted patients in institutions for the mentally retarded. *Danish Medical Bulletin*, **17**, 148–152.

Warburg, M. (1982). Why are blind and severely impaired children with mental retardation much more retarded than sighted children? Symposium on Early Visual Development. *Acta Ophthalmologica* **157** (suppl.), 72–81.

Weale, R.A. (1982). *A Biography of the Eye.* London, Lewis.

Wiley, J.A. (1971). A psychology of auditory impairment. In W.M. Cruickshank (ed.), *Psychology of Exceptional Children and Youth* (3rd edn). Englewood Cliffs, N.J., Prentice-Hall.

Woodruff, M.E. (1977). Prevalence of visual and ocular anomalies in 168 non-institutionalized mentally retarded children. *Canadian Journal of Public Health*, **68**, 225–232.

Woodruff, M.E. (1986). Differential effects of various causes of deafness on the eyes, refractive errors, and vision of children. *American Journal of Ophthalmology and Physiological Optics*, **63**, 668–675.

World Health Organization (1980). *International Clarification of Impairments, Disabilities and Handicaps*. Geneva, WHO.

Yuodelis, C. and Hendrickson, A. (1986). A qualitative and quantitative analysis of the human fovea during development. *Vision Research*, **26**, 847–855.

Zadnik, K., Mutti, D.O., Fusaro, R.E. and Adams, A.J. (1995). Longitudinal evidence of crystalline lens thinning in children. *Investigative Ophthalmology and Vision Science*, **36**, 1581–1587.

2

The importance of early visual assessment

INTRODUCTION

In the previous chapter we outlined aspects of the development of the eye and visual system and how these relate to the maturation of visual functions. Currently, researchers are expanding knowledge in this field and techniques have been refined for the measurement of visual function.

This accumulating knowledge of normal development allows us to deduce with more certainty when development is not normal. Our increased knowledge also highlights the importance of the early assessment and management of visual problems. This is because impaired vision not only puts at risk a child's overall development, as outlined in the previous chapter, but may also compromise future visual functioning; research has shown that the first few years of life are critical for visual development, and any obstruction to the visual pathways during this time results in profound effects on visual performance. It seems that infants must both 'see to learn' and, in some respects, 'learn to see'.

In this chapter we examine the importance of assessing vision and managing problems early. As in any medical condition, the earlier defects are detected and remedied the better the prognosis, both in terms of minimizing permanent visual impairments and giving the child with visual difficulties the best possible chance of utilizing vision effectively in fulfilling their developmental tasks. Early screening is therefore important. Some visual problems, if detected early enough, are treatable with glasses, or by patching one eye. Others can be minimized through the provision of low vision aids. At other times surgical or pharmaceutical intervention is required. Yet other problems, if undetected, may be lethal, such as the childhood eye tumour retinoblastoma. If severe visual impairment proves to be inevitable, then special services can be brought into play at an early stage so that alternative, non-visual routes to development can be fostered.

In early visual assessment we wish to detect the following:

1. Ocular pathology which may have a life- or sight-threatening potential and which may require medical or surgical intervention, such as retinoblastoma.

2. Threats to binocular vision development. One example is the presence of strabismus, or eye turn, which will result in loss of stereopsis (perception of small differences in depth) and usually in amblyopia (reduced acuity not correctable with glasses). Another threat to binocular vision development is anisometropia, in which the refractive status of the two eyes differs; this may also result in loss of stereopsis and in amblyopia, either directly or through a secondary strabismus.

3. High refractive errors. In the case of astigmatism, the result may be amblyopia along one axis of vision (meridional amblyopia). High hyperopia may result in headaches and poor school achievement and may also cause bilateral amblyopia. High myopia may cause social difficulties.

4. Other threats to the normal development of visual acuity, such as congenital cataract. Any such blockage which prevents a clear retinal image prevents the development of normal visual acuity. Intervention should be as early as possible, even within a few days of birth, since this is probably the most important factor in visual outcome.

5. Visual impairment which cannot be treated. Early detection is important so that management strategies can be implemented. Important issues to consider are the assessment of functional vision and the important role of parents as rehabilitators (or, to be more accurate in the case of prevention, habilitators).

LIFE- AND SIGHT-THREATENING DISEASES

There are a few conditions in which ocular abnormalities are the first indication of systemic disease which may require immediate investigation and treatment. These include tumours, neurological diseases and infections.

Tumours

One of the most extreme and urgent examples is that of tumours of the eye or adnexa (nearby structures) which may metastasize to other parts of the body. For example, retinoblastoma is a childhood ocular tumour which, if left untreated, will spread to the optic nerve and thence to the brain with almost 100% fatality (Moore, 1990). If caught before optic nerve involvement the mortality rate is less than 8%, while if the lamina cribrosa (where the optic nerve enters the eye) is involved this rises to 15%; once it has spread further back in the optic nerve it spirals to 65% (Kanski, 1989). Another example of a tumour is rhabdomyosarcoma, the most common tumour arising from the orbit (eye socket) and the third most common tumour amongst children. When treated early (when the tumour is confined to the orbit) survival rates are around 90%, but if left until it has invaded the bone they fall to 65%.

Neurological diseases

Other cases requiring immediate investigation are neurological conditions, which may present with an ocular manifestation. For example, neurological involvement may present as an abnormality of eye movements. After congenital anomalies, the most common causes of third and sixth nerve palsies in children are trauma, inflammation, and tumour (Tomsak and Dell'Osso, 1995).

Papilloedema is a swelling of the optic nerve head which can be detected on ophthalmological examination as a blurring and elevation of the optic disc. It is caused by raised intracranial pressure which can be caused by brain tumour, brain haemorrhage or haematoma (bruising), or infections (e.g. meningitis), all of which may require immediate treatment or intervention. Papilloedema is thus a neurological emergency. One other cause of papilloedema is hydrocephalus which, if left untreated, will almost inevitably result in widespread brain damage and loss of vision due to optic atrophy.

Infections

Systemic infections may occasionally be detected in the eyes. Congenital toxoplasmosis is a disease caused by a protozoan infection which may cause an inflammation of the choroid and retina. This is the most frequently recognized feature of the disease. If detected in neonates it should be treated and, likewise, in older children if the lesion is in a sight-threatening area of the retina. Toxocariasis is another parasitic infection which can endanger sight if untreated; 80% of untreated cases will eventually have visual acuity poor enough to be registered as legally blind. Interstitial keratitis (corneal inflammation) together with inflammation of the iris can result from congenital syphilis. Anterior uveitis (inflammation of the iris) can be the first manifestation of ankylosing spondylitis.

Infections of the eyes may require treatment in order to preserve vision. Chronic infections such as conjunctivitis or blepharitis (inflammation of the eyelids), if left untreated, may lead to more serious disorders, such as corneal ulcer, corneal opacity and/or perforation, iritis or even cellulitis.

Although this is not an exhaustive list, it is apparent that a number of eye and systemic diseases can be detected by routine eye examinations, resulting in earlier referral, more effective treatment and thereby retention of normal vision or even retention of life. In Chapter 4 we discuss the more common conditions and their management in more detail. It should also be noted that physical abuse in children results in ocular complications in 20% of cases (see Chapter 3).

THREATS TO THE DEVELOPMENT OF BINOCULAR VISION

The two most common types of strabismus (a lack of alignment of the two eyes) in early childhood are infantile esotropia (an inwards eye turn), which occurs in the first year of life and accommodative esotropia, which occurs between 30 and 40 months (Graham, 1974). It should be noted that children do not grow out of an eye turn. In many cases its presence is obvious to lay observers and the child will be brought in for examination as a result. However, in some cases it may occur intermittently or be a fairly small angle and thus go undetected. An eye turn will result in decreased binocularity, including decreased depth perception, and usually in monocular amblyopia. In the case of accommodative esotropia, binocular vision, including stereopsis, will have developed normally and there is a good prognosis for acuity and normal binocularity if treated early, typically with glasses and occlusion (patching) therapy. In the case of infantile esotropia, the expectation to regain full, normal binocular vision is lower, but good acuity in each eye and anomalous binocular co-operation can be obtained in most cases (von Noorden, 1988) if treated early with a combination of glasses, occlusion therapy, prisms and, sometimes, surgery.

HIGH REFRACTIVE ERRORS

Apart from the risk of amblyopia (discussed in more detail below), undetected and uncorrected high refractive errors can cause psychological and emotional difficulties, can be a factor in learning difficulties and can impact on the child's social functioning. For example, high uncorrected hyperopia has been linked to reading difficulties (Simons and Gassler, 1988). In addition, high uncorrected hyperopia may be a causative factor in esotropia.

THREATS TO THE DEVELOPMENT OF VISUAL ACUITY

Amblyopia can occur in any young eye which for any reason does not receive a clear retinal image during the critical period of visual system development. Blocks to a clear retinal image may be congenital or acquired. Uncorrected refractive errors in one or both eyes can give rise to unilateral or bilateral amblyopia. In other cases a clear image is not obtained because the ocular media through which light should pass are opaque rather than transparent, as in cataracts and corneal opacities. Light may also be prevented from entering the eye by ptosis (drooping eyelid) or haemangioma (a tumour affecting the eyelid). In all such cases, if there is no intervention, deprivation amblyopia occurs.

Refractive causes of amblyopia

Uncorrected anisometropia (significantly different refractive error in each eye), high hyperopia, and high persistent astigmatism may all result in either unilateral or bilateral amblyopia. These refractive errors are described in Chapter 5.

Uncorrected anisometropia can result in monocular amblyopia because only one eye can be in focus at a given time. Which eye is used will depend on the relative refractive errors and the distance of the object of regard. Commonly, the result is that one eye is used consistently over the other, which develops a cortical deficit so that, even when corrected at a later time in life, normal acuity cannot be attained. The amblyopia which develops in cases of anisometropia is usually more severe than that in cases of bilateral high hyperopia and astigmatism because of the competitive cortical interaction between inputs from the two eyes.

In the case of high uncorrected hyperopia there may be consistent defocus of the retinal image of both eyes, resulting in slight bilateral amblyopia. The loss of visual acuity may not be as severe as in anisometropia, but because both eyes are affected, the functional ramifications can be more serious.

Meridional amblyopia (confined to one axis of vision) occurs in cases of uncorrected persistent astigmatism, because only one meridian of an astigmatic eye can be focused on the retina at one time. The eye will choose which meridian to focus according to the relative refractive errors of the meridians and the distance and the configuration of the object, i.e. whether it is composed chiefly of vertical, horizontal or oblique components. In many cases one meridian will be consistently blurred and, in all cases, meridians between the major meridians will never receive a clear image. The result is a blur ellipse which will cause a cortical neurological deficit in one meridian compared with others. When the refractive error is corrected in later life, acuity will remain poorer in that meridian. Acuity for complex targets involving all meridians will be compromised.

Cataract

A cataract is an opacity in the lens of the eye. Congenital cataracts are one of the leading causes of blindness in children. According to the American Academy of Ophthalmology (1994, p. 90) blindness resulting from cataracts accounts for 15–20% of students in schools for blind children. Cataracts may affect one or both eyes, and may be inherited, associated with a disease syndrome, or of unknown cause. Cataracts that are dense, occupying more that 3 mm of the central lens, cause profound effects on vision, resulting in irreversible amblyopia if they are not treated. Cataracts that are small (1–2 mm), occupying the anterior surface of the lens, may not interfere with vision to any significant extent. The American Academy of Ophthalmology (1994, p. 94) recommends that congenital cataracts should be detected and removed during the first 2–3 months of life. A refractive correction should be given immediately for optimal visual outcome. Delay in the treatment of monocular cataracts results in severe monocular deprivation. Delay in the treatment of binocular cataracts results in binocular deprivation and nystagmus, a continual jiggling and unsteady fixation of the eyes.

Ptosis and haemangioma

Ptosis is a drooping of the upper eyelid. It may be congenital or acquired. If the lid is completely closed during the first few months then deprivation amblyopia results. Usually the ptosis is partial; amblyopia in these cases is more likely to result from accompanying refractive error and strabismus than from the ptosis itself.

Ptosis may also result from capillary haemangioma, a tumour of the orbit, which occurs in approximately 1 in 200 infants (American Academy of Ophthalmology, 1994, p. 149). Capillary haemangioma is usually benign, but any child with acquired ptosis and/or proptosis (an eye protruding abnormally from its socket) must have an ophthalmological examination to rule out rhabdomyosarcoma. Most capillary haemangiomas involve the upper lid, but there may be an intra-orbital component evidenced by displacements to the globe (eyeball). About 30% of haemangiomas are evident at birth and 95% by 6 months of age (American Academy of Ophthalmology, 1994). They may be very small initially and then grow rapidly, reaching their maximal size between 6 and 12 months. In about 40% of children the tumours regress completely by 4 years of age, and in most children by 8 years of age. About 50% of children with lid or orbital haemangiomas develop amblyopia, usually from anisometropic astigmatism; that is, the two eyes have different refractive status, with the misshapen eyeball causing blurred vision in one eye, resulting in a loss of visual acuity. Strabismus develops in about one-third of children with haemangioma. It is important to monitor visual acuity in children with ptosis and/or haemangioma to determine that visual acuity is not affected. The child should also be refracted (have their refractive status checked) at regular intervals. Ptosis is discussed further in Chapter 4.

Corneal opacities

Corneal opacities can also cause deprivation amblyopia if they significantly interfere with vision and are not treated quickly. Corneal opacities may result from trauma occurring during a forceps delivery, from a temporary growth called a dermoid or they may be diffuse opacities resulting from metabolic disease or glaucoma. It is important that children recovering from corneal injuries, or corneal surgery, are refracted. This is because dermoids, corneal surgery or trauma during forceps delivery may result in changes to the refractive error, in particular, astigmatic changes. It is important not to risk the development of amblyopia secondary to an uncorrected refractive error as well as that resulting from deprivation arising from the corneal opacity itself.

UNTREATABLE VISUAL IMPAIRMENT

There are some ocular disorders for which there is no treatment and which result in low vision. Early diagnosis is still required in order to counsel, institute habilitation and set required support in place for the future. Some of these conditions are non-progressive and congenital. Examples are: albinism, in which the eye lacks pigmentation leading to problems such as poor acuity and extreme sensitivity to light (photophobia); coloboma, in which a portion of the eye structure, such as the iris or lens, is missing; and achromatopsia, in which the child cannot see colours. Other conditions develop during the first or second decade of life, such as cone dystrophy, Stargardt's macular dystrophy and retinitis pigmentosa, all of which cause deteriorating vision.

Usually a child with visual impairment will have been diagnosed before being seen by the optometrist, but there are occasions when an optometrist is the first to suspect the problem. In this case referral will be necessary for differential diagnosis and other testing. However, an optometrist should be involved in providing any necessary aids to optimize existing visual performance, such as refractive corrections and tinted lenses. In addition, early counselling of the child's parents and environmental adaptations at home and at school are critical in such cases.

The importance of early assessment for development

As discussed above, there is clear evidence relating to the importance of early visual assessment for the sake of a child's future visual functioning and, in some cases, general health. However, the early detection of severe visual problems also has very broad implications given the role that vision normally plays in a child's general development (Chapter 1). It is timely at this point to remind ourselves of the WHO's distinction between disorder, impairment, disability and handicap. All too often, disorder and impairment lead to unnecessary disability and handicap because of lack of appropriate assessment and treatment as well as societal attitudes towards those with impairments.

What is the proper role of eye professionals when it comes to severe visual impairment? Lovie-Kitchin and Bowman (1985), discussing the role of the optometrist, see this as being at the level of impairment and disability, with handicap being the province of other professionals, such as social workers and psychologists. Hill (1987) has deplored the lack of interest of eye professionals in blindness as compared with vision, and Shute (1991) has argued that the vision care specialist has a wide role to play. Certainly, the central role of eye professionals lies in assessment and in reducing impairment and disability. However, vision care workers are also part and parcel of general society which influences degree of handicap in various ways – by the provision or otherwise of appropriate services to those who need them, by the degree of understanding of the importance of visual functioning for an individual's development, and by the very way they communicate with those with impairments and their families. Communication will be considered in the following chapter, while here we discuss the importance of early low vision assessment for the general development of children with and without additional impairments.

Children with low vision

It can be argued that the most basic right of the child with low vision is accurate assessment of the problem (Hill, 1987), yet children who display no visual behaviour are often diagnosed as cortically (and thus 'hopelessly') blind without confirmatory electrophysiological evidence (Allen and Fraser, 1983). A child who is labelled as 'blind' and treated as such is destined to live the life of a person without vision regardless of their true visual potential. There is ample evidence from psychological research that people live up (or down) to the labels placed upon them (e.g. Giles, 1991), and Shute (1991) has given anecdotal examples of children not using their remaining visual capacity because of labels put upon them by professionals and, indeed, themselves ('I can't do that–I'm blind').

Legal definitions of blindness can cause a problem here. Someone who is legally blind may have some usable residual vision which the label obscures. An important aspect of visual assessment of children with severe visual impairment is to move beyond the labelling and specify whatever visual capacity remains so that appropriate interventions can be implemented. The assessment of functional vision is discussed later.

As stated in the previous chapter, Hyvarinen (1994) considers that children with severe visual impairments should be considered as 'developmental emergencies', and that intervention should start immediately. The severity of the developmental impact is almost certainly correlated with the severity of the visual loss. It is also related to timing: the child who has had some months or years of visual experience before adventitious vision loss will have the advantage over the child with congenital impairment, as some degree of normal development will have taken place and is not subsequently lost (although such a child and family will have to adjust to the different challenge of the loss of a sensory faculty that the child once had).

Habilitation consists of trying to minimize the impact of visual impairment through education of the parents and by early intervention programmes (the critically important role of parents is discussed further below).

Physical development may be aided by the involvement of a physiotherapist. Parents may need encouragement to let the child take reasonable risks with regard to rough and tumble and playground activities, perhaps with the use of safety glasses. Participation in appropriate sports will also enhance physical co-ordination, strength and self-esteem. Sports should be chosen according to the level of vision: cycling, judo, dance, gymnastics and swimming are some that can be considered. Children with less severe impairments can take part in those ballsports that use a large ball or which take place on a small pitch or court, such as soccer, basketball and netball. The child may need to be shown around the pitch in advance to ensure understanding of the concept of the game. One exception is the child at risk of retinal detachment, for whom most sports will be risky; however, even these children can take part in non-contact, non-ball activities such as swimming.

Various professionals, such as special needs advisers, psychologists and teachers, are able to assist in aiding parents to promote their child's social and cognitive development and later their educational attainment. Much of this assistance will be of a preventative nature. To take examples mentioned previously, parents may be encouraged to use touch instead of vision as an indicator of turn-taking with their child, and to warn the child verbally about their intentions and actions. If problems do develop, the interventions can be put in place to help to solve them. For example, referral to a psychologist might be indicated if the child engages in the practice of eye-poking to a concerning degree (as many as three-quarters of 'blind' preschoolers do this at least weekly; Troster, Brambring and Beelmann, 1991).

The value of early assessment and interventions with children with severe visual impairments is suggested by the increase in abilities of 'blind' children noted in recent years. Although studies have shown that children with little or no vision may be severely delayed in many aspects of development, much of the research which demonstrated this was carried out in the days before early intervention was commonly implemented. Developmental delay has now been reduced and Leung and Hollins (1989) have noted the need to revise upwards the developmental norms for children without vision. Nor, they caution, must average attainment necessarily be considered adequate, as children with high IQs have the potential to perform at a level above the average.

Interventions to promote development in the case of low or absent vision continue to be refined. For example, as we saw in the previous chapter, children without vision have difficulty in coming to understand spatial concepts. Nielsen (1992) has developed a 'little room' for infants – a small space with hanging objects in reach – and demonstrated an improvement in spatial skills as a result of experience in this specially-designed setting.

Intervention programmes are thus demonstrably effective, and the vision care specialist has a vital role to play in helping children to fulfil their potential, through the assessment of visual strengths and weaknesses, by providing education and advice to the family, by prescribing visual aids as necessary and by ensuring that other appropriate services are brought into play at an early stage. It is helpful to build up a file of useful leaflets on various topics and contact information about other relevant agencies such as hospitals, schools, psychologists and special education advisers.

Good communication and co-operation with others working with the child is invaluable. For example, information should be provided about whether central vision is normal and whether there are field losses. The implications of these factors should be made clear, such as the degree of detail the child will be able to see and the likely effects on mobility.

Sadly, the potential value of good vision care for children with severe visual impairment is not always matched by reality. This is indicated by a study on low vision aid usage by children in England and Wales, which found that many children do not receive low vision aids or even regular visual assessments (Leat and Karadsheh, 1991). A similar story emerges in other wealthy industrialized nations. In a US study, Hofstetter (1985) discovered that nearly half of a sample of 60 students with severe visual loss had not received appropriate visual aids and guidance, and many had inappropriate corrective prescriptions. In the light of similar inadequacies within the Canadian context Hill (1987) has proposed that eye practitioners have an advocacy role to play for children with low vision.

Children with multiple impairments

It is vital that a child who has a non-visual impairment, such as hearing loss or intellectual impairment, receives visual assessment. We saw in the previous chapter the various ways in which such impairments can inhibit a child's development, and how visual problems in addition can compound the disadvantage.

Although non-visual impairments are frequently associated with visual problems, it does not follow that a corresponding level of priority is afforded to those so affected. At particular risk of neglect are those with intellectual impairment, despite their high chance of experiencing ocular problems, with the most profound intellectual impairments being associated with the most severe visual deficits (Warburg, 1970, 1982). Jacobson (1988) found that many with intellectual and visual impairments reach adulthood without any assessment of their vision, and Harries (1989) reported that certain London ophthalmologists felt unable to accept any more intellectually impaired people for routine services. These are clear examples of disability and handicap being added to impairment because of societal attitudes.

Such neglect is often justified on the grounds that time and effort expended on intellectually impaired people are unlikely to translate into an improved quality of life for them. Jacobson's (1988) study, following up adults in an institution 6–12 months after the provision of refractive corrections, has disproved this. Although those with hyperopia did not respond very favourably to their spectacles, those with myopia tolerated their spectacles well, and were reported by staff to be more mobile and interested in activities, while those with bifocals participated more in close work. Intraocular surgery (mainly cataract extractions) resulted in improved vision in 8 out of 14 patients (the remainder having optic atrophy or retinal damage). One can only speculate about the quality of life these people might have experienced if their visual problems had been identified and treated at an earlier age. We should also note the fact that people without intellectual impairments expect vision care as a right without having to justify it in terms of improved quality of life.

Early oculovisual assessment of those with intellectual impairments facilitates remediation, whether by the provision of refractive corrections, the supply of low vision aids, the provision of surgery or orthoptic treatment and giving relevant information to parents and others working with the child, so that the child's developmental potential can be reached. Children with Down syndrome are a case in point: whereas expectations used to be low for them, it is now known that many are capable of learning to read, pass examinations and gain employment (e.g. Feuerstein, Rand and Rynders, 1988). However, they are likely to experience age-related visual problems earlier than the general population (Jacobson, 1988), so it is particularly vital that their vision is monitored to enable them to keep up early progress. They are also likely to have reduced accommodative capacity (Meades, Woodhouse and Leat, 1990) and so may need reading glasses or bifocals at an early age.

Children with profound multiple impairments present perhaps the greatest challenge in terms of visual assessment. They may have some or all of the following problems: intellectual impairment, mobility problems, co-ordination problems, communication difficulties, hearing impairment, low vision, behavioural problems and perhaps additional health problems. Indeed, as noted in the previous chapter, trying to disentangle the abilities of such children is extremely difficult, so that it is often not even clear whether a child has an intellectual impairment or high intelligence.

Despite the high risk of visual problems in those with multiple impairments, this group has traditionally been ignored by the average eye professional and is often excluded from vision screening programmes (Cress et al., 1981) and denied treatment such as surgery and corrective lenses (Hill, 1987). In the study by Orel-Bixler, Haegerstrom-Portnoy and Hall (1989), only 37% with significant refractive error were wearing their proper correction, and uncorrected refractive errors from -10 to $+20$ D were found.

This lack of service provision is all the more serious given evidence that the prevalence of children with multiple impairments is increasing (Brennan et al., 1992). These are commonly children where perinatal complications are the causative factor, improved medical technology leading to increased survival rates.

If low vision is determined, then a functional visual assessment is indicated for the same reasons as for those who only have visual impairments, with clear and usable information being sent to parents and other involved professionals (Brennan et al., 1992; Michael and Paul, 1991). In fact, the necessity for a functional assessment may be greatest with these clients who are less able to communicate for themelves what they can or cannot see.

A further reason for assessment is that early visual function may well be predictive of the final intellectual outcome in certain disorders, such as in the case of perinatal complications (Miranda et al., 1977) and Down syndrome (Miranda and Fantz, 1973, 1974).

Lastly, as in the case of those who only have visual impairments, it is important to monitor changes in visual function. Some infants with severe multiple impairments display little or no visual behaviour and are thus regarded as 'blind'. However, Rogow et al. (1984) have noted that some do become more capable visually at a later age. This observation is supported by more recent work by Groenendaal and van Hof-van Duin (1992), who noted visual improvements up to the age of 16 years as a result of vision stimulation in a group of children with severe perinatal hypoxia.

Rogow et al. (1984) take issue with the common belief that the visual behaviours observed in the early days of life are innate, suggesting that there is a large learned component. They maintain that the infant who has reduced vision in addition to other impairments is at a particular disadvantage, since restricted mobility reduces the chances of changing visual input and integrating information coming in from the various senses.

Rogow et al. (1984) and associates counsel against the early assumption of blindness in the absence of functional eye disease, so that interventions to promote the development of any visual capacity can be introduced. This would include optometric and ophthalmological interventions as well as advice from special educators to break the vicious circle of developmental disadvantage that can occur. Harrison (1985) has also argued for early visual assessment as part of the process of avoiding the establishment of 'disabled' patterns and attitudes. As with children who have visual impairment alone, then, it is vital that multiply-challenged children are monitored regularly and that information about changes in visual function is provided to care workers, educationists and parents.

The lack of vision care provided for these children results from the fact that many eye practitioners have been frustrated by their lack of response to standard subjective testing procedures (Hill, 1987). Yet there is now a wealth of data which shows that most of these children are testable, making use of preferential looking techniques which have now been available for a number of years (Lennerstrand, Axelsson and Andersson, 1983; Mohn and van Hof-van Duin, 1983; Hertz, 1987; Hertz and Rosenberg, 1988; Orel-Bixler et al. 1989). If training in the expected response is given between clinic visits, the percentage of testable children increases (Geruschat, 1992). Aitken and Buultjens (1991) also emphasize the need for visual assessments of children with multiple impairments; in a questionnaire survey of ophthalmologists and their testing procedures it was found that the majority appear to use the Sheridan Gardiner test (a matching test – see Chapter 7) and, when that fails, to rely on electrophysiological testing. Only two reported using preferential looking techniques.

To summarize, the reasons for visual assessment in multiply-challenged children are:

1. The high incidence of visual defects and need for correction.
2. The need for a functional assessment in the case of low vision.
3. The need to give advice regarding environmental adaptations and simple low vision aids.
4. The need to implement vision stimulation.
5. The predictive value of visual assessment for intellectual potential.
6. The possibility of improvements in vision.
7. The need to break the cycle of disadvantage.

SCREENING

Programmes for detecting visual problems

We have established the importance of detecting and treating children's visual problems as early as possible for the sake of both future visual functioning and general development. There are a number of ways in which this could be done.

1. A full oculovisual examination for all infants by an eye care practitioner.
2. A modified clinical examination.
3. A screening programme which may be carried out by professionals who are not vision care specialists. A limited number of tests would be included.

Most practitioners would agree that the ideal would be for all children to have a full oculovisual examination. This would include taking a history and assessing ocular health, refractive error and oculomotor and sensory systems in order to detect variations from the normal and establish a diagnosis and management plan. There may be some disagreement about the age at which this should be done, but there is little doubt that this would result in the correct detection of almost all visual problems. However, this ideal is unlikely to be mandatory as the financial burden must either fall on the state or the family. Although a number of countries do have health plans which cover children's eye examinations, there would be a significant cost implication of making such eye examinations mandatory. Thus it remains up to the parents to take a child for an examination, and this is frequently done in response to an observed vision difficulty or concern, rather than for a routine examination. Increasing the numbers of children brought by parents for routine assessment, through the use of health education programmes, is one avenue for catching children with visual disorders. The other avenue is vision screening of all children, in order to detect those who might have a visual problem and who should therefore have a complete examination.

One form of screening is through a modified clinical examination. This is a scaled down version of a full examination and includes assessment of the following:

1. Visual acuity (VA). This will show whether a child's visual development is falling within the normal range, meaning that the development of amblyopia is unlikely and eliminating conditions which give rise to congenitally low VA. It is also important to compare the VA in each eye.
2. For the presence of strabismus, or squint. This may be undertaken using the cover test, Hirschberg test or 5 D prism test (Chapter 9), in which deviations of one eye are detected directly. Alternatively, stereopsis may be measured; if there is a manifest squint stereopsis will be absent or only grossly present.
3. Refractive error which is outside the normal limits of infant populations (Chapter 5) and which may need to be corrected with spectacles.
4. Ocular examination by ophthalmoscopy. This technique examines the media of the eye (the refractive components) for clarity, thus eliminating conditions such as congenital cataract. The retina and optic nerve head are also examined.

Screening may also include a test for normal ocular movements (motility) and examination of pupil reactions and external areas of the eyes (lids, conjunctiva, lashes) using a hand magnifier.

These tests require the considerable involvement of skilled eye professionals. For this reason, and because this is not a particularly rapid screening method, it may be expensive to implement. It is therefore unlikely to be widely adopted, despite being favoured by the American Optometric Association and having been shown to be effective (Schmidt, 1990).

The third alternative, rapid screening by non-specialists, is more usually adopted. It is typically implemented through schools because the importance of good vision for education is recognized and also because, since education is mandatory, it is easy to reach all children of a given age. However, there are still a number of anomalies and loopholes in this system.

One example is that, in Britain, vision screening is mandatory for all children except those in private schools (as though poor vision did not matter, nor had any long-term consequences for those children).

Screening through schools in Australia has also been described as unsatisfactory (Rooney, 1992). Screening methods vary from state to state and are essentially aimed at detecting reduced distance acuity and strabismus, which is inadequate for detecting many of the visual anomalies which lead to learning problems at school. Rooney notes that reading problems at school are the commonest reason for a child to present for optometric assessment, with disorders at near making up 90% of disorders detected.

Although it is easier to undertake screening of the whole population at school, it is almost universally agreed (and there is much evidence to suggest) that screening should occur before school age is reached

(Ingram et al., 1986; Atkinson 1993; Marsh-Tootle et al., 1994), possibly as early as 1 year or 6 months of age, since treatment before the age of 2 years is more effective than later. Vision screening at around the first birthday is indicated in order to detect infantile strabismus and any signs which suggest a risk of later strabismus. Since other vision problems, such as myopia, increase after the age of 6 years, rescreening in the early school years is also indicated. The Hall Report in Britain recommended screening at 21 and 39 months and 5, 8 and 11 years (Hall, 1989). Recently, certain states in the USA have introduced mandatory screening of preschoolers, and yet there are virtually no studies or guidelines regarding which tests should be used for this age group.

Validity and efficiency of screening programmes

Vision screening is normally recognized as being a test, or series of tests, designed to identify the maximum possible number of children with visual problems, but to pass those children with normal vision, and which is cheaper to administer than a full oculovisual examination. The test should therefore be quick (so as to reduce costs), be administerable by non-vision professionals and be designed to specifically pick out the most prevalent vision difficulties which need treatment. The test should also be as valid as possible, in other words we want the smallest number of children with normal vision failing the test and being referred for further oculovisual assessment, and the smallest number of children with vision problems managing to pass the test and going undetected. There are four categories of results which emerge from any type of testing for abnormalities.

1. Those who pass and have normal vision (true negatives).
2. Those who pass but have a disorder (false negatives).
3. Those who fail and have a disorder (true positives).
4. Those who fail but have normal vision (false positives).

Sensitivity is the proportion of children who fail the test (are identified as having a vision problem) who actually do have vision problems (true positives divided by the total number of positives). The specificity is the proportion of children who pass the test who actually do have normal vision (true negatives divided by total number of negatives). A good test will have high sensitivity and specificity. A poor test will have low sensitivity (failing too many children) or low specificity (it misses too many children who have vision problems) or both. In order to calculate the sensitivity and specificity of a screening procedure, a full examination (as the gold standard) on both those who pass and those who fail must be done, otherwise the numbers of false and true negatives will never be known. Very few studies of screening tests have done this.

Vision screening does not result in a diagnosis and only indicates the need for further investigation. Low sensitivity and specificity result in increased costs, either due to too many referrals for further examination or in terms of the health- and education-related costs (to say nothing of the personal costs) of undetected visual problems. If there are signs which give reason to suspect a vision difficulty, a child should still be referred for a full examination, even if he or she passed the screening.

It is sometimes difficult for parents to comprehend the difference between a screening test and a full examination. If their child has passed a screening test but there is nevertheless some sign that indicates the need for referral, parents may find this hard to understand. It may be similarly difficult for them to appreciate why children who have passed a screening test are occasionally found at some later date to have a visual problem. Conversely, parents may wonder why it is that their child can fail a screening test but be found on subsequent examination to have normal vision. The poorer a screening test is, in terms of sensitivity and specificity, the greater the likelihood of disillusionment and misunderstanding. However, if we have to choose between the two, high sensitivity is preferable to high specificity. It is better with a condition which has low prevalence, and when the implications of over-referral are not too severe, to over-refer than to miss disorders.

Screening protocols

What are the commonest vision disorders which may require treatment, correction or monitoring at an early age, and which may not lead to signs that are noticed by parents, and which we therefore wish to detect with any vision screening procedure? The most common disorders are high refractive errors, strabismus and amblyopia. We also wish to detect organic disorders. The tests used should therefore be specifically designed to quickly detect the majority of such conditions.

Efficiency can be increased by only presenting targets at the criterion level, plus a few initial targets to familiarize the child with the task. For example, if 6/9 is the criterion for passing, we do not need to show larger or smaller acuity symbols. We are not trying to measure acuity, but to determine if it falls below a certain value.

A number of screening methods which have been developed are described below.

Distance visual acuity only

This is the current method of screening in British schools. It is undertaken at an age when the majority of children can read letters, which is, of course, late in terms of the visual development period. A letter chart is used and children often line up for the test, which means that they may learn the letters from listening to others read them aloud (this problem could be alleviated by having alternative charts available). If the letters are read with both eyes open vision loss in one eye only will be missed, while subsequent monocular testing using the same chart will not be valid. Even in the absence of these shortcomings, measuring visual acuity alone will only detect some refractive errors (myopia and astigmatism beyond 1–2 D), depending on what fail criterion is chosen (Figure 2.1). Low to medium hyperopia, which may well need correction, is likely to go undetected, as may strabismus and anisometropia.

Visual acuity with plus lenses

If a visual acuity measure through plus (converging or convex) lenses (+2 to +2.5 D) is added to the test of distance acuity alone, then significant amounts of hyperopia can also be detected. If the child has 2 D or more hyperopia, VA will be similar (or better) with the positive lenses. Passing the test thus involves demonstrating poorer acuity with the positive lenses. This approach is used in Massachusetts, together with a test of phoria (tendency to misalignment of the eyes) at distance and near (Rosner and Rosner, 1990).

Vision screening instruments

Various screening instruments have been developed which simulate distance vision by means of positive lenses. Most are based on the stereoscope principle. These include the Keystone and the Ortho-Rater. These measure a number of visual functions and were developed for industrial vision screening in adults rather than for children, although some include targets adapted for children (North, 1993). Therefore many of the tests are inappropriate for young children and the procedure is more time-consuming than is necessary. Most measure such functions as distance and near acuity, visual acuity under blur (with plus lenses), depth perception, colour vision, visual fields and alignment of the eyes. These instruments have an unacceptably high rate of over-referrals (low specificity) when used with children (Hammond and Schmidt, 1986).

Fig. 2.1
The relationship between refractive anomalies and Snellen visual acuity in 1920 eyes in the Orinda Study. Lines for each mean acuity level are plotted against refractive error. If a referral criterion of 6/12 (20/40) is taken, all the children with refractive errors inside the shaded area would not be referred. Some of these, e.g. those with +2.00 D of hyperopia or more, would be false negatives, i.e. they are not referred although they need correction. (From Blum, H., Peters, H.B. and Bettman, J.W. 1959, Vision Screening for Elementary Schools: The Orinda Study. Berkeley, CA, University of California Press.)

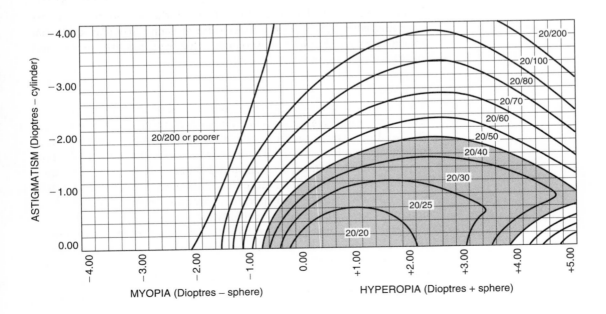

Stereopsis

Stereotests, which assess the ability to detect small differences in depth, have been suggested as a means of detecting strabismus, amblyopia and poor visual acuity. However, it has been shown that people with small squints and medium refractive errors are able to pass certain tests. It seems that the choice of test and the pass/fail criterion are critical. Testing stereopsis is discussed further in Chapter 9.

Photorefraction (or videorefraction)

This technique, described in Chapter 5, has been suggested as a screening tool for refractive error. It is very quick and non-threatening to administer and it is reputed that it can be administered by non-professionals with minimal training. A disadvantage is that it may miss hyperopia unless cycloplegic drops (drug to reduce accommodation) are used, which is far from ideal in the screening situation. Also, it may miss small angle strabismus as it relies on the Hirschberg test (measurement of the symmetry of reflection of light from the two corneas). The only study to investigate its sensitivity and specificity is that of Fern (1991) who found a sensitivity of 65% and a specificity of 93%. These figures show that the test has some potential, although the precise figures will be unique to the particular photorefractor and the sensitivity is much lower than would be desired.

Screening: conclusion and suggestions

As stated above, there are three main types of disorder that we wish to detect: refractive errors (any myopia, moderate astigmatism and hyperopia), strabismus and amblyopia, as well as some organic disorders. A different approach may be indicated depending on the age of testing and a battery of short tests is likely to be more effective than any single test. However, there is much that we do not yet know regarding which tests are the most valid at each particular age, what referral criteria should be used and what resultant sensitivity and specificity can be obtained.

At 1 year

Almost no studies have been done to assess the effectiveness of screening for this age group. The use of preferential looking to assess VA has been suggested, but this may miss myopia (as the test is undertaken at close distances) and its validity for detecting amblyopia is questionable (Mayer, Fulton and Rodier, 1984); it is also time-consuming. Stereoacuity is difficult to measure at this age and failure may indicate inability to perform the test rather than lack of stereopsis, resulting in low specificity.

There is a great need for additional data before any definite proposals for screening this age group can be made, but at present it seems that photorefraction/videorefraction is the only realistic and time-efficient candidate, the moderate sensitivity reported above perhaps being increased by adding a VA test. Photorefraction will detect myopia greater than the camera distance. It will also successfully detect anisometropia, astigmatism and high hyperopia, but moderate degrees of hyperopia will be missed. The more recent videorefractors can detect strabismus larger than 8 prism dioptres (see Chapter 9) by measuring the symmetry of the corneal reflection (Bobier et al., 1997). Although some small-angle strabismus will be missed, most strabismus at this age is of large angle and is therefore likely to be detected.

In the early school years

Measurement of VA will detect myopia, high astigmatism, amblyopia and some organic disorders. Hyperopia, moderate astigmatism and strabismus may be missed. With the addition of a VA test through plus lenses, hyperopia can be detected. If we add a stereotest such as the RDE (Chapter 9) most strabismus and monocular amblyopia will also be detected (N.B. a test of phoria could be used instead). Rooney (1992) recommends also examining accommodation (Chapter 5) and convergence (Chapter 9) as problems at near can cause difficulty with schoolwork.

VISUAL IMPAIRMENT

Early assessment of functional vision

For children who are already diagnosed as visually impaired early testing is still important, but it will take on a different emphasis. The focus is no longer on detecting abnormality, but on functional assessment and, at the appropriate developmental stage, the provision of low vision aids. Parents and teachers will need to know as early as possible the functional visual capabilities of the child. In other words, they need to know what environmental modifications can be made in order that the child's performance is not limited by lack of vision. Now we must think in terms of habilitation, that is, helping the child to keep up, as much as possible, in developmental milestones, rather than to be allowed to fall behind and then require rehabilitation.

The information regarding visual function should be made available to those who work with the child. It may be considered the right of the parents to have this information and, ideally, any professional who is working with the child should have it too (parents will very rarely refuse permission for information to be given which will benefit their child). Parents and teachers will also need counselling regarding the educational impact of a particular eye condition, its prognosis for functional vision and its stability or otherwise. Parents are also likely to benefit from counselling for the range of emotions associated with the news that a child has reduced vision (see also the section in the final chapter on 'breaking bad news'). Genetic counselling should also be offered in the case of hereditary conditions so that, should parents want more children, the risks of a similar condition occurring again can be explained.

A functional visual assessment aims to describe the visual capabilities as fully and as practically as possible. Acuity measures will still be important but will have to be described in terms that can be interpreted by lay persons. If quantitative acuity is not attainable, then the ability to fixate and track a stimulus or to make fixation movement towards a stimulus indicates some degree of visual function and vision stimulation programmes may be considered (see final chapter). However, other aspects of visual performance are as important, if not more important, than VA. Some idea of the extent of the visual field, contrast sensitivity and colour vision are also needed to fully describe functional vision. In fact, these factors can have more impact on the child's vision for functional purposes than VA; it is well accepted for adults that reduced fields or contrast sensitivity will impair performance far more drastically than the same logarithmic decrease in VA (Marron and Bailey, 1982; Pelli, 1986).

After the first functional assessment, the information must be updated regularly. There are several reasons for this:

1. As the child grows the ability to respond to different tests generally increases so that more (and more reliable) information becomes available.
2. Functional vision may actually improve either of its own accord or in response to specific visual stimulation programmes.
3. Some ocular disorders are progressive.

Assessing functional vision, then, is a primary reason for testing the vision of children with visual impairments.

A second reason is that early visual acuity measurement can be predictive of eventual visual outcome in certain disorders. For example, Birch and Spencer (1991) have shown that forced choice preferential looking acuity is predictive of both the visual and anatomical outcome in retinopathy of prematurity (ROP).

A third reason for functional assessment is that advice about environmental modifications needs to be given as early as possible. People who work with the child should be made aware of how to increase visual contrast in the home and at nursery or preschool/kindergarten, what colour combinations to use and what type of pens. For example, the surround of doors and the edges of steps and stairs can be marked with a contrasting colour. Felt tip pens (or textas, for our Australian readers) provide better contrast than pencils or wax crayons. Picture information should be simple and uncluttered. However, many of the materials and toys for preschoolers are within the visual capabilities of visually impaired children, but parents may need to be encouraged to allow the child to do puzzle books and play with educational toys which are within the visual capabilities of the child. In fact, a more systematic approach to their learning of visual processing skills may be necessary. Information regarding appropriate lighting should be given, e.g. does the child need more or less light than normal and is glare a problem? Written information and ideas can be given to the parents and the child should be linked with relevant organizations who will become involved with the child in their own setting, such as the Royal National Institute for the Blind, UK. The eye professional should ensure that the child is registered as visually impaired or blind and that the family is linked with all necessary and desired support organizations.

A fourth reason for regular assessment of children with low vision is so that low vision aids can be introduced at the appropriate point. Hats with wide brims, tinted glasses and side shields for glare control can be introduced from a very early age for infants with conditions known to result in photophobia. Contact lenses with opaque iris imprints should also be considered in cases such as albinism as they may help control glare more effectively than glasses. Visual demands increase as the child goes through school owing to decreased print size, decreased available accommodation (with age) and increased volume of work and, at some point, low vision aids may be required (preferably as early as the child can learn to use them). Ritchie, Sonksen and Gould (1989) recommend that stand magnifiers should be introduced when a child reaches the level of development and attention of a sighted 2–3 year old. This can result in an increase in visual experience, allowing the child to gain an appreciation of detail otherwise not seen (for example, small objects or detail on postage stamps), and may even improve unaided visual functioning. The exact developmental level at which children can benfit is dependent on visual acuity: the poorer the vision, the greater the developmental age required. Telescopes should be considered as soon as the child has sufficient hand-eye co-ordination so that an appreciation of distance detail such as birds and animals can be gained. However, as we noted earlier, many children with visual impairments are certainly not obtaining regular low vision aid assessments. In fact many are not receiving assessments at all (Leat and Karadsheh, 1991) and are consequently being supplied with low vision aids by teachers; this is unlikely to result in a child receiving the optimum aids for his or her own particular needs and level of visual function. Brennan et al. (1992) found that several children with aphakia had either not been prescribed bifocals or had bifocals positioned too low to be used (having no lens in the eye, these children definitely need some sort of separate reading prescription – see Chapter 5). If visual impairment is diagnosed, the child should be referred to a low vision clinic or to an optometrist who undertakes low vision work where the child should be monitored yearly.

Cosmetic considerations are also important. It should not be thought that this is only important to teenagers and adults. Children's interactions with each other and adults are highly dependent on looks, so that a child's social integration and even emotional development may be dependent on appearance. We should always consider and offer the options for best cosmesis, whether this be strabismus surgery for a child with developmental delay or contact lenses to get rid of glasses which are very thick and heavy or have an unusual tint. Contact lenses should be considered for cosmetic reasons for very high prescriptions, as in high myopia and in aphakia, and when very dark tints or red tints are necessary, as in achromatopsia. However, it must also be remembered that contact lenses are not necessarily the best cosmetic option. Some children with unusual eyes may look better, and feel less self conscious, with glasses. For example, a child was seen who had a very hyperopic, amblyopic and microphthalmic right eye while the left eye was normal; although she did not benefit visually from the refractive correction in the right eye, it was decided to prescribe a high plus lens which magnified the appearance of that eye, making it look more similar to the left.

In summary, early and regular visual assessment of children with visual impairments is important to enable:

1. Functional vision to be assessed (with counselling to the parents).
2. Acuity to be assessed – early acuity may be predictive of final acuity in some disorders.
3. Advice to be given regarding environmental adaptations.
4. The child to be linked with appropriate support organizations.
5. The introduction of low vision aids when required.
6. The tracking of changes in visual function.
7. A consideration of cosmetic factors.

The role of parents in visual impairment

On the question of habilitation or rehabilitation, we have already noted that since early intervention has been encouraged, children without vision have demonstrated more developed abilities. Leung and Hollins (1989) have drawn attention to the particular role of parents in intervention programmes. Whereas it was once usual to send children away to residential 'schools for the blind', with minimal involvement of parents, now many more are educated in mainstream schools, with parents continuing to play a central role.

Guralnick (1991) has reviewed the effectiveness of early intervention programmes for children with developmental disabilities (such as Down syndrome) and at biologic risk (such as very low birth weight). In some instances developmental problems were eliminated, while in others the degree of decline as the children matured was minimized. It is now thought that one of the most vital elements of such programmes is involvement of families. In particular, it is thought important to foster 'normal' parent–child relationships, given that disruption can occur in various ways (e.g lack of eye contact if the baby is blind, lack of a close early relationship with a preterm infant in an incubator). The precise mechanisms are unknown as yet, but Greenstein (1975) found that deaf children's language development was related not so much to the mother's linguistic style but to the warmth of the mother–child relationship. Conner (1976) suggests that the amount of mutual looking may be a vital link here. If so, this suggests an important reason for assessing whether a child's visual potential will permit, or can be improved enough to permit, parent–child visual contact or, if not, to explore alternatives, such as using touch to indicate conversational turn-taking as mentioned previously.

Part of the vision care professional's role is to educate families about their child's condition and the services available to them. Although some parents do indeed become experts on their child's particular condition – the film 'Lorenzo's Oil' representing the most remarkable case – others know very little, because previous attempts at education have been ineffective or non-existent. A parent may, for example, be able to say that the child has had an operation, but be unable to say precisely what the nature of it was. Also, they may not realize if the condition is a genetic one. Hill (1987) points out that they, and later the children themselves, are entitled to genetic counselling, as well as vocational guidance to avoid the building up of plans which are unrealistic, whether aimed too high or too low.

There are numerous reasons, then, why it is vital that professionals working with children with disabilities establish good collaborative relationships with parents. Good communication skills are essential for this, and communicating with both parents and children will be discussed in detail in the next chapter. At this point, we can note that establishing good relationships with parents of children with disabilities is not always easy, and there is often a tendency for parent and professional to adopt an adversarial stance. Seligman and Seligman (1980) have identified five negative attitudes of professionals which foster conflict. They are feeling pity, fear or hostility towards child or parents, feeling hopeless about the situation, reinforcing family denial of the problem, viewing the family's observations as untrustworthy and viewing the family members as emotionally disturbed. There are perhaps two underlying roots to these unhelpful attitudes.

The first is frustration arising from dealing with clients who are difficult to assess and/or whose problems seem insurmountable. This can be alleviated by increasing practitioner knowledge about children with special needs and ways to adapt standard procedures for them (these issues are addressed throughout this book). It also has to be recognized that where 'cure' is not an option, the professional still has a role to play in helping child and family to cope.

The second kind of difficulty faced by the professional is a lack of understanding of the family's viewpoint and the particular expertise they themselves bring to the situation. Recognizing and respecting parental expertise is fundamental to developing good relationships with parents. The days of the old 'doctor knows best' relationship in health care are numbered (Shute, 1991), and the expertise of the vision care worker cannot be effective without parental co-operation. As Davis (1993) has said in a book about communicating with the parents of children with disabilities, 'the effects would be compromised if the parents disagreed, were not consulted or were distressed or dissatisfied' (p. 38). As we noted above, some parents gain expertise on their child's condition which outstrips that of the professionals, and all parents are experts about the needs of their particular family as well as invaluable advocates and rehabilitators for their child. The major exception is when the eye professional suspects that a child has been abused, in which case it may be necessary, in the interests of the child, to take action contrary to the wishes of the family (dealing with child abuse is discussed in detail in the next chapter).

CONCLUSION

This chapter has established the importance of assessing children's vision and managing any problems early in life, in the interests of future vision, health and overall development. We have given particular attention to the vision care of those children who are the most profoundly at risk in terms of being unable to fulfil their developmental tasks because of low vision or multiple impairments. However, we should not forget the many children who are the 'bread and butter' of vision care practice. Their visual problems may be mild by comparison, but are nevertheless of great importance to the individuals concerned. Even relatively mild visual defects may put a child at some disadvantage. Examples given by Chapman and Stone (1988) include the child with uncorrected myopia who does not realize that stars exist, or that trees have separate leaves (also noted by Leat; personal communication); the child with undiagnosed hyperopia who is unable to concentrate on close activities; the child with defective colour vision who does not understand reactions to his strangely-painted pictures; and the child with unclear vision who misses out socially by not quite grasping what is going on. Good vision care has an important part to play in the lives of the many with such mild problems as well as the few whose needs are greatest.

REFERENCES

Aitken, S. and Buultjens, M. (1991). Visual assessments of children with multiple impairments: a survey of ophthalmologists. *Journal of Visual Impairment and Blindness*, **85**, 170–173.

Allen, J. and Fraser, K. (1983). Evaluation of visual capacity in visually impaired and multi-handicapped children. *Rehabil. Optom.*, **1**, 5.

American Academy of Ophthalmology (1994). *Basic and clinical science course in pediatric ophthalmology and strabismus. 1994–1995. Section 6.*

Atkinson, J. (1993). Infant vision screening: Prediction and prevention of strabismus and amblyopia from refractive screening in the Cambridge photorefraction program. In K. Simons (ed.), *Early Visual Development, Normal and Abnormal*. Oxford, Oxford University Press.

Birch, E.E. and Spencer, R. (1991). Visual outcome in infants with cicatricial retinopathy of prematurity. *Investigative Ophthalmology and Vision Science*, **32**, 410–415.

Bobier, W.R., Guinta, A., Kurtz, S. and Howland, H.C. (1997). Identification of convergence accommodation in infants aged 2 to 6 months. *Vision Science and its Applications*, Vol. 1, OSA Technical Digest Series. Washington DC: Optical Society of America. pp. 108–111.

Brennan, V., Miller, K.B., Ryu, F. and Lolli, D. (1992). A model to provide outreach low vision services to children with deaf-blindness. *Journal of Visual Impairment and Blindness*, **86**, 65–67.

Chapman, E.K. and Stone, J.M. (1988). *The Visually Handicapped Child in your Classroom*. London, Cassell.

Conner, L.E. (1976). New directions in infant programs for the deaf. *The Volta Review*, **78**, 8–15.

Cress, P.J., Spellman, C.R., DeBriere, T.J. et al. (1981). Vision screening for persons with severe handicaps. *JASH*, **6**, 41.

Davis, H. (1993). *Counselling Parents of Children with Chronic Illness or Disability.* Leicester, BPS Books.

Fern, K.D. (1991). A comparison of vision screening techniques in preschool children. *Investigative Ophthalmology and Vision Science*, **32**, 962.

Feuerstein, R., Rand, Y. and Rynders, J.E. (1988). *Don't Accept Me as I Am: Helping "Retarded" People to Excel.* New York, Plenum.

Geruschat, D.R. (1992). Using the acuity card procedure to assess visual acuity in children with severe and multiple impairments. *Journal of Visual Impairment and Blindness*, **86**, 25–27.

Giles, H. (1991). "Gosh, you don't look it!" A sociolinguistic construction of ageing. *The Psychologist: Bulletin of the British Psychological Society*, **3**, 99–106.

Graham, P.A. (1974). Epidemiology of strabismus. *British Journal of Ophthalmology*, **58**, 224–231.

Greenstein, J.M. (1975). *Methods of Fostering Language in Deaf Infants.* Final report to HEW, Grant no OEG-0-72-5339, June, 1975.

Groenendaal, F. and van Hof-van Duin J. (1992). Visual deficits and improvements in children after perinatal hypoxia. *Journal of Visual Impairment and Blindness*, **86** (5), 215–218.

Guralnick, M.J. (1991). The next decade of research on the effectiveness of early intervention. *Exceptional Children*, **58**, 174–183.

Hall, D.B.M. (1989). *Health for all Children. Report of the Joint Working Pary on Child Health Surveillance*, Oxford, Oxford University Press.

Hammond, R.S. and Schmidt, P.P. (1986). A random dot E stereogram for the vision screening of children. *Archives of Ophthalmology*, **104**, 54–60.

Harries, D. (1989). Multi-handicapped people and service development. *British Journal of Visual Impairment*, **VII**, 43–46.

Harrison, W. (1985). Assessment and stimulation of vision in multiple-handicapped children. *British Orthoptic Journal*, **42**, 26–31.

Hertz B.G. (1987). Acuity card testing of retarded children. *Behavioral Brain Research*, **24**, 85–92.

Hertz, B.G. and Rosenberg, J. (1988). Acuity card testing of spastic children: preliminary results. *Journal of Pediatric Ophthalmology and Strabismus*, **25**, 139–144.

Hill, J.L. (1987). Rights of low vision children and their parents. *Canadian Journal of Optometry*, Summer 1987, **49**, 78–82.

Hofstetter, H.W. (1985). Unmet vision care needs. *Journal of Vision Rehabilitation*, **3**, 16.

Hyvarinen, L. (1994). Assessment of visually impaired infants. *Low Vision and Vision Rehabilitation*, **7**, 219–225.

Ingram, R.M., Walker, C., Wilson, J.M. et al. (1986). Prediction of amblyopia and squint by means of refraction at age 1 year. *British Journal of Ophthalmology*, **69**, 851–853.

Jacobson, L. (1988). Ophthalmology in mentally retarded adults. *Acta Ophthalmologica*, **66**, 457–462.

Kanski, J.J. (1989). *Clinical Ophthalmology.* London, Butterworths.

Leat, S.J. and Karadsheh, S. (1991). Use and non-use of low vision aids by visually impaired children. *Ophthalmic and Physiological Optics*, **11**, 10–15.

Lennerstrand, G., Axelsson, A. and Andersson, G. (1983). Visual acuity testing with preferential looking in mental retardation. *Acta Ophthalmologica*, **61**, 624–633.

Leung, E. and Hollins, M. (1989). The blind child. In M. Hollins (ed.), *Understanding Blindness.* New Jersey, Lawrence Erlbaum.

Lovie-Kitchin, J.E. and Bowman, K.J. (1985). *Senile Macular Degeneration.* Boston, Butterworths.

Marron, J.A. and Bailey, I.L. (1982). Visual factors and orientation-mobility performance. *American Journal of Optometry and Physiological Optics*, **59**, 413–426.

Marsh-Tootle, W.L., Corliss, D.A., Alvarez, S. et al. (1994). A statistical analysis of modified clinical technique vision screening of preschoolers by optometry students. *Optometry and Vision Science*, **71**, 593–603.

Mayer, D. L., Fulton, A.B. and Rodier, D. (1984). Grating and recognition acuities of pediatric patients. *Ophthalmology*, **91**, 947–952.

Meades, J., Woodhouse, J.M. and Leat (1990). Assessment of accommodation in children. *Ophthalmic and Physiological Optics*, **10**, 413.

Michael, M.G. and Paul, P.V. (1991). Early intervention for infants with deaf-blindness. *Exceptional Children*, **57**, 200–210.

Miranda, S.B. and Fantz R.L. (1973). Visual preferences of Down's syndrome and normal infants. *Child Development*, **43**, 555.

Miranda, S.B. and Fantz R.L. (1974). Recognition memory in Down's syndrome and normal infants. *Child Development*, **45**, 651.

Miranda, S.B, Hack, M., Fantz, R.L. and Fanaroff, A.A. (1977). Neonatal pattern vision: predictor of future mental performance? *Journal of Paediatrics*, **91**, 642–647.

Mohn, G. and van Hof-van Duin, J. (1983). Behavioural and electrophysiological measures of visual disorders in children with neurological disorders. *Behavioural Brain Research*, **10**, 177–187.

Moore, A. (1990). Retinoblastoma. In D. Taylor (ed.), *Ophthalmology*. Boston, Blackwell Scientific Publications.

Nielsen, L. (1992). *Space and Self: Active Learning by Means of The Little Room.* Copenhagen, SIKON.

von Noorden, G.K. (1988). A reassessment of infantile esotropia. XLIV Edward Jackson Memorial Lecture. *American Journal of Ophthalmology*, **105**, 1–10.

North, R. (1993). *Work and the Eye.* Oxford, Oxford Medical Publications.

Orel-Bixler, D., Haegerstom-Portnoy, G. and Hall, A. (1989). Visual assessment of the multi-handicapped patient. *Optometry and Vision Science*, **66**, 530–536.

Pelli, D.G. (1986). The visual requirements of mobility. In G.C. Woo (ed.), *Low Vision; Principles and Applications.* New York, Springer-Verlag.

Ritchie, J.P., Sonksen, P.M. and Gould, E. (1989). Low vision aids for preschool children. *Developmental Medicine and Child Neurology*, **31**, 509–519.

Rogow, S.M., Hass, J. and Humphries, C. (1984). Learning to look: Cognitive aspects of visual attention. *Canadian Journal of Optometry*, **46**, 31–34.

Rooney, K. (1992). *Strategies of Early Intervention for Literacy and Learning for Australian Children.* Submission to House of Representatives Standing Committee on Employment, Education and Training, South Australia.

Rosner, J. and Rosner, J. (1990). *Pediatric Optometry*, 2nd edn, Boston, Butterworths.

Schmidt, P.P. (1990). Vision screening. In A.A. Rosenbloom and M.W. Morgan (eds), *Principles and Practice of Pediatric Optometry.* New York, Lippincott.

Seligman, M. and Seligman, P.A. (1980). The professional's dilemma: learning to work with parents. *Exceptional Parent*, **10**, 511–513.

Shute, R.H. (1991). *Psychology in Vision Care.* Oxford, Butterworth-Heinemann.

Simons, H.D. and Gassler, P.A. (1988). Vision anomalies and reading skills: A review of the literature. *American Journal of Optometry and Physiological Optics*, **65**, 893–904.

Tomsak, R.L. and Dell'Osso, L.F. (1995). Eye movement disturbances in children. In R.L. Tomsak and J. Lawton-Smith (eds), *Pediatric Neuro-ophthalmology.* Boston, Butterworth-Heinemann.

Troster, H., Brambring, M. and Beelmann, A. (1991). Prevalence and situational causes of stereotyped behaviors in blind infants and preschoolers. *Journal of Abnormal Child Psychology*, **19**, (5), 569–590.

Warburg, M. (1970). Tracing and training of blind and partially sighted patients in institutions for the mentally retarded. *Danish Medical Bulletin*, **17**, 148–152.

Warburg, M. (1982). Why are blind and severely impaired children with mental retardation much more retarded than sighted children? Symposium on early visual development. *Acta Ophthalmologica*, **157** (suppl.), 72–81.

3

Opening the consultation

INTRODUCTION

In this chapter we consider a number of issues which are of importance at the opening of a consultation with a child's family: risk factors for various disorders, presenting signs and symptoms and effective communication skills.

Initially, we need to be aware of the risk factors for various ocular and visual disorders in children, as well as those for systemic disorders which have an ocular impact. The types of presenting problems will also vary between different types of practice. Parents are likely to take a child with an ocular injury to an emergency facility, while a child with a red, sticky eye may be taken to the family doctor. The optometrist in a university clinic or hospital setting will see a different population of children from those who work in private practices. Eye practitioners who provide services to those with special needs will see a large number of children with multiple challenges and with ocular disorders which result in visual impairment.

Information about risk factors needs to be considered in association with the presenting signs and symptoms. Signs are the objective evidence of a disorder and may include the observations of parents, other carers and the examiner. Symptoms are the subjective observations or complaints by the child, including pain or discomfort associated with the use of their vision. When working with preverbal children (or older non-verbal children) signs will be more readily available (and will usually be given more weight) than symptoms. In fact, often we will have to rely on objective information regarding discomfort or difficulty occurring when the child engages in visual tasks since children, even those who can speak, are less likely to complain of symptoms than are adults. They assume that their own visual experience is normal and even symptoms such as headaches after reading may simply lead the child to abandon the task rather than to complain. Poor vision may only become evident when an adult observes some unusual reaction. The signs noticed by parents and other adults are therefore critically important, usually being the reason for the child's being brought for examination.

Parents are usually good judges about whether there is a visual problem present or not. Occasionally, however, a parent's concerns prove unfounded or, conversely, a child's vision appears poorer on testing that the parent believes it is. This can happen because some children, particularly those with cortical visual impairment and/or multiple impairments, perform better at home than in the unfamiliar and possibly threatening environment of the consulting room.

Taking an effective history from the family is a crucial element of the consultation. The goals for the examiner during initial discussion with parent and child will include determining the chief concern of the parents and eliciting information about general background history and specific signs and symptoms. The ability to communicate well and to provide an atmosphere conducive to an effective examination is therefore essential, so later in the chapter we look in detail at ways of promoting effective communication with parents and children.

RISK FACTORS

Risk factors can be separated into four categories: genetic, prenatal (arising between conception and birth), perinatal (arising during birth or in the first week of life) and postnatal (occurring any time after the first week of life). Often, these influences will interact with one another to determine the outcome, e.g., if a child is born with a visual impairment eventual visual capacity will be further compromised if a suitably stimulating environment is not provided.

The purpose of this section is not to describe each condition in depth, but rather to alert the eye professional to the factors which most commonly give rise to ocular disorders and to the most common associated ocular disorders in each case. The interested student is referred to books on paediatric ophthalmology for further detail, such as that by Taylor (1990) (see also Chapter 4 on ocular health assessment).

Genetic risk factors

There are many eye disorders which show a Mendelian inheritance pattern. For example, albinism (lack of pigment in hair, skin and eyes) is usually autosomal recessive while ocular albinism (affecting the eyes only) is usually X-linked recessive, thus affecting more boys than girls. The most clear and common example of X-linked recessive inheritance is colour deficiency, affecting 8% of white boys. Other conditions behave with a Mendelian pattern but with variable penetrance (frequency of expression of a gene) or expressivity (severity of condition). For example, X-linked retinoschisis has high penetrance with variable expressivity (Kanski, 1988), so that some people have the mutated gene but not the condition. Best's macular dystrophy, which is autosomal dominant, has variable penetrance and expressivity. Other conditions show a variety of inheritance patterns. For example, retinitis pigmentosa can be autosomal recessive, autosomal dominant or X-linked recessive.

Many other disorders, such as moderate and low myopia and infantile esotropia, are multifactorial (Fatt, Griffin and Lyle, 1992). This means that a number of genes determine the condition together with environmental factors. Gwiazda et al. (1993) found that if one parent is myopic there is a 22.5% chance of the child developing myopia whereas if both parents are myopic the chances increase to 42%. Retinoblastoma is inherited in some cases but not in others; genetic investigations can determine whether or not subsequent siblings are at risk and therefore in need of screening (Gallie, 1993).

Consanguinity results in a much higher incidence of many types of disorders, ranging from cerebral palsy to rare syndromes to specific ocular disorders such as Stargardt's disease. The practitioner needs to ask whether the parents are blood relatives if genetic eye disease is suspected.

Hughes and Newton (1992) suspect that many cases of cerebral palsy may be genetic in origin and that the number of cases caused by perinatal asphyxia or infections is lower than previously thought. A low Apgar score at birth (denoting a developmentally delayed infant, see Chapter 1) may not mean that the damage occurred as a result of birthing difficulties, but may rather indicate that the infant was already developmentally damaged prior to birth. (See below and Chapter 1 for descriptions of cerebral palsy.)

Although this book cannot include a comprehensive coverage of the many genetic syndromes (some very rare) which have ocular repercussions, we have provided below a brief description of two of the commonest, Down Syndrome and Fragile X Syndrome.

Down syndrome (Trisomy 21)

This is due to an additional, or an additional part of, chromosome 21. It is the most common genetic cause of intellectual impairment and may be becoming more common as the age at which people have children is increasing. The incidence is 1 in every 600–800 births, but this increases dramatically as the age of the mother increases, e.g. to 1 in 40 at the age of 40. Older fathers are also more likely to have a child with Down syndrome (e.g. Hook, 1980). Ocular abnormalities and complications in Down syndrome are as follows (Millis, 1987).

1. Short, oblique palpebral apertures (gap between eyelids when eye is open) and epicanthus (fold of skin over nasal junction of lids).
2. Brushfield's spots (white or yellow raised speckles on iris) in 85%. These have no functional significance.
3. High refractive errors (myopia, hyperopia and astigmatism).
4. Strabismus.
5. Congenital nystagmus.
6. Cataract.
7. Blepharitis (inflammation of the eyelids).
8. Colour vision abnormalities (Perez-Carpinell et al., 1994; de Fez and Climent, 1994).
9. Exposure keratitis (inflammation of the cornea) due to incomplete closure of lids while sleeping.
10. Keratoconus (abnormal cornea) in 6%.
11. Reduced accommodation (Woodhouse et al., 1993; see also Chapter 5 on refractive error).

12. Slightly reduced visual acuity. Acuity is often somewhat reduced even in the absence of ocular anomalies. Commonly, values between 6/30 and 6/9 are found for children between the ages of 6 and 12 years (Courage et al., 1994).
13. Unusual vessels at the optic disc (more cross the optic discs).
14. Reduced contrast sensitivity has been reported (Perez-Carpinell et al., 1994) but this involved the Vistech charts for which the repeatability has been questioned.

Fragile X Syndrome

This has only fairly recently been recognized, yet it is second only to Down syndrome as a genetic cause of intellectual impairment and is its most common familial (inherited) cause (Maino et al., 1990). Frequencies are estimated at 1/1000 for males and 1/2000 for females and the penetrance is high. Diagnosis used to be based on testing for sites in the X chromosomes that were liable to breakage in certain cultures. The current method of diagnosis consists of molecular testing for trinucleotide repeats. The condition results in a large range of physical signs, speech and language difficulties, perceptual anomalies and behavioural disorders. Poor eye contact, strabismus and refractive error are the eye signs associated with this disease.

Prenatal risk factors

Since prenatal defects arise so early in development, multiple defects are common. In fact, the finding of three or more structural anomalies (e.g. of hands, face, eye, mouth or ear) indicates that the origin of the anomaly is prenatal. Unexplained intellectual impairment also indicates a prenatal developmental cause.

Prenatal risk factors fall into the following three classes:

1. Infection, e.g. cytomegalovirus (CMV), toxoplasmosis.
2. Insult (anoxia, drugs or trauma) → cerebral palsy ± epilepsy, IUGR (see below), fetal alcohol syndrome.
3. Ideopathic, developmental, e.g. spina bifida, hydrocephalus, cerebral palsy.

These factors are interactive with each other and with genetic and environmental factors.

Toxoplasmosis

This results in chorioretinitis, or inflammation of both the retina and choroid (both resolved and active), strabismus (where the chorio-retinal scarring occurs at the macula), papillitis (inflammation of the optic nerve head), papilloedema, intellectual impairment, hydrocephalus, microcephaly (small head), and epilepsy.

Cytomegalovirus

This is the most common of intra-uterine infections. There are many complications, including microcephaly, optic atrophy, chorioretinitis, microphthalmos, cataracts and keratitis.

Rubella (German measles)

Infection in the first trimester results in a more complete syndrome, i.e. evidencing more of the signs. Infection in the fourth month results in fewer effects. Congenital rubella syndrome includes intellectual impairment, heart defects, growth retardation, hearing loss, cataract, microphthalmos, pigmentary retinopathy with slightly reduced acuity, keratitis and glaucoma.

Hydrocephalus

This is an increased pressure in the cerebrospinal fluid (Rosenbloom and Morgan, 1990). It can be due to developmental abnormalities or be caused by infection, haemorrhages resulting from prematurity (see below), tumours or meningitis. It is treated by the surgical insertion of a shunt between the ventricles of the brain and either the heart or the peritoneal cavity. If untreated, or not treated in time, it results in intellectual and physical impairments, optic atrophy and cortical visual loss. In fact, it is rare for diagnosis to occur and for a shunt to be installed before some cortical damage has occurred. The shunts can lose patency due to mechanical blockage or infection which can result in further brain damage including optic atrophy. Strabismus may be secondary to optic atrophy or due to nerve palsies. Gaze palsies and nystagmus are common.

Spina Bifida

This is a developmental abnormality of the spinal cord in which there is incomplete closure of the cord posteriorly (Rosenbloom and Morgan, 1990). The most serious form of this is myelomeningocoele in which the nervous tissue protrudes through the unclosed spinal cord and results in physical disabilities in the lower limbs and lack of function in some organs. Hydrocephalus is associated with spina bifida. Strabismus is common in hydrocephalus. It can be con-comitant due to loss of acuity because of optic atrophy or incomitant due to nerve palsies. It may be secondary to encephalitis or meningitis resulting from the exposed neural tissue. Various patterns of ocular motility have been reported.

Cerebral palsy (CP)

It is now thought that the most common causes of CP are prenatal and genetic (Nelson, 1991; Hughes and Newton, 1992), although it can also result from perinatal and postnatal influences. Causes include, anoxia, toxaemia, maternal thyroid abnormality, prenatal maternal infection (e.g. herpes zoster, influenza), postnatal infection in the child (e.g. meningitis, mumps), prematurity and trauma (including non-accidental injury). The incidence of ocular disorders is high, estimated at 56–75% (Jones and Dayton, 1968). The frequency of ocular disorders is as follows:

1. Significant refractive errors: 40–76% (Maino, 1979).
2. Strabismus: 34–60% (Duckman, 1979), esotropia being more common than exotropia, and 43% having an additional vertical component.
3. Incomitant eye movements or difficulty tracking a target: 40% (Leat, 1996).
4. Reduced visual acuity: 12–24%.
5. Ocular pathology (most commonly optic atrophy) 28%.

There is some evidence that most of these ocular disorders are approximately twice as common amongst those with spastic rather than athetoid cerebral palsy (See Chapter 1). Reduced accommodation has been reported in 100% using a subjective test and 42% using objective dynamic retinoscopy (Duckman, 1979; Leat, 1996). Other reported disorders are visual perceptual difficulties (Duckman, 1979) and nystagmus (Evans et al., 1985).

Intra-uterine Growth Retardation (IUGR)
This is diagnosed if a child weighs less than the 10th percentile for his/her gestational age. The most common causes are fetal alcohol syndrome, maternal malnutrition and viral disease (e.g. cytomegalovirus, rubella). Children classified with IUGR are likely to have intellectual and physical impairments. Low birth weight infants are more prone to visual impairment, myopia, strabismus (esotropia), retinopathy of prematurity and visual perceptual problems.

Fetal Alcohol Syndrome (FAS)
This can occur if the mother has abused alcohol during pregnancy (Rosenbloom and Morgan, 1990). Abuse of alcohol means drinking several measures of alcohol per day in the first few months (Maino, 1995). There may be a resultant central nervous system dysfunction of the child. Most commonly this includes microcephaly, intellectual impairment and growth deficiency. The eyes are widely spaced with a short palpebral aperture. There is also a high prevalence of myopia, strabismus, ptosis, astigmatism, steep corneal curvature and retinal and optic nerve abnormalities, as well as anterior segment anomalies (e.g. corneal opacities, anterior chamber anomalies and iris defects).

Other recreational drugs
There is no clear pattern of either systemic or ocular effects in mothers who use recreational drugs during pregnancy (Giese, 1994). The difficulty in establishing patterns is partly due to the fact that many are multiple drug users. The use of recreational drugs is also associated with poor nutrition which would then become a confounding factor which in itself can lead to IUGR. There seem to be more data on the use of cocaine than other drugs and the following ocular complications have been named: optic nerve anomalies, delayed visual maturation, eyelid oedema, nystagmus, strabismus,

retinal coloboma and microphthalmia (see also Block et al., 1997). The use of marijuana has been implicated in causing myopia, strabismus, abnormal oculomotor function and optic nerve head anomalies. Heroin has been implicated in causing low birth weight, prematurity and small head circumference. The most consistent findings for all drug use is that of neurobehavioural defects such as difficulty attending to and engaging in stimuli and difficulty in changing states of arousal.

Perinatal risk factors

Risk factors occurring around birth can be grouped into three categories:

1. Prematurity.
2. Fetal distress resulting in antepartum haemorrhage or neonatal asphyxia. This often results in spastic cerebral palsy.
3. Infections, e.g. herpes simplex.

The Apgar score gives an index of the baby's health status straight after birth (see Chapter 1).

Preterm infants

Children who are born preterm (before 37 weeks gestation) are frequently low in birth weight also (less than 2500 g or 5.5 lb). Birth weights between 1500 and 2500 g can occur in full-term babies, being then due to intrauterine growth retardation. Very low birth weight is defined as 1500 g (3.3 lb) to 1000 g (2.2 lb) and extremely low birth weight is less than 1000 g. The incidence of low birth weight infants in Britain in 1979 was 6.9% and of very low birth weight was 0.9%. Figures in European countries are similar. Of the very low birth weight babies, 74% of live births survive the first 28 days and the survival rates are improving dramatically (Fielder et al., 1993).

Preterm birth is associated with higher prevalence and larger amounts of myopia (see Chapter 5). As gestational age and birth weight of premature infants decrease, the risk of retinopathy of prematurity (ROP), and the risk of greater severity of ROP, increases (Ng et al., 1988). ROP is also associated with a further risk of myopia (see also Chapter 4).

Birthweight and associated ROP risk are as follows.

Birth weight	Percent with ROP
< 1000 g	53–88.5
1300 g	55.6–75.4
1500 g	35–60

(Figures from Fielder et al., 1993).

Visual acuity is lower in preterm babies (without other complications) but they catch up by 8 months, i.e. rate of development seems to be faster in preterm infants. If corrected for postconceptual age, they have slightly better or similar acuity (van Hof-van Duin and Mohn,

1986). It is thought that the vision stimulation of being out of the womb may speed up development.

Bilateral posterior subcapsular symmetrical lens opacities are sometimes seen in preterm infants. These often resolve with no residual abnormalities.

Periventricular and intraventricular haemorrhages often occur during hypoxic insults or hypertensive episodes and the most common time is 38 hours after birth. These frequently result in hydrocephalus, motor and intellectual disability, cerebral palsy, epilepsy, cortical blindness (due to damage of the optic radiations or visual cortex) and strabismus (esotropia, where one eye turns in, or hypotropia, where one eye turns down when the other fixates). Porencephaly (cavities or cysts in the brain) commonly develops in areas where the haemorrhages spread. The more premature the baby, the greater the risk of these complications.

Fetal Distress

Groenendaal and van Hof-van Duin (1992) measured a number of visual functions in children who had suffered severe perinatal hypoxia and who had a range of intellectual, neurological and/or physical impairments. They found that all the children had some ocular or visual defect ranging from slight to severe, e.g. abnormalities of pupils, ocular motility and visual fields and loss of visual acuity.

Herpes simplex

Infection is transmitted to the child from a mother with genital herpes at the time of vaginal delivery. Complications are encephalitis resulting in neurological impairment, blepharoconjunctivitis, occasionally retinitis or vitritis (inflammation of the vitreous) resulting in secondary cataracts.

Postnatal risk factors

1. Infection and inflammatory diseases (e.g. meningitis).
2. Trauma (accidental and non-accidental) → haemorrhage → cerebral atrophy, optic atrophy (see later in this chapter for the effects of non-accidental injury).
3. Tumour.
4. Environmental (e.g. malnutrition, socio-economic status, passive abuse; see below).

Malnutrition, although rare in Western societies, must be recognized as one of the world's leading causes of blindness in children, often in combination with infections (Sandford-Smith, 1986). Children are more susceptible to vitamin A deficiency and the ocular effects are conjunctival and corneal dryness, Bitot's spots (raised spots resulting from hardening of the exposed conjunctiva), corneal ulceration, night blindness and retinal changes. Protein deficiency makes the effects of vitamin A deficiency more devastating.

Socio-economic status is a factor in the prevalence of prematurity and low birth weight (being higher in lower socio-economic groups) and possibly in the prevalence of some types of cerebral palsy even when the confounding effect of low birth weight has been factored out (Dowding and Barry, 1990).

Passive abuse, or neglect, involves failing to provide for a child's physical and emotional needs. It will have severe consequences on the child's emotional and behavioural development. Severe lack of stimulation may result in lack of development of cognitive and visual processing skills. Abuse is dealt with below in some detail.

CHILD ABUSE

This is not a subject that any health care professional dealing with children can ignore. There has been a dramatic increase in reported cases of child abuse with, for example, an average increase of 6% per year in America between 1985 to the early 1990s (Giese, 1994). In one Ontario urban area of population 200 000, there were 4000 reported suspected cases in 1991. Of these, there were 196 cases of physical abuse, 600 children considered to be at high risk of physical abuse, 270 cases of founded sexual abuse, 300 cases which were at high risk of sexual abuse and 125 cases of neglect. This means that of the total reported cases, 15% were founded and 22.5% were high risk. Therefore, we must be aware that when we examine children's vision we will sometimes see children who have been, are being, or are at risk of being, abused and we must be cognizant of the signs. Laws have now been passed in all states of the USA and provinces of Canada that all suspected cases must be reported. Failure to report is considered a crime. The same applies in South Australia for certain professionals who are mandated to report suspicions of abuse which arise in the course of their professional work. Health professionals must be aware of the legal requirements in their particular country, province or state. It could also be argued that all individuals, regardless of legal obligations, have a moral responsibility to report suspected cases of child abuse to the appropriate children's care organization.

Legal definitions of abuse vary somewhat between jurisdictions. The following description is based loosely on current Ontario law. All forms of abuse can occur actively (commission) or passively (omission), for example, by shaking a child or by failing to prevent a partner from shaking a child.

Types of abuse

1. Physical abuse. This is non-accidental injury, e.g. hitting a child hard enough to leave bruises, shaken baby syndrome.
2. Emotional abuse. This is continuous criticism, verbal harassment or other acts which undermine a child's self-esteem, e.g. constantly saying that the child is not loved or wanted, or is worthless or useless.

3. Sexual abuse. This falls into two categories: molestation (touching a child with sexual intent) and exploitation (exposing the child to sexual stimuli, e.g. pornographic pictures).
4. Neglect. This occurs when the genuine physical or emotional needs of the child are not met. *Emotional neglect* is the continual withholding of love, nurturance, communication or stimulation from a child, e.g. if the child receives little or no affection on an ongoing basis. *Physical neglect* is failure to provide the basic needs of food, clothing and shelter. *Lack of medical treatment* (not providing consent for medical treatment to cure, prevent or alleviate physical suffering or harm) constitutes a form of neglect.

The use of recreational drugs during pregnancy may also be considered a form of child abuse.

A child is considered to be in need of protection where abuse has already happened or there is considered to be a substantial risk of its happening. Suspicion should be founded on reasonable evidence. In law, the responsibility to report suspected abuse may transcend other legal responsibilities such as acts which deal with confidentiality. In other words, we do not have to obtain the parents' consent to release information or even inform them that we are going to make a report, although it may be preferable to do so (see Chapter 14 for a discussion of ethical and legal issues in child vision care).

Ocular signs

Table 3.1 gives a summary of the signs of the different types of abuse, based upon Smith's (1988) account. Physical abuse is the easiest to detect, but the other types of abuse are more common. It is estimated that 40% of all physically abused children have ocular complications, the most common sign being intraocular haemorrhage which is associated with brain injury in the shaken baby syndrome. However, 20% of ocular complications are due to direct trauma and occur mostly at the points of structural weakness of the eyes (e.g. lens dislocation, scleral ruptures at the insertions of the extra-ocular muscles and tearing at the root of the iris). Functional disturbances of vision (i.e. those occurring with no definable organic, structural or pathological disorder, Tomsak, 1995) or other functional symptoms such as blinking, photophobia, micropsia (objects appearing small) and transient visual obscurations sometimes occur in children. They typically result from stress which could have many causes such as sexual abuse, school difficulties or family problems.

Shaken baby syndrome

Formerly known as whiplash shaken child, this is the largest cause of death from child abuse. External injuries are minimal or absent, but multiple bone fractures are not infrequent and repeated violent shaking is the primary cause of intracranial haemorrhages in children under 2, causing permanent brain damage. Sometimes repeated small

Table 3.1   Signs of child abuse and neglect

Ocular signs	General signs	Behavioural signs
Retinal haemorrhages, particularly in child > 6 weeks and < 3 yr	Bruises around cheeks, jaw, eyes, ears, mastoid area	Frozen watchfulness
Cortical blindness	Soft tissue bruises	Fear of strangers
Ruptured globe	Hand prints, four or five small bruises	Fear of parents or of going home
Retinal detachment	Human (round) bite marks	Sad affect, depressed, apathetic
Chorioretinal atrophy	Suspicious lesions in various stages of healing (important sign)	Indiscriminate attraction to strangers
Papilloedema		Low intellectual performance
Optic atrophy	Hair loss	Low self-esteem
Cataracts	Torn upper lip	Impaired ability to enjoy life
Dislocated lens	Torn floor of mouth	Social withdrawal
Glaucoma	Burns on any posterior part of the body	Learned helplessness
Angle recession	Stocking glove burns	Suicidal thoughts or attempts
Iris tears (iriodialysis)	Poor hygiene	Drug and alcohol abuse
Pupil anomalies	Loop mark (from whipping)	Misconduct in school
Hyphaema (haemorrhage into anterior chamber)	Small lesions round ankle, wrist or neck (rope burns)	Academic failure
		Low school attendance
Corneal scars, oedema	Lesions at mouth corners (from gag)	Aggressive behaviour
Conjunctival/subconjunctival haemorrhages	Poor general health	Sleeping problems
	Signs of malnutrition	Running away
Periorbital ecchymosis (bruising)	Unexplained fractures	Low level of activity
Lid lacerations	A history of recurrent injuries	Weight fluctuation
Ptosis	Failure to thrive	Fatigue
Strabismus	Growth failure	Generalized acting out
Nystagmus		Sexual acting out
Incomitant eye movements		Speech disorders
Eyelashes: crab louse		Appears normal but unable to learn learned functions
		Habits, e.g. sucking, biting, rhythmic motion
		Will not play

Adapted from Smith, S.K. (1988). Child abuse and neglect: a diagnostic guide for the optometrist. *Journal of the American Optometric Association,* **59,** 760–765. Reproduced with permission of the American Optometric Association. N.B. It is not usually a single sign, but a cluster of behavioural and physical signs, which indicates abuse.

intracranial haemorrhages result in mild intellectual impairment. Retinal haemorrhages occur in 50–80% and are usually bilateral (Levin, 1990). Retinal haemorrhages inflicted by shaking can be flame-shaped, dot or blot haemorrhages. Occasionally vitreous haemorrhages are seen. The severity of retinal haemorrhages is a likely indicator of the degree of neurological damage.

The reported incidence of retinal haemorrhages in newborns varies widely, from 2.5 to 50%: this figure will depend on the timing of the eye examination, since the haemorrhages often resolve quickly, usually disappearing within a few days and rarely lasting longer than 4–6 weeks. Other causes of retinal haemorrhages in children are blood disorders, post cataract surgery and meningitis. It is no longer thought that cardiopulmonary resuscitation causes retinal haemorrhages; they are only caused by accidental injury when this is life-threatening (and there will be no doubt about this cause). In the absence of these other causes, physical abuse should be suspected. In fact, retinal haemorrhages may be almost pathognomonic of abuse in the absence of other causes.

General physical signs

Bruises are often seen, but these are different from those sustained by children during the normal course of play, which frequently results in bruises on the knees, shins and elbows, especially after a child has started walking. Suspicious bruises and other lesions are as listed in Table 3.1.

Burns or scalds accidentally caused by flames or spilled hot liquid often occur down the front of a child. Liquids often leave a central severe burn with surrounding splash marks. Because of reflex withdrawal, such accidental burns are usually only partial thickness, whereas inflicted burns are often deeper, causing damage to the dermis (deep layer of skin). They may be inflicted by cigarettes or a heater (the latter causing a linear or grid pattern), typically on the hands, feet or back. If a child's hand or leg is held in excessively hot water there is a typical 'stocking glove appearance' where the scald marks come part way up the hand or leg. Burns in various stages of healing or in association with bruises are suspicious.

Behavioural signs may be observed in the way that the child interacts with the eye professional or other adults and in the interaction between parent and child. Generally, a parent will be more restrained in public than in private, therefore excessive punishment or verbal abuse of a child in public usually indicates that worse things are happening at home (see example below).

Case history

Great care must be taken with signs (in particular, behavioural signs) which could indicate abuse but which could also have other causes. The whole clinical picture must be considered and a careful history taken. If suspicious signs are noted, we should ask the parent what caused them and listen to see if the explanations are plausible and immediate. Hesitation, vagueness or inconsistency are supicious. Note, therefore, if the story differs between the two parents or if it changes during or between examinations, or whether the child's story differs from that of the parent. Children will rarely lie to get the parent into trouble (they are more likely to cover up if they think that something wrong or shameful has occurred). Determine also whether the story is consistent with the location, severity and type of injury. Multiple visits for accidental injuries are suspicious, as is a delay in seeking medical attention.

Factors which increase risk

Anything which adds stress to a family increases the risk of abuse. Such factors include a child who is preterm or has a disability, financial and marital problems, conditions of poverty, social isolation, alcoholism and drug abuse. It is important to recognize, however, that abuse can and does occur in families in all socio-economic groups, including the well-educated and financially well-off. It is mostly, but not always, the biological parents (usually mothers) who inflict physical abuse. Almost all abusers were abused as children.

What to do

Avoid a confrontation with the parents and avoid blame. For example, say that 'someone may have done something to your child and I think that you would like to find out who. In any case I am legally bound to let the [appropriate authority] know about this.' Accurately record all observations, both behavioural and clinical. If you are unsure about whether the observations you have made are sufficient grounds to make a report, call a social worker, a child psychologist or other specialist worker in this area. In some jurisdictions the child protection agency can be contacted directly by a person who feels unsure and the organization will determine whether or not there are sufficient grounds to proceed. If the grounds are not sufficient to make a report at that time you might choose to schedule the child for re-examination fairly soon.

A report, probably by telephone for speed, should be made as early as possible, preferably the same day. The agency should investigate soon. Unfortunately, reporters may not receive any feedback as to whether their suspicions were correct, but may become further involved if there is a court case in which their evidence is important in establishing that abuse happened – hence the importance of keeping accurate and detailed records.

An example

Two brothers aged 4 and 6 were brought for examination by their mother. There was no medical history of developmental delay, yet the 4 year old was not talking, failing to reach the expected milestones for his age and, at one point during the consultation, hid in the corner (this behaviour demonstrated a fear of strangers far in excess of, and at a later age than, the normal 'stranger anxiety' exhibited by infants). In the course of the attempted examination the mother commented that he was afraid of all strangers and also his father. The 6 year old demonstrated incoherent speech and lacked the normal ability to perform in testing. It was not possible to perform a full examination (as expected for their age) with either boy.

At one point during the examination the mother shouted at the 6 year old (who cowered and was unable to respond to the mother) and hit him (most parents will not hit their child in the consulting room). She made no effort to comfort the children when they were wary of the test situation.

After the family had left, all these observations were documented and, after discussion with a colleague and a psychologist, the local child protection agency was telephoned and the observations described.

SIGNS AND SYMPTOMS

Reported signs

Signs can be distinguished into two categories: reported signs (observations made by the parents/carers) and observed signs (as observed by the examiner). Reported signs include the chief concern of the parents and signs which are elicited on further questioning during the case history. Usually, the first question in the case history is regarding the chief concern: why has the child been brought for examination? In most cases this will be answered in a straightforward manner and Table 3.2 shows the most frequent signs for presenting a child to a primary eye care provider and their most common causes. In some cases there may be a hidden agenda and the first-mentioned concern may not be the one which is uppermost in the parents' minds. This is discussed later, in the section 'Communicating with parents'.

Although the majority of information is obtained in the initial interview (case history) there are times when the eye professional has to check and refine his or her understanding, or to ask for more information about things which become apparent during the testing. For example, a medium degree of hyperopia may be measured, or a convergence insufficiency be determined. The examiner may then probe more thoroughly regarding difficulty with near tasks, school work or attention span.

Table 3.2 Common presenting signs

Signs	Most common visual causes
Parent or someone else has noticed an eye turn, head turn or the eyes 'don't look right'	Strabismus, pseudostrabismus, incomitancy (Chapter 9), nystagmus
Child rubs eyes, blinks a lot, screws up eyes	Refractive error, photophobia, binocular anomalies
Child shuts one eye when doing close work or in bright sunlight	Phoria (Chapter 9), refractive error (anisometropia)
Itching, watering or red eyes, discharge from eyes	Conjunctivitis, allergy, poor punctal patency (poor tear drainage), blepharitis (Chapter 4)
Child brings books close to the eyes, or sits close to the television	Refractive error, poor visual acuity
Child appears to have difficulty seeing the blackboard at school or some other distance object, or is not able to see the same detail as someone else	Myopia, astigmatism, high hyperopia, low vision due to ocular disorder or CNS involvement
Child is having difficulty learning to read at school, has been identified as having a specific learning difficulty, is behind peers at school or exhibits some behaviour or habit associated with school work, e.g. untidy writing	Many visual factors have been associated with reading difficulties. The most likely to be associated are: hyperopia, vertical phoria, anisometropia, aniseikonia (ocular images differing in size) (Simons and Gassler, 1988), convergence insufficiency, accommodation dysfunction, low fusional reserves (a measure of compensation for a phoria), and near exophoria (Chapter 9) (Evans and Drasdo, 1990)
Child has reduced attention span at near	Hyperopia, accommodative dysfunction
Child seems to trip over, has poor co-ordination or bumps into objects	Refractive error, constricted visual fields, binocular anomalies, CNS involvement
Less common, but very important signs	
White pupil (leukocoria)	Congenital cataract, retinoblastoma, coloboma, retinopathy of prematurity (Chapter 4)
Large eye(s)	Congenital glaucoma, buphthalmos (Chapter 4)
Small eye(s)	Microcornea, microphthalmos (Chapter 4)

Symptoms

Children will occasionally complain of symptoms which may be similar to those of an adult: headaches, diplopia (double vision), tired and sore eyes, blurred vision, visual distortions, difficulty seeing at distance or near. The cause of these symptoms is then likely to be similar to that in adults. It must be remembered that children may be less accurate in their recall than adults regarding frequency and duration of symptoms and the examiner should question both the parent and the child. A different point of view is often gained from each party. Frequently, parents may not have specifically questioned the child regarding details of the symptoms and are surprised when questioning elicits certain information, e.g. 'You didn't tell me that, Johnny'. However, children are suggestible and may give the answers which they believe the examiner wants to hear. Therefore more accurate information may be gained from the observations and recall of the parent, for example, regarding how often the child complains of headaches.

Chief concern

One of these signs or symptoms may be mentioned as the chief concern. Others may be elicited with further questioning. However, the chief concern may be neither a sign nor a symptom. Other reasons for bringing the child for examination are as follows.

1. The child has failed a screening test.
2. The child will be starting school and an eye examination is sought to ensure normal visual function.
3. The child has been involved in an accident, e.g. trauma to the head or the eye.
4. There is a family history of eye turn, refractive error or other eye disorder.
5. The parents may have heard of the likelihood of vision difficulties in children with another known condition, e.g. Down syndrome.
6. The parents may have heard about new treatments for certain conditions and want to know if this would be relevant for their child.
7. The parents may want a second opinion regarding a previous diagnosis or treatment plan, e.g. another optometrist or doctor has prescribed glasses or has said that the child has a strabismus.

For the chief concern, the eye professional will seek to fully understand details about the sign or symptom: the frequency, severity, duration (both the total duration over which the sign/symptom has been occurring and the time which it lasts when it does occur) and conditions under which it occurs, such as visual tasks being undertaken at the time, distance of fixation, time of day and day of the week. When symptoms which are likely to be associated with near work are mentioned, the examiner should ask whether they occur on school days or weekends, in the holidays or term time. A pattern of headaches which occur more frequently on school days is likely to be vision related (although headaches occurring regularly before school could be associated with school phobia).

Once the main reason for bringing the child has been elicited and described, questioning will proceed in a scanning and a probing manner (Rosner and Rosner, 1990), covering areas not initially mentioned by the parent/carer. Then, with each sign or symptom which is positive, the examiner will probe in order to gain a full understanding of it, as in the case of the chief concern. Scanning should cover the following areas, if not already mentioned as part of the chief complaint.

1. Vision: does the child appear to have normal vision and visual function for his/her age?
2. Appearance of eyes: do the eyes look normal and healthy and aligned?
3. Apparent eye-related pain/discomfort: does the child show any signs of discomfort?

Children with visual impairment or multiple disabilities

In cases where a visual impairment or other disability has already been diagnosed, the most common chief concerns are different, as follows:

1. Parents want a functional assessment of the child's visual ability. In other words, 'what or how much can my child see?'

   Visual acuity may not have been measured previously, therefore parents/carers may have no idea whether the child's poor performance is because of a lack of vision or a lack of understanding. They may have no idea what to expect of the child nor what size to make visual material. This is especially true for nonverbal children with multiple impairments.

2. Parents want information about how to encourage the best use of vision. What helpful adaptations can be made in the school setting? Will low vision aids or glasses help?
3. What is the prognosis? Is the vision going to get worse or better?
4. Parents want more information about the eye condition in order to understand it better.

There is other information to be gathered in the case where a diagnosis has already been made. It would obviously be important to know what the diagnosis is, who made it, how long ago, what treatment, if any, has been given or will be given and what explanation was given about the eye condition and the prognosis. Lastly, an optometrist should determine whether the child is still being seen regularly by an ophthalmologist or paediatrician and how often. This information will be used to determine the following:

1. Likely visual function and management of the condition.
2. Whether dilated fundus examination is necessary.

3. The counselling given regarding the eye condition and its prognosis.

If the child is under an ophthalmologist's care, dilated examination is probably not indicated, unless recent symptoms indicate it. If the parents have little understanding of the eye condition (which may be because they were not told, or did not understand or remember the explanation given) then further counselling will be needed.

Gathering general background information

As we discuss further at the beginning of the following chapter, the examination of a child (or, indeed, an adult) does not consist of a process of gathering all possible data for eventual analysis; not all tests are performed on all children (this would be impossible), but background information and results obtained as testing progresses indicate the direction that subsequent testing should take. For example, if the case history indicates that the parents are concerned that the pupil of one eye has a white appearance in certain lighting conditions, this will lead to a very different examination than in the case of the child whose parents have requested a routine examination before the child starts attending school. Other examples are given below.

- There is a strong family history of esotropia and the child has moderate hyperopia, but with no strabismus. We may prescribe glasses or decide to re-examine the child more frequently than if there is no family history.
- The history indicates that the child was preterm and had been on oxygen. A dilated fundus examination would be indicated.
- A boy is non-strabismic, but has a family history of colour vision defects. Colour vision testing would therefore be important; however, if an anisometropia is detected with amblyopia, this would be of more immediate concern and the testing would be directed towards dealing with the more pressing problem first.

Some background information sought is the same as asked of an adult:

1. Current general health – current medical treatment and medications, including planned future treatment. Known allergies (food, medications, environmental).
2. Past general health – serious illnesses or hospitalizations.
3. Ocular history – previous spectacle wear, occlusion therapy, surgery, infections, medications.
4. Family history – general and ocular.

Other information is particularly relevant to the examination of a child, including prenatal and birth history, general developmental history and information about school.

Prenatal

How was the mother's health during pregnancy? Were there any complications or infections? Did the mother drink excessive alcohol, smoke or use any medications? It is often difficult to obtain an honest response to some of these questions.

Birth history

Was the child full-term or preterm (if the latter, how many weeks preterm?). What was the child's weight at birth? It is also useful to ask the Apgar score; in cases of a difficult or unusual birth, the parents are likely to know this. In the case of prematurity, was oxygen necessary and for how long? Was the birth natural, caesarian or a forceps delivery?

General development

Is the child keeping up with the expected developmental milestones, physically, cognitively, behaviourally, and socially?

School information

Is the child working at the expected grade level, or lagging behind at school? Are there any concerns expressed by the teachers or are there any specific areas of concern regarding the child's progress? One good way of wording this is to ask if the parent is happy with the child's progress at school. Also determine if the child is being given any extra tuition in any areas, or is receiving physical, occupational, or speech therapy.

Since there is so much information to be gathered, especially on the first visit, it may be helpful to ask the parents to complete a form while in the waiting room. This is an easy way of gathering much of this general background information. However, if this approach is used, it will still be necessary to verbally review and clarify the information, especially any factors which are unusual. An example of such a form is given in the Appendix to this chapter.

Clinical (observed) signs

We should also observe the child and this observation should start even before the child walks into the examination room and should certainly continue while the case history is being taken. The observant examiner will notice unusual visual behaviours when the child is playing in the waiting room. For example, observe the child looking at a book or playing with a toy. Does the child use a normal working distance or bring the toy exceptionally close to examine it? Is there a head tilt? While case history is being taken, observe the child for any signs of strabismus which may be intermittent and displayed during interaction with the parent. Watch the child's eye movements (are they full or is there any appearance of incomitancy?), ability to make eye contact, and head position. Does the child use visually guided reach for a toy of interest or 'lose' a toy when it rolls out of reach? If you offer the child a toy will he or she reach out to take it? Will the child crawl towards something of interest or sit passively on the floor? Does the child take an active visual interest in the environment or seem to be sitting still and attending to sounds? Is there a greater response to hearing than to vision or is there not much response at all? This latter case would suggest that a child has a severe visual disability with possible hearing loss in addition.

This observational information has enormous initial value. It may be difficult to obtain further information in some children who are very difficult to test because of behavioural problems and it gives a useful guideline regarding the expected level of visual function and the size of initial stimuli or acuity symbols with which to start the testing procedure.

It is also invaluable to make initial general observations about the child. Does the child make normal body movements or are movements floppy or jerky? Is the child of apparently normal size for his or her age? Is the child in a pushchair/stroller even though seeming big enough to be walking or crawling? Does the child walk confidently or hesitatingly? A child with a severe vision loss will be more hesitant and posture may be affected. Does the child's head hang rather than being kept upright (another sign of severe visual impairment)? Does the head look a normal shape and size (in many syndromes it may be abnormal)? Are eyes in a normal position, are they sunken, smaller or larger than normal? Blind and severely visually impaired eyes are often sunken due to their small size (microphthalmia, microcornea) or eye poking behaviour. Note the hair and skin colour. Watch also for signs of disturbed behaviour such as hand-flapping, head-rocking or biting/sucking the hand.

COMMUNICATING WITH PARENTS

Relationship between professional and parent

In paediatric consultations, the identified client/patient is not the only one with whom the practitioner must communicate. A parent (or other caregiver) generally acts as a 'broker' between health care professional and child (Garbarino and Stott, 1990). This is not to imply that the practitioner should only communicate with the child through the parents (indeed, this has probably happened far too much in the past), but it is a fact that the parent is often the one who is identifying a visual problem, rather than the child, that the parent will be giving much of the history in the case of a young child, and will also have a strong influence on the success of any intervention programme. The parent may also be much more worried about the situation than the child.

Health care practitioners spend much of their working lives communicating with those who present for vision care, so it might be assumed that they must be good at it. However, research shows that communication breakdown is the rule rather than the exception in health care consultations (Dickson and Maxwell, 1985; Bourhis,

Roth and MacQueen, 1989). A study of client perceptions of optometrists revealed two main factors, the strongest being concerned with support and understanding of clients' feelings, and the second concerned with task-related issues (Thompson, Hearn and Collins, 1992). Given the importance to clients of emotional issues, it is unfortunate that health care workers are generally more comfortable with task-related matters (Byrne and Long, 1976), which presumably reflects the kind of professional training typically given.

People are often dissatisfied after a consultation with a health care professional, even when the practitioner believes all has gone well. Research has shown that poor communication can lead to people feeling that they receive insufficient information and that the practitioner is not really interested in them; they are also likely to show poor recall of information and advice. The practitioner, on the other hand, may fail to elicit necessary information and have to face the consequences when their advice is not followed and people express their dissatisfaction (Dickson, 1989). This type of scenario was shown to occur specifically in paediatric consultations in a study by Korsch and Negrete (1972), who found that in more than a quarter of paediatric interviews the mother's main concerns were never covered because no opportunity was given to discuss them. Furthermore, as discussed in the previous chapter, parent–practitioner relationships often become antagonistic when the child has a disability.

One way of looking at communication problems in interviews is in terms of three facets of the interview – its structure (such as sequence of questions), and characteristics of the respondent and the interviewer (Young et al., 1987). However, recent research suggests that interview outcome is most heavily dependent on the social roles of the participants (Garbarino and Stott, 1989). This takes us back to our discussion in the previous chapter about the importance of recognizing the vital role that parents play in rehabilitation programmes, and the fact that the old 'doctor knows best' days are disappearing. In many aspects of health care the professional is becoming not so much *in* authority, but *an* authority, someone whose expertise can be drawn upon in the context of a collaborative relationship (Gardner and McCormack, 1990; Shute, 1991). Some optometrists' preference for the word 'client' rather than 'patient' results from this shift in approach, whereby the professional takes on more of a counselling than a dictatorial role. Although other practitioners prefer to retain the word 'patient' because they feel that it has a more caring connotation than 'client' and is more appropriate in medical and paramedical contexts, there seems to be broad agreement that, whatever the terminology, a co-operative approach to consultation should be the aim. There is a great deal of evidence which indicates that this approach is successful in terms of positive outcomes, including greater practitioner and client/patient satisfaction.

The nature of communication

Communication can be regarded as a skilful activity, and therefore as something which, fortunately, can be learned and improved, and success in training health care workers in communication skills has been demonstrated (Dickson, Hargie and Morrow, 1989). If a client/patient is to be viewed as more than a passive recipient of treatment, then communication must be much more than a simple process of extracting some kinds of information from them and pouring in other kinds. Both participants simultaneously transmit and receive messages, not all of which are overt.

Communication in health care can also be seen as purposeful and goal-directed (Dickson, 1989), and a vision care worker's communicative skill can be regarded as the ability to achieve goals set during a consultation. The practitioner's goals in consulting with a parent and child will in general be as outlined earlier (for example, to determine the chief concern and to elicit information about ocular history). However, these goals may need to be modified in the light of information which emerges during the course of the consultation, and new goals may arise as specific concerns of parent and child become apparent. The practitioner can also assist the parents in the goal-setting process (for example, if parents have come in search of an impossible 'cure' for their child's problem they may need assistance to move towards a goal of coping). Above all, communicative skill involves listening and encouraging parents to tell their stories in their own way.

Non-verbal communication

One very important aspect of communicative skill is an awareness of the importance of hidden, or covert, messages. Regardless of what is actually said, nonverbal ('body language') indicators such as posture and tone of voice carry messages about dominance and submissiveness, friendliness and hostility, interest and boredom, which the skilful communicator emits and interprets accurately (Argyle, 1988).

Components of non-verbal communication include orientation and distance, eye contact, 'paralinguistic' cues (such as voice tone and pauses in speech) and body movements. The following account is necessarily limited, and can only give a flavour of what is a complex subject. It must also be borne in mind that there is some degree of cultural variation in matters such as eye contact and the acceptable distance apart for communicating individuals to be.

The orientation of interactants to one another and their distance apart reflects the intimacy of the situation. A practitioner who sits at a great distance or behind a desk will not be sending out signals conducive to a friendly atmosphere which encourages client participation. Thought should be given, therefore, to the layout of furniture in the consulting room. Sitting at a 45–90 degree angle to the other person about one-and-a-half metres apart is generally recommended, while if several family members are present, chairs should be roughly in a circle and of a similar height so that one person does not tower over the others (Davis, 1993).

Posture gives clues to how willing a person is to be involved in communication. Leaning slightly forward indicates a positive attitude (although leaning very far forward can indicate aggression). A parent who leans away with arms and legs crossed may indicate that a difficult topic has been touched upon. This is, of course, a two-way process, with the parent also monitoring the examiner, who will appear uninterested in the interaction if such a posture is adopted.

Eye contact is another important component of non-verbal communication. It helps to regulate turn-taking, with the speaker generally making relatively little eye contact until the end of the utterance, then looking steadily at the listener to 'hand over the floor'. Prolonged eye contact indicates strong emotion, affection or hostility, depending upon the context, while aversion of gaze indicates anxiety or embarassment. In fact, in an optometric context, practitioner eye contact is not as important as good listening skills are in demonstrating personal warmth (Thompson, Hearn and Collins, 1992).

Paralinguistic cues include features such as tone of voice and rate of speech, which are important both for regulating turn-taking and for indicating emotion. Dropping the voice, for example, indicates a readiness to hand over the floor, while a lack of readiness is indicated by raising the voice if interrupted. The practitioner can encourage a parent to continue speaking by using so-called 'grunts' (such as 'uhu').

Movements of the body and face are another important aspect of communication. Facial expression indicates the kind of mood, such as happiness or depression, while other body movements reflect intensity – at the extreme, someone may leap up and down with either joy or anger. Hand gestures are used as an accompaniment to speech, reflecting what is said and emphasizing important points; the practitioner can use these to impress important points upon the parent, and also note emphatic gestures (and intonation) by the parent to detect points which he or she regards as important. 'Self-manipulative' movements, such as fiddling with clothing and other items can indicate increased anxiety or distraction (Shute, 1986). Subtle 'mirroring' of another person's body position, such as sitting cross-legged when they do, also gives out the signal that one is in accord with them.

Although there are individual and cultural differences in nonverbal communication, and we cannot read body language like a book (Burnard, 1989), it is an important feature of communication and one in which it is well worth developing skills. Playing back videotapes of our own typical nonverbal style is particularly helpful, but simply becoming aware of the nature and importance of nonverbal signalling may help us to become better communicators (Weinmann, 1987).

Health beliefs

Even within the older type of patient–practitioner relationship, the recipient of health care services was not a passive being, obediently following practitioner instructions. For years health care workers have torn out their hair over patients who do not 'comply'. It is now known that one important aspect of this is that health-related messages and information are filtered through the recipient's own belief system and subsequently forgotten, dismissed as irrelevant or impractical, or never even understood in the first place because their frame of reference is so different from that of the practitioner.

A psychological model which has proved helpful in trying to understand these issues is the Health Belief Model (Rosenstock, Derryberry and Carriger, 1959). Various aspects which have been identified, and which the practitioner may find helpful to address, concern the following:

1. Trigger – what prompted the parent to bring the child for health care at this time? (This will often be identical with the chief concern.)
2. Vulnerability – how vulnerable does the parent see the child as being to a particular condition? (For example, the parent may be concerned about the possibility of squint because of family history.)
3. Seriousness – if a child turns out to have a particular problem, how serious does the parent consider this? (For example, a parent who always hated wearing spectacles may consider a prescription for their child to be disastrous.)
4. Barriers – what barriers to action does the parent perceive? (In addition, the practitioner may have to detail potential drawbacks of a particular course of action – Chapter 14.)
5. Benefits – what benefits are there to the proposed course of action (the practitioner may have to outline these).
6. Efficacy – does the parent believe the prescribed course of action is feasible and likely to be effective?

Research has suggested that the best approach is for the practitioner to determine an individual's idiosyncratic health beliefs, and good communicative techniques are necessary to do this. In their early years children develop their health beliefs under family influence, so discovering parental health beliefs may help to clarify the child's beliefs also. We can also note here that achieving good communication can be very important from a legal perspective. For example, if a child suffered some negative consequence as a result of a particular procedure or treatment, a parent might be successful in a suit for negligence if the practitioner had not made clear any likely risks of that course of action (Chapter 14).

Effective history-taking from parents

As we have already discussed, there are certain topics about which the practitioner will be seeking background information, such as the child's developmental history, signs which the parents have observed and their chief concern. Taking histories is a vital aspect of health care consultations yet, as with communication skills in general, learning

Fig. 3.1
Taking histories is a vital aspect of
health care consultations, yet
learning how to do it effectively is
often left to chance.

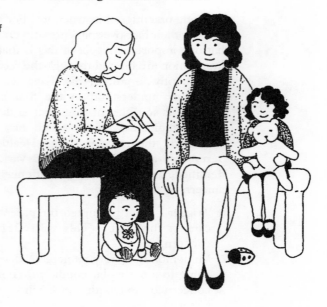

how to do it effectively is often left very much to chance (Dickson,
1989) (Figure 3.1). Even experienced practitioners are often lacking
in skill (Maguire, 1984) and thus do not provide good models for
students. They often neglect important areas when interviewing, or
collect data in ways likely to be inaccurate and incomplete. Poor use
of questioning skills has been found, together with failure to exercise
appropriate control over the interview and failure to check whether
interpretation of what the client says is accurate.

It is vital to establish good rapport from the outset, perhaps
beginning by personally fetching the clients from the waiting area if
practicable (Davis, 1993); this also provides the opportunity for initial
observations of the child. Rapport is helped by looking at the family
members and knowing and using their names; it is highly advisable to
check how they would like to be addressed (e.g. first name or last,
Miss, Mrs or Ms) to avoid offence. It is important to introduce
yourself and explain your role, also, as parents are often not clear
about this, especially if they have been taking their child to a range of
different professionals: the job descriptions of optometrists, ophthalmologists and orthoptists are not self-evident to the uninitiated! The
exchange of a few pleasantries is helpful in setting a friendly tone and,
ultimately, in promoting improved adherence to advice.

A pro forma (see Appendix 3:1 for an example) for recording
history is a useful guide for ensuring that all necessary areas are
covered, and for recording information, but should not be followed
slavishly from A to Z. It can also be used as a way of gathering initial
information prior to the examination. In this case, as we discussed
earlier, the practitioner will review the important points arising from
the form completed by the parent (for example, the chief complaint)

in order to gather more detail and gain a better 'feel' for the parents' concerns than would be obtained from the answers on a form.

Initial routine questions, like name and address, can be useful for easing into the interview and continuing the process of establishing rapport. Such questions, with fixed answers, are known as 'closed questions', and should not be overused, for two reasons. First, they may steer the interview down a particular path and close off other avenues for exploration and, second, the parents may drop into a mode of responding by only answering questions rather than being forthcoming about their own viewpoint.

The aim should be to achieve a two-way flow of communication, using near the beginning of the interview an 'open-ended' question such as 'Did you have a particular reason for bringing Sophie to see me just now?' This gives parents the opportunity for putting across their problems as they see them. A further opportunity can be offered later in the interview by a further open-ended question, such as 'Is there anything else you'd like to discuss?' or 'Have you any queries we haven't covered yet?' A good two-way flow of communication is facilitated by the development of an awareness of the difference between closed and open questions and the achievement of a good balance between them.

As we noted earlier, parents may not initially mention what is, in fact, their true chief concern. It is difficult for people to talk about topics which are very sensitive and personal at the outset of a consultation, but once some rapport has developed the concern may be mentioned, especially if we explicitly offer further opportunities. We should listen and be sensitive to clues regarding any hidden concerns, which may come forth later in the examination. For example, in the case of a child with a visual impairment, the initial chief concern may be given as wanting to know how much the child can see, but a hidden concern may be whether the child is going to lose all his or her vision, or to know whether the child will ever be able to obtain a licence to drive a car.

Even silence can be used effectively to encourage a parent who seems reluctant to discuss a problem. This must be an attentive silence, accompanied by nonverbal signals which indicating a willingness to listen, including looking at the parent, readiness to make eye contact, looking interested and giving little nods and grunts when the person does begin to respond.

If this strategy fails one option is to go back to some direct questioning. The other, which can be used if there is a suspicion of an emotional response which the parent is not expressing, is to use 'confrontation'. Despite its name, this should be in no way aggressive; it consists of the practitioner suggesting his or her perception of the parent's feelings, such as by saying, 'You seem concerned about something at the moment'. This is often enough to enable the parent to say what the problem is. If not, his or her decision not to open up should be respected and the interview should move on. Sometimes it may be the case that a parent is not willing to openly discuss certain concerns with the child present. Equally, children are often very protective of their parents, and may refrain from discussing matters they believe will upset them. Honest and open communication between all parties concerned should be the aim, but there may be circumstances under which separate interviews would be beneficial. However, this may, in practice, be difficult to organize.

Clarification is a useful technique for ensuring understanding of the parent's viewpoint. It consists of the practitioner offering a summary of what he or she understands the parent's view to be, and offering the opportunity to correct it. This should not be overused, however, as it can give a 'mechanical' feel to the interview, or even suggest that the parent should not add anything further (Burnard, 1989).

These techniques form part and parcel of effective listening by the practitioner. Important components of the parents' 'story' include their understanding of the child's condition, their concerns about it and what they expect to gain from the consultation. The practitioner will then be in a better position to evaluate the situation and to offer information and advice in useful ways. This will be discussed further in the final chapter.

COMMUNICATING WITH CHILDREN

Children's communicative competence

In some respects, communicating with children is very similar to communicating with adults. In both situations, we aim to set up a warm and trustful relationship which facilitates a two-way flow of communication, and this entails us in trying to gain insight into the worldview of the other person. However, there are special considerations when working with children. As we saw in Chapter 1, young children understand the world in different ways from adults, so it can be especially difficult to see things from the child's viewpoint. Children's thinking, although it often seems cute to adults, has a logic of its own if only we can discover it. Adults may also be reluctant to give children the opportunity to discuss sensitive matters because of a need to see children as happy and innocent creatures, which leaves adults protected but children isolated (Irizarry, 1987). A child, like an adult, will want to know clearly and simply what is going on and why an interview is being held.

Just as with adult clients, the process of communication depends heavily on the relationship between child and practitioner, and the rules and goals of the interview are renegotiated as it proceeds, not just in words, but nonverbally. Children's 'communicative competence', therefore, is not simply a matter of language skills, but depends on their psychological resources, their cognitive development and their grasp of sociocultural conventions. We will now consider each of these in turn, this discussion being based on points raised by Garbarino and Stott (1989).

Psychological competence

This refers to issues of self-esteem and coping. For preschoolers in particular, their self-esteem is highly dependent on approval from adults, so they will be reluctant to give answers which they believe will lead to disapproval. The practitioner should demonstrate interest in what the child says, and let the child take some control. If the child feels stressed, there may be crying, aggression, withdrawal or lethargy. Although these behaviours may make us feel under attack, it is more helpful to simply regard them as the child's attempts to express discomfort, and try to ascertain the cause of the discomfort and ways to alleviate it. For example, in the case decribed above, a small boy's extreme withdrawal behaviour was judged, in the light of other evidence, to result from abuse.

Cognitive competence

The question of a child's cognitive competence is complicated. A general rule of thumb is to try to understand the situation from the child's point of view. This is no easy matter, but an understanding of child development will certainly help. In this regard, it is helpful to bear in mind the likely developmental tasks the child is facing and to have some insight into how children's understanding of health-related matters develops (this will be examined in detail in the next section). Until a child is 10 or 11, he or she may not be capable of expressing a lack of understanding or lack of knowledge, and may fabricate an answer to please the questioner. A nonjudgemental attitude, and giving the child 'don't know' as an explicit alternative answer to questions can help (this is especially important when asking the child which of two lenses gives a clearer image, since such fine judgements can create anxiety even in adults).

Language competence

Preschoolers are more proficient in using language in familiar settings with familiar adults than in new places, undertaking new activities with strangers, which is precisely the situation when their vision is being assessed. We should not take anything for granted, but try to use modes of communication familiar to the child, being constantly alert to the possibility of misunderstandings, in both directions. Note the level of the child's speech, vocabulary and grammar and adjust your own communications accordingly, to something rather above the child's level of expression (children generally understand more than they can express themselves).

Understanding of sociocultural conventions

This is another important feature of communicative competence. For example, in some cultures it is rude for a child to contradict an adult, or to look an adult in the eye. Children pick up these rules as quickly as they acquire vocabulary and grammar, as illustrated by the son of one of the authors who, at the age of 3, was attempting to communicate with a shy 5 year old whose eyes were fixed firmly on the ground: he thrust his face into the older boy's, demanding, 'Look at me when I'm talking to you!' If the adult and child have different understandings of the unspoken conventions applicable to the situation, then the way is open for misunderstandings. For example, the child might want to please the adult by supplying 'correct' answers to questions, and hesitate to mention symptoms not covered by the interview.

An important sociocultural feature of communication is the use of questions to children by adults. As we noted in Chapter 1, carers' questions to young children are not generally intended to elicit information, but to gain compliance ('Are you coming with me?') or to direct attention ('Can you see the ball?') (Wood and Wood, 1983). This feature of adult-to-child questioning continues into school age, when teachers' questions are most often used to check out the child's knowledge, and both child and teacher assume the teacher knows the answer already. An interview is different: the adult really does want to glean information from the child, who may not realize this, and therefore respond with one-word or very brief answers, or even no answer at all. Very young childen may also have difficulty in producing detailed answers to questions about the past or their daily routines. The tester therefore needs to make the purpose of the interview and assessment procedures very clear, and be prepared to use extra prompts and follow up on initial questions rather than accepting brief responses as final. Some children as young as 2 are able to give detailed answers to questions in response to careful prompting (Fivush, Gray and Fromhoff, 1987).

When interviewing a child, it is helpful to know something about their experience to latch on to, such as the journey to the clinic or a toy the child has brought along. Discussing this helps to build rapport, and can lead in to relevant questions or tests. For example, it is possible to move smoothly from looking at a picture book to looking at letters in an acuity test. Use the child's own terms for items. If the child appears not to understand a question or instruction, repeating it is not likely to help – it is better to put it another way. Asking 'Do you understand?' is useless (a positive answer is likely, regardless). Rather, ask the child to repeat back to you what you asked.

It is worth, finally, noting Garbarino and Stott's (1989) point that it is not possible to produce a cookbook of how to interact effectively with children, as any inflexible technique will fall short. The health care professional needs an understanding of child development and a willingness to communicate with the child in a flexible way which will vary depending on the child and adult concerned, the relationship between them and their respective understanding of the setting in which the interaction takes place. Adaptability is therefore the keyword. In particular, it is important to understand children's motivation for their behaviours – if we ever find ourselves considering a child's behaviour to be irrational or meaningless, feeling we want to say, 'don't be silly' – we should think again!

Children's understanding of vision care

In this section, we will look at what is known about the development of children's understanding of health-related issues, and apply this in particular to the vision care context. Just as health care practitioners have been shown to be not particularly adept at communicating well and at taking histories effectively, so they are not especially accurate at judging the likely knowledge levels of children of various ages. Perrin and Perrin (1983) asked physicians, nurses and students of child development to estimate the ages of children on the basis of their answers to health-related questions; they tended to underestimate the age of 12–15 year olds, and overestimate the age of 4–7 year olds. This lack of knowledge could lead to a practitioner talking down to or over the heads of children. However, age alone is only a guide to a child's level of understanding, and Garbarino and Stott (1990) make the general point that the practitioner should neither assume nor discount a child's ability to understand, and that co-operation from a child is more likely when he or she is included in discussions and when appropriate explanations are given.

Infants

Obviously, an infant's understanding of vision testing will be severely limited, and testing depends in the main on observing responses which occur automatically to certain visual stimuli. However, verbal interactions become increasingly possible, and many older infants (12 months or even less) can understand a simple request to find a visual stimulus (for example, in the Frisby stereopsis test, 'Where's the ball?'), and respond by looking at the target or touching it (Shute et al., 1990). Even before this stage, however, it would be wrong to regard the infant as somehow passive. Throughout Chapter 1 emphasis was laid on the infant as an active participant in his or her own development, and the infant brought for vision care will be busily trying to make sense of this new situation.

One task for the examiner will be simply trying to keep the baby's attention long enough for testing to take place in the face of competing stimuli. Streamlined procedures and the use of attractive toys (especially those which move or make a noise) are helpful. A dummy (pacifier) or bottle of milk or fruit juice supplied by parents can also be invaluable at times, such as during retinoscopy, not only to maintain attention, but to calm a child who reacts negatively to the testing situation.

There are ways, however, to try to avoid such negativity from arising. As mentioned previously, it is helpful in the first place to try and schedule the appointment at a 'good' time for the child.

The level of social development of the infant is also important because it affects the way in which the optometrist can relate to the baby. Wariness of strangers can create difficulties for a health care worker who is seeking an infant's co-operation. Most vision testing can be carried out successfully with the infant on the parent's lap. Ideally, preferential looking tests are best carried out with an assistant holding the baby, as parents sometimes have a tendency to turn the child towards the target, but this is not always possible with babies who have become wary of strangers, and one then has to remind parents not to give inadvertent signals to the baby (you could try asking them to look away from the targets themselves, but this may not work as it is difficult for parents to distance themselves from their child's 'performance').

Attempting to keep the infant comfortable with the social situation is one way of facilitating visual assessment. Aspects of the physical environment are important too in ensuring that fear responses do not interfere with testing. Since looming objects and sudden, unexpected happenings are fear-provoking for babies it is advisable to move smoothly. It is useful to have a dimmer switch in the testing room, so that if the lights need to be turned off the baby isn't suddenly plunged into darkness. This is also helpful with older infants, who are increasingly likely to be afraid of the dark (parents can provide information about the child's likely response during history-taking, so that you can prepare for it).

New experiences may be fear-provoking for toddlers, so experiences such as eye-patching for monocular testing and wearing red-green goggles for certain stereo tests can create problems. For example, Shute et al. (1990) found that the success rate for testing monocular acuity dropped from 63% during the first year to 22% during the second, and noted that between the ages of 12 and 24 months infants seem to be particularly sensitive to prolonged or difficult test procedures. It seems to be sound advice with this age group to begin testing with whatever seems to be the most important test given the child's history, and to be prepared for full assessment to take more than a single session.

Preschoolers

Preschoolers who are brought for sight testing may have very little idea what it is all about. Young children's reasoning abilities are best demonstrated in familiar situations, so the unfamiliar context of the health care consultation is a difficult one for them to understand and cope with. This is illustrated by the case of the child who took seriously an optometrist's joke about nailing on a slipping trial frame and responded by leaping down from the chair and grasping her mother in fear (Shute, 1991). Despite their limited understanding of vision and vision testing, preschoolers are better able than infants to co-operate actively with testing procedures, provided a child-friendly atmosphere is established and explanations are given in a way the child can understand. This is again illustrated by the study of Shute et al. (1990), in which almost 100% of children over the age of 3 years were successfully given full visual assessments, including stereopsis and monocular acuity testing.

Establishing a child-friendly atmosphere means dispensing with white coats and having some suitable posters and toys in the waiting area. The more play-like the testing situation can be made to be, the better co-operation is likely to be achieved. The practitioner who is prepared to spend time on the floor with a child, even performing some aspects of testing there, is likely to build better rapport with the child and therefore to achieve good results.

It is important to establish a non-judgemental atmosphere, where the child receives praise for effort and where there is no suggestion of being 'on trial'. Strange as it may seem to adults, young children frequently feel to blame for their own physical afflictions, and may regard them, and their treatment, as punishment for some real or imagined wrongdoing (Kister and Patterson, 1980). So, for example, a child whose parents have repeatedly admonished her or him to sit further away from the television screen may feel to blame for a visual problem. Unfortunately, also, some parents use the authority figure of a health care practitioner as a way of controlling children's behaviour (overheard in a doctor's waiting room – 'If you don't sit still the doctor will come out and give you an injection'). The eye care practitioner should therefore be alert to, and rectify, these kinds of misunderstandings by children. One particular example is the use of the term 'lazy eye', which may carry the unintended implication that it would work well if only the child tried harder (a suggested substitute explanation could be in terms of one eye not being as strong as the other – patching could then be described as giving the eye exercise to make it stronger).

The child, like the parents, has a right to know what is happening and, indeed, will co-operate better if suitable explanations are given. Tell the child your name, and explain simply that you are going to see how well the child's eyes are working. Do not confuse the child with more detail at the start, but take matters a step at a time as they arise. It can be difficult to decide what level of explanation to offer to a child, but it is helpful to have a general idea of the way in which children's ideas about health and their bodies develop as they grow older.

Young children's ideas about health matters often turn out to be surprisingly vague or mistaken from the adult and professional point of view. They often use external cues as to their state of health, so that a 4 year old may know he or she is ill because of being kept home from nursery school rather than because of the way they feel (Wilkinson, 1988). Young children are therefore likely to have great difficulty in explaining or appreciating any visual problems they have; as we noted earlier, they will probably accept them as normal, only realizing they are not if adults observe and label unusual behaviour on their part. A young child with an identified disorder may wrongly believe it has been caught from contact with someone or something, may feel guilty about it, or may have distorted ideas about his or her body, so such misunderstandings should be corrected.

The impact of the experience of vision care on the young child may ultimately depend more on what happens to them, in terms of sensory experiences, than on what is said (Robinson, 1987), although suitable explanations can help to moderate such experiences. Many children fear sight tests because of previous experiences with 'drops'. Bright lights, the big chair and strange equipment can be similarly intimidating. Basically, the child should be prepared for each such experience as it comes, not by glossing over any likely discomfort, but equally by not setting up expectations which are too negative by an unfortunate choice of words. Thus drops 'may sting a little' or 'feel a bit funny for a minute but then it will feel OK' (if you say that it will not hurt a bit, trust will be destroyed). The big chair can be described as 'fun' and the child given a ride up and down in it. Eye patches can be modelled by the examiner, a parent or a toy animal, and the child should be warned that the light of the ophthalmoscope will be very bright. Do not deny any discomfort the child reports, such as watering eyes – acknowledge it, and say that it will feel better in a minute. Indeed, one could even add that making tears is a clever way the eye has to make itself feel better.

Use a play format as far as possible, and allow even the youngest child to retain a degree of control over a situation. So, for example, rather than saying 'Now I'm going to put a patch over your eye', offer two patches (perhaps with different designs on them) and ask which they would prefer.

Older children and adolescents

By about 6 years old children think of their bodies in functional terms (Crider, 1981), so explanations about their eyes helping them to see and glasses helping them to see better will be understood. There seems little harm in saying this to younger children also, but they are less likely to understand them. It is only towards the teenage years that most children can appreciate abstract ideas about how their bodies work, and explanations about long and short sight and so on are appropriate then. Below this age, more concrete explanations are needed, and carefully-chosen metaphors may be useful (for adults as well as children), such as describing the astigmatic eye as being shaped more like a rugby ball than a soccer ball.

Young children do not see their health as being in their own control, but as they grow older they increasingly do so (Burbach and Peterson, 1986). Older children are therefore capable of understanding, and may want a say in, what is going on. Older children and adolescents become increasingly able to give their own histories and to co-operate with vision testing, using methods which are similar to those used with adults. However, it must be remembered that even at these ages the child may harbour misunderstandings about vision care, may want to give pleasing answers to questions and may be anxious. Suitable explanations of what is happening should be offered at all stages, and the child given plenty of opportunity to express concerns and ask questions. Since one of the developmental tasks of older children is the laying down of attitudes towards social groups and institutions, the eye professional has the opportunity to play a part in developing young people's understanding of, and a positive attitude towards, vision care.

CONCLUSION

In this chapter we have covered issues that are of particular concern early in a consultation about a child's vision. Knowledge about risk factors and clinical signs need to be blended with good communication skills so that an effective history (in terms of background information, signs and symptoms) is taken. Good groundwork is essential at this stage of the consultation so that the clinical examination will be appropriately targeted and so that good rapport can be established with parents and child. Establishing a positive atmosphere in the early stages helps to ensure that a child will co-operate with testing and that parents will feel that they have been listened to, thus increasing their likelihood of being satisfied with the consultation and co-operating with any later management programme. Communication skills will be equally valuable later in the consultation, including the closing stages, when information and advice are to be imparted, and this will be discussed further in the last chapter.

REFERENCES

Argyle, M. (1988). *Bodily Communication*. London, Methuen.

Block, S.S., Moore, B.D. and Scharre, J.E. (1997). Visual anomalies in young children exposed to cocaine. *Optometry and Vision Science*, **74**, 28–36.

Bourhis, R., Roth, S. and MacQueen, G. (1989). Communication in the hospital setting: a survey of medical and everyday language amongst patients, nurses and doctors. *Social Science and Medicine*, **28**, 339–346.

Burbach, D.J. and Peterson, L. (1986). Children's concepts of physical illness: A review and critique of the cognitive-developmental literature. *Health Psychology*, **5**(3), 307–325.

Burnard, P. (1989). *Counselling Skills for Health Professionals*. London, Chapman and Hall.

Byrne, P. and Long, B. (1976). *Doctors Talking to Patients*. London, HMSO.

Courage, M.L., Adams, R.J., Reyno, S. and Kwa, P. (1994). Visual acuity in infants and children with Down syndrome. *Developmental Medicine and Child Neurology*, **36**, 586–593.

Crider, C. (1981). Children's conceptions of the body interior. In R. Bibace and M. Walsh (eds). *New Directions for Child Development, No. 14. Children's conceptions of health, illness and bodily functions*. San Francisco, Jossey Bass, pp. 49–65.

Davis, H.D. (1993). *Counselling Parents of Children with Chronic Illness or Disability*. Leicester, The British Psychological Society.

Dickson, D.A. (1989). Interpersonal communication in the health professions: a focus on training. *Counselling Psychology Quarterly*, **2**, 345–366.

Dickson, D., Hargie, O. and Morrow, N. (1989). *Communication Skills Training for Health Professionals. An instructor's handbook*. London, Chapman and Hall.

Dickson, D. and Maxwell, M. (1985). The interpersonal dimension of physiotherapy: implications for training. *Physiotherapy*, **71**, 306–310.

Dowding, V.M. and Barry, C. (1990). Cerebral palsy: social class differences in prevalence in relation to birthweight and severity of disability. *Journal of Epidemiology and Community Health*, **44**, 191–195.

Duckman, R.H. (1979). The incidence of visual anomalies in a population of cerebral palsied children. *Journal of the American Optometric Association*, **50**, 1013–1016.

Evans, B.J.W. and Drasdo, N. (1990). Review of ophthalmic factors in dyslexia. *Ophthalmic and Physiological Optics*, **10**, 123–132.

Evans, P., Elliott, M., Alderman, E. and Evans, S. (1985). Prevalence and disabilities in 4 to 8 year olds with cerebral palsy, *Archives of Disease in Childhood*, **60**, 940–945.

Fatt, H.V., Griffin, J.R. and Lyle, W.M. (1992). *Genetics for Primary Eye Care Practitioners*, 2nd edn. Oxford, Butterworth-Heinemann.

Fielder, A., Foreman, N., Moseley, M.J. and Robinson, J. (1993). Prematurity and visual development. In K. Simons (ed.), *Early Visual Development, Normal and Abnormal.* London, Oxford University Press, pp. 485–504.

Fivush, R., Gray, J.T. and Fromhoff, F.A. (1987). Two-year-olds talk about the past. *Cognitive Development,* 2(4), 393–409.

Gallie, B.L. (1993). The misadventures of RB1. In I. Kirsch (ed.), *Causes and Consequences of Chromosomal Aberrations.* Boca Raton, CRC Press.

Garbarino, J., Stott, F. and Faculty of the Erikson Institute (1989). *What Children can tell us.* San Francisco, Jossey Bass.

Gardner, A. and McCormack, A. (1990). *The potential role of communication in developing self efficacy in the patient.* Presented to 5th European Conference of Rehabilitation International, Dublin, May.

Giese, M.J. (1994). Ocular findings in abused children and infants born to drug abusing mothers. *Optometry and Vision Science,* 71, 184–191.

Groenendaal, F. and van Hof-van Duin, J. (1992). Visual deficits and improvements in children after perinatal hypoxia. *Journal of Visual Impairment and Blindness,* 86, 215–218.

Gwiazda, J., Thorn, F., Bauer, J. and Held, R. (1993). Emmetropization and the progression of manifest refraction in children followed from infancy to puberty. *Clinical Vision Science,* 8, 337–344.

Hook, E.B. (1980). Genetic counseling dilemmas: Down syndrome, paternal age and recurrence risk after remarriage. *American Journal of Medical Genetics,* 5, 145.

Hughes, I. and Newton, R. (1992) Genetic aspects of cerebral palsy. *Developmental Medicine and Child Neurology,* 34, 80–86.

Irizarry, C. (1987). *The Inner World of the Child.* Paper presented to conference on the Social Context of Child Abuse, sponsored by S. Australian Office of the Govt Management Board & Dept. of Premier & Cabinet, Dec. 1987.

Jones, M.H. and Dayton, G.O. (1968). Assessment of visual disorders in cerebral palsy. *Archivio Italiano di Pediatria,* 25, 251–264.

Kanski, J.J. (1988). *Clinical Ophthalmology,* 2nd edn. London, Butterworths.

Kister, M.C. and Patterson, C.J. (1980). Children's conceptions of the causes of illnesses: understanding of contagion and use of immanent justice. *Child Development,* 51, 839–846.

Korsch, B.M. and Negrete, V.F. (1972). Doctor-patient communication. *Scientific American,* 227, 66–74.

Leat, S.J. (1996). Reduced accommodation in children with cerebral palsy. *Ophthalmic and Physiological Optics,* 16, 375–384.

Levin, A.V. (1990). Ocular manifestations of child abuse. *Pediatric Ophthalmology,* 3, 249–264.

Maguire, P. (1984). Communication skills and patient care. In A. Steptoe and A. Matthews (eds), *Health Care and Human Behaviour.* London: Academic Press.

Maino, D.M. (1995). *Diagnosis and Management of Special Populations,* Mosby's Optometric Problem Solving Series. St Louis, Mosby, p. 194.

Maino, D.M., Schlange, D., Maino, J.H. and Caden, B. (1990). Ocular anomalies in fragile X syndrome. *Journal of American Optometric Association,* 61, 316–323.

Maino, J.H. (1979). Ocular defects associated with cerebral palsy: A review. *Rev Optom (Oct),* 69–72.

Millis, E.A. (1987). Ocular findings in children. In D. Lane and B. Stratford (eds), *Current Approaches to Down's Syndrome,* London; Holt, Rinehart & Winston, pp. 103–119.

Nelson, K.B. (1991). Prenatal origin of hemiparetic cerebral palsy: How often and why? *Pediatrics,* 88, 1059–1062.

Ng, Y.K., Fielder, A.R., Shaw, D.E. and Levene, M.I. (1988). Epidemiology of retinopathy of prematurity. *The Lancet,* Nov., 1235–1238.

Perez-Carpinell, J., de Fez, M.D. and Climent, V. (1994). Vision evaluation in people with Down's syndrome. *Ophthalmic and Physiological Optics,* 14, 115–121,

Perrin, E.C. and Perrin, J.M. (1983). Clinicians' assessments of children's understanding of illness. *American Journal of Diseases of Children,* 137, 874–878.

Robinson, C.A. (1987). Preschool children's conceptualisations of health and illness. *Children's Health Care,* 16, (2), 89–96.

Rosenbloom, A.A. and Morgan, M.W. (1990). *Pediatric Optometry.* New York, Lippincott.

Rosenstock, I., Derryberry, M. and Carriger, B.K. (1959). Why people fail to seek poliomyelitis vaccination. *Public Health Reports,* 74, 98–103.

Rosner, J. and Rosner, J. (1990). *Pediatric Optometry.* Boston, London, Butterworths.

Sandford-Smith, J. (1986). *Eye Diseases in Hot Climates.* Bristol, Wright.

Shute, R. (1986). 'It's worse than going to the dentist'. Identifying and dealing with anxiety in optical practice. *Optical Management*, Oct., 10–12.

Shute, R.H. (1991). *Psychology in Vision Care.* Oxford, Butterworth-Heinemann.

Shute, R., Candy, R., Westall, C. and Woodhouse, J.M. (1990). Success rates in testing monocular acuity and stereopsis in young children. *Ophthalmic and Physiological Optics*, **10**, 133–136.

Simons, H.D. and Gassler, P.A. (1988). Vision anomalies and reading skill: a meta-analysis of the literature. *American Journal of Optometry & Physiological Optics*, **65**, 893–904.

Smith, S.K. (1988). Child abuse and neglect: a diagnostic guide for the optometrist. *Journal of the American Optometric Association*, **59**, 760–765.

Taylor, D. (1990). *Pediatric Ophthalmology.* Boston, Blackwell Scientific.

Tomsak, R.L. (1995). *Pediatric Neuro-ophthalmology.* Boston, Butterworth-Heinemann.

Thompson, B.M., Hearn, G.N. and Collins, M.J. (1992). Patient perceptions of health professional interpersonal skills. *Australian Psychologist*, **27**, (2), 91–95.

van Hof-van Duin, J. and Mohn, G. (1986). The development of visual acuity in fullterm and preterm infants. *Vision Research*, **26**, 909–916.

Weinmann, J. (1987). *An Outline of Psychology as Applied to Medicine.* Bristol, Wright.

Wilkinson, S.R. (1988). *The Child's World of Illness.* Cambridge, Cambridge University Press.

Wood, H. and Wood, D. (1983). Questioning the pre-school child. *Educational Review*, **35**, (2), 149–162.

Woodhouse, J.M., Meades, J.S., Leat, S.J. and Saunders, K.J. (1993). Reduced accommodation in children with Down syndrome. *Investigative Ophthalmology and Vision Science*, **34**, 2382–2387.

Young, J.G., O'Brien, J.D., Gutterman, E.M. and Cohen, P. (1987). Research on the clinical interview. *Journal of the American Academy of Child and Adolescent Psychiatry*, **26**, (5), 613–620.

Appendix 3.1

History form. This is adapted from forms used at the Paediatric and Special Needs Clinic, School of Optometry, University of Waterloo (by permission). A form such as this can be used as a pro-forma by the clinician, or the parent/guardian can be asked to complete the form while waiting for their appointment in the waiting room, or it could be sent to the parents in advance by mail. However, a form alone should not be used for taking history (see text).

Details relating to the institution and details of the child (name, address, date of birth, names of parents, etc.) should precede the following:

Reason for today's appointment:

_____

_____

_____

_____

Child's Personal History (please answer those questions which apply, and give details)

yes ☐ no ☐   any complaints of blurred or double vision?

yes ☐ no ☐   does your child have an eye turn (strabismus)?

yes ☐ no ☐   has your child ever had one eye patched to improve her/his other eye?

yes ☐ no ☐   have you, or your child's teachers, identified a reading problem?

yes ☐ no ☐   has your child ever been in hospital? Please give details

_____

_____

yes ☐ no ☐   has your child ever had eye surgery? please give details

_____

_____

yes ☐ no ☐   has your child been registered as visually impaired or legally blind?

yes ☐ no ☐   is your child taking any medication? Please list

_____

_____

yes ☐ no ☐   any serious health-related problems since birth?

_____

_____

yes ☐ no ☐   any known allergies? Please list.

_____

_____

yes ☐   no ☐   is child achieving expected developmental milestones
                for his/her age?
yes ☐   no ☐   other relevant history or comments:

_____

_____

Mother's Pregnancy (circle or fill in the blank, or check here _____
if history not known).
general health of mother during pregnancy:
good _____ fair _____ poor _____
pregnancy was considered:

               full-term _____

               premature _____ by how many weeks _____

               postmature _____ by how many weeks _____

labour considered: normal _____ difficult _____
delivery was by: forceps _____ caesarian _____ natural _____
any serious eye or general health problems at birth?: yes ☐ no ☐
Please describe:

_____

_____

birth weight:_____

Date of child's last visual examination: _____

by (name and address): _____

_____

Date of child's last medical examination: _____

by Dr (name and address): _____

_____

_____

Family Eye History (please tick box if present, or check here _____ if history not known).

Condition	**Person with it** (relationship to child)

yes ☐ no ☐   eye turn (strabismus)   _____

yes ☐ no ☐   ever had one eye patched to improve other eye   _____

yes ☐ no ☐   colour vision problems   _____

yes ☐ no ☐   eyes shake constantly (nystagmus)   _____

yes ☐ no ☐   glaucoma   _____

yes ☐ no ☐   eye-related surgery   _____

yes ☐ no ☐   poor vision or legal blindness   _____

yes ☐ no ☐   cataract   _____

yes ☐ no ☐   other   _____

Family General Health History (please tick box if present, or check here _____ if history not known).

Condition	**Person with it** (relationship to child)

yes ☐ no ☐   allergies (drug)   _____

yes ☐ no ☐   allergies (other)   _____

yes ☐ no ☐   asthma   _____

yes ☐ no ☐   diabetes   _____

yes ☐ no ☐   high blood pressure   _____

yes ☐ no ☐   low blood pressure   _____

yes ☐ no ☐   thyroid   _____

yes ☐ no ☐   epilepsy   _____

yes ☐ no ☐   stroke   _____

yes ☐ no ☐   heart problems   _____

yes ☐ no ☐   genetic syndromes (please give name)   _____

_____

yes ☐ no ☐   other conditions

_____

Are the child's parents related by blood? yes ☐ no ☐

When completed, please return this form and any supporting information to:

(address to which form should be posted here)

4

Ocular health

INTRODUCTION

We recognize that ophthalmologists will be very familiar with ocular health assessment in children and with eye disorders which are common in this population. We have therefore directed this chapter to primary eye care practitioners such as optometrists and paediatricians. Other readers unfamiliar with ocular health assessment may be able to gain a broad picture (with the help of the brief definitions which we have provided) but parts of the chapter are likely to be too technical. Further information may be found in Millodot's (1997) *Dictionary of Optometry* and Taylor's (1990) text on paediatric ophthalmology.

The chapter commences with a description of methods for the examination of the eyes of infants and children and then describes the most common eye diseases in children, together with their management. We will not describe the fundamental principles of commonly used techniques, for example, the optics of ophthalmoscopy; the interested reader is referred to other texts for this information. We will, rather, describe how these techniques may be modified and made appropriate for use with children. In the case of more unusual techniques, a more detailed description is given.

THE PROBLEM SOLVING APPROACH

Young children often do not respond well to prolonged testing, and how far we push a child in terms of carrying out a detailed examination will depend on the results obtained as the examination progresses. We do not just collect and analyse all possible data, but remain aware of possibilities throughout the examination and eliminate differential diagnoses along the way. Hypotheses are formed and tested. Some are rejected, and further possibilities may be considered. In this way, we act as clinicians and not as technicians or assistants, who would simply collect information for future analysis, possibly by another person.

The tests which the clinician wishes to perform may change in the light of emerging results. Sometimes tests may be left to a later date because others become more important. For example, measuring stereopsis may not yield particularly useful information when congenital glaucoma is suspected; intraocular pressures, corneal evaluation and the fundus examination become much more important. Conversely, if strabismus is suspected, stereopsis would be more relevant than intraocular pressures. In the case of a child brought in for a routine examination with no signs or symptoms, with normal acuity for his or her age and normal refractive error, an ocular health examination would still be undertaken, but probably without dilation and not in as much detail as in the case of a child with reduced acuity in one eye and symptoms of headache and fever. This is, of course, no different from the approach one takes with adults, but since a child's attention span and possible duration of co-operation are shorter, it becomes more crucial to gain the critical information first, leaving other tests until later.

Along with a problem solving approach we must also keep in mind a sensible and efficient method for collecting information which is also sensitive to the child's developmental level and mood. For example, binocularity tests are generally performed before monocular acuities are attempted, not only because occlusion (patching) may change the appearance of an intermittent strabismus into a constant one, but because patching is also more likely to upset a child. Once the child's confidence has been gained somewhat, occlusion can be attempted. Similarly, ophthalmoscopy, which requires getting close to the child and invading their 'personal space', is frequently left until the end of the examination. Procedures which require drops are also left to the end, so other measurements which would be affected by their administration must be done earlier.

Thus we can think in terms of the following two levels of testing:

1. Standard, in which tests are performed in a screening fashion. It may be considered unethical to put a child through extended unnecessary testing.
2. Investigative, in which there are signs, symptoms or other findings which indicate that an abnormality may be present or in which a differential diagnosis between two or more possibilities must be reached.

EXTERNAL EYE EXAMINATION

As soon as the child enters the consulting room the external examination starts with simple observation, and this continues during the consultation. As described in Chapter 3, clinical (observed) signs about the child's visual and general behaviour are noted during the case history taking, including how the child relates to and communicates with parents and the clinician, general physical characteristics, apparent motor ability and appropriateness of these characteristics for the child's age. The external eye appearance is also noted. Any gross abnormalities of lids, lashes, globes, corneae, conjunctivae or eye position are noted. Do the eyes look abnormally large, or too small? Is the interpupillary distance abnormally large? Is there a difference in size between the two eyes, which may be indicative of buphthalmos (abnormally enlarged eye as a result of glaucoma) in the larger eye or microcornea or microphthalmos in the smaller eye. Unilateral ptosis (see below) can sometimes give rise to the appearance of buphthalmos in the other eye. It is important to distinguish between ptosis of one eye and proptosis (bulging) of the other and to distinguish between true ptosis and pseudoptosis as, for example, in cases of reduced orbital volume or hypertropia (an upwards eye turn). In order to determine which is the abnormal eye, we must measure visible iris diameter, lid position and proptosis.

Normally, the upper lid covers 2 mm of the upper cornea (Kanski, 1989) and the normal corneal diameter is 10 mm in neonates, increasing to 12 mm (adult size) by 2 years of age. Proptosis can be detected by observing the child from above his or her head, or by measuring with a ruler from the lateral orbital rim to the apex of the cornea, in which case differences between the two eyes of 2 mm or more are considered abnormal.

Look at the symmetry of the orbits and, if there is any asymmetry, palpate around the orbits and lids, checking for any areas of bony protrusion, soft tissue masses or pain (as judged by the child's response). The lids and lashes should be examined for signs of blepharitis or mucous discharge. Observe the colour of the conjunctiva and sclera. Observe any epiphora (watery eyes) or abnormal photophobia.

Pupil reactions can be measured in the same way as for adults. Direct and consensual pupil responses are present at birth in full-term and in most premature babies, the pupil light response developing between 30–35 weeks gestational age (Isenberg et al., 1990; Robinson and Fielder, 1990). Up to 6 months postnatal age, the pupil diameter is miotic compared with adults, being around only 2–3 mm, and the pupil response is slower and smaller in magnitude. It is thought that the dilator muscle develops strength later than the sphincter and that smaller pupil diameters contribute to the larger depth of focus in infants. It is not unusual for the pupils of neonates to be unequal in size (anisocoria) and this may persist up to 3 years of age. Up to 1 mm anisocoria is not of concern if there are no third nerve defects such as ptosis. Hippus (physiological fluctuations in pupil size) is also more common in younger individuals and in those with lighter iris coloration (Day, 1990).

Note also the regularity (roundness) and centration of the pupils, the iris colour and the presence of any heterochromia (different coloured irides).

In young babies examination of the cornea, anterior chamber and lens can be accomplished with a penlight (the best type being a slit penlight) and a loupe. This allows the gross clarity of the cornea and anterior chamber to be established. In cases where the integrity of the corneal surface must be assessed, fluorescein can be instilled and staining assessed with the Burton UV lamp usually reserved for contact lens assessment (Figure 4.1). Oblique illumination of the anterior chamber from the temporal limbus with a penlight allows estimation of the depth of the anterior chamber.

Fig. 4.1
The Burton lamp.

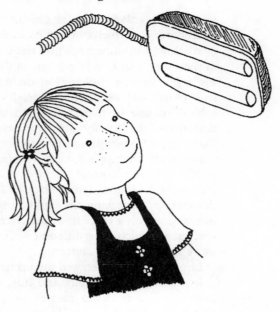

Hand-held slit lamps are available, providing magnifications up to 16×, and models are currently marketed by Kowa, Clement Clarke and Amtek. With these, a reasonable examination of the anterior segment can be achieved in most infants. For both handheld slit-lamp examination and ophthalmoscopy, the child can be held supine, with his or her head on a parent's knees and, for a larger child (3 years or more), their legs around the parent's waist. The child's head is held by an assistant if it is necessary to restrain the child (Figure 4.2).

Fig. 4.2
Infant in position for ocular examination.

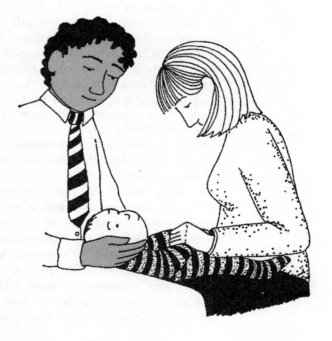

Children of 3 years and upwards can sit or stand for a short time for examination at the table slit-lamp. Positioning the child at the correct height can be challenging and this can either be done with the child on a parent's lap, kneeling on the chair or standing at the slit lamp. Even an infant can be tested, being held by an adult so that the child is prone with his or her forehead against the band. A quick examination is usually in order, but otherwise the same illumination and examination techniques are used as for adults. Grading the angles may be difficult as children find it difficult to maintain steady fixation. However the angles on all normally formed eyes should be open.

INTERNAL EYE EXAMINATION

Awareness of the reflex during retinoscopy can give valuable information. For example, any irregularity or darkened portions indicates media or retinal abnormalities. A brief glimpse of a white reflex may occur in retinoblastoma or any disease which results in large areas of retinal atrophy or missing retina, as in coloboma. The reflex may change colour at different angles to the visual axis. These signs are not diagnostic, but indicate that further examination, including a dilated fundus examination, is in order. Irregularities of the reflex may be indicative of keratoconus, or other abnormalities of the cornea such as cornea plana (unusually flat cornea).

Ophthalmoscopy is usually undertaken last in the examination, as by then a trust and rapport will hopefully have developed between the child and the practitioner. Ophthalmoscopy is undertaken in a similar way to adults, although it is more difficult, not because of the pupil size but because of lack of fixation and attention. For example, children often have difficulty keeping their eyes still or else they look directly at the ophthalmoscope light, so that a good view of the fovea is obtained, but nothing else. In these situations the binocular indirect ophthalmoscope is particularly useful as a view of the disc can also be obtained while the child fixates the light. In general, several quick views will result in greater co-operation than one extended look. Some further points to help with fundus examination are given below.

- For babies, undertaking the fundus examination while the child is bottle feeding usually gives rise to good co-operation and the child should be made comfortable on the parent's lap before starting. Alternatively, lay the child with the head towards the examiner (Figure 4.2). This latter method may have to be used for the more restless child.
- For toddlers, the practitioner must have a supply of interesting toys (such as hand puppets), a video, or some projected interesting light. The distance of these fixation targets is less important than during retinoscopy. Alternatively, fundus examination can be made into a game, for example, some examiners say they are 'going to see what the child had for lunch or breakfast' (although this could give the

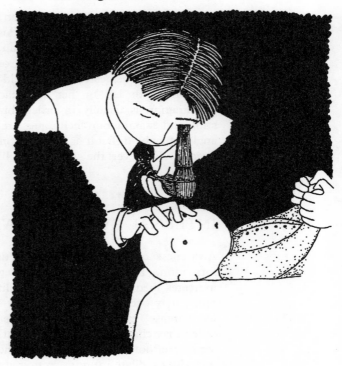

Fig. 4.3
Indirect ophthalmoscopy of infant.

child some inaccurate ideas about anatomy!), or the child is given
a task to do such as telling the examiner what is happening on
the television screen or how many fingers the child's parent is
holding up.

- Use the monocular indirect (MIO) or binocular indirect ophthalmoscope (BIO) for the initial view, assessing the disc (colour, size,
  and distinctness of the edge) and the peripheral retina, detecting
  any areas which require a more magnified view with the direct
  ophthalmoscope. In comparison with the direct ophthalmoscope,
  both the MIO and the BIO have a longer working distance (and are
  thus less threatening) and a larger field of view, allowing more
  complete and faster coverage of the retina and minimizing the
  effects of eye movements due to poor fixation by the child. Both of
  these instruments should usually be used on reduced brightness
  setting. Both, particularly the BIO, require practice and the
  paediatric eye care practitioner should first develop expertise with
  adults (these are invaluable instruments for examining any age
  group).
- Ask a parent to help by holding an illuminated finger puppet in the
  appropriate direction in order to view the periphery. It is possible
  for the parent who is holding the child to help in this way.
- Use a direct ophthalmoscope to assess the media (focusing from the
  anterior to posterior surfaces), estimate the cup to disc ratio and
  assess the fovea in more magnification plus any areas of concern
  identified with indirect ophthalmoscopy. Children will often con-
  veniently look at the light.

Differences between the infant and adult fundus

Retinal haemorrhages may be present in newborns and may be unilateral or bilateral. They may be intraretinal or preretinal and vary considerably in extent from slight to extensive over a large percentage of the retinal area (McCormack, 1994). Intraretinal haemorrhages usually resolve completely in a few days or weeks (seldom persisting beyond 1 month). The retinal vessels are more dilated and tortuous in neonates. Similarly, there are frequently conjunctival haemorrhages and the conjunctival vessels are tortuous and prominent in normal neonates for the first hours or day of life. These are not normally noticed because the eyes are often closed and the cornea is large in comparison with the palpebral aperture.

In general, the infant fundus is more shiny than the adult fundus, i.e. there are more reflections from around the vessels. It generally has a 'wetter' appearance, but this is not due to the presence of extra fluid. During the first six months there is less pigmentation, so that the choroidal vessels stand out more clearly and the retina appears paler. One can usually start to detect the foveal reflex around 2 weeks after birth although in some infants it may not be visible until 6 weeks (Isenberg, 1994). Up to the first year, the disc is slightly paler in an infant, the disc margins more indistinct and the cupping increases in depth and width (Rosner and Rosner, 1990). The lamina cribrosa becomes more apparent during this period and the retinal vessels move nasally, whereas at birth they arise more from the centre of the disc. However, the relative distance between the disc edge and the fovea does not change, being 2–2.5 disc diameters.

Dilated fundus examination

It is much easier, and sometimes necessary in order to achieve a complete and reliable examination, to undertake the internal eye examination of a child with the pupils dilated. This can be achieved by the use of suitable pharmaceutical mydriatic agents. However, in many cases, pupil dilation alone in a child is not an issue, as a full cycloplegic examination will be necessary in order to accurately measure the refractive error. Cycloplegic agents inhibit the effect of the cilary muscle on the lens and thus reduce the effects of accommodation and allow an accurate measurement of the full refractive error (Chapter 5). Since a secondary effect of cycloplegic drops is pupil dilation, this allows dilated fundus examination on the same occasion. However, if cycloplegia is not undertaken and if there is any reason for concern, either from the case history, visual functional tests, presence of strabismus or other observations of the child, the optometrist should not hesitate to dilate the pupils.

Different eye care practitioners will have their preferred technique for the instillation of eye drops. The following guidelines are used by the Visual Electrophysiology Unit at the Hospital for Sick Children in Toronto. Techniques used vary from child to child. Children between the ages of about 3 and 7 years sit on a parent's or caregiver's knee, with their head resting back against the adult's shoulder. Older children sit on their own. The child is told that a drop is going to be put into her or his eye, and that it will sting a little. Children under 3 years of age are laid horizontally, on a parent's/caregiver's knee (Figure 4.4). Alcaine (proparacaine hydrochloride 0.5%), a local anaesthetic, is used first. For dilation, in babies, cyclopentolate 0.5% is necessary and can be used in combination with phenylephrine 2.5% to obtain even better dilation. In very low birthweight or preterm infants phenylephrine should NOT be used. Also note that, in infants under 3 months of age, the maximum dosage of cyclopentolate is two drops of 0.5% (Moore, 1990), i.e. 1% concentration should NOT be used in this age group. In dark-skinned children, two drops would be necessary separated by 5 minutes. Fundus examination can take place after 30 minutes. In toddlers and pre-schoolers, tropicamide 0.5% or 1% is usually sufficient to obtain good dilation for fundus examination and can also be used in combination with phenylephrine 2.5%.

Which drugs are available for use by eye care practitioners varies widely throughout the world and even between some states and provinces of the same country. The eye care practitioner must be aware of, and abide by, the regulations governing his or her profession locally. This may mean the use of a different drug, or a drug in a lower concentration, than we have recommended here. The eye care practitioner must also be aware of the laws governing consent to treatment. For most eye care optometric procedures this is not a great issue. For example, most of the acts which an optometrist performs are not covered by the law controlling consent to treatment in Ontario, Canada, but when eye drugs are used, the optometrist must

Fig. 4.4
Instillation of eye drops.

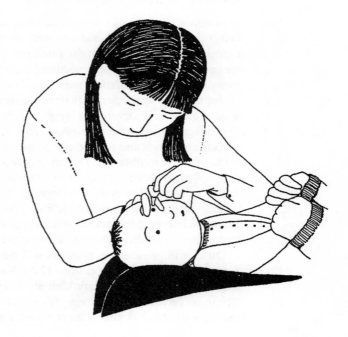

be aware of relevant laws regarding who can give consent in the case of a child or other person who cannot make an informed choice, such as people with mental challenges. In general, it is important to explain to the person giving consent the purpose, side-effects, duration and any risks of the drugs so that an informed choice can be made. The risks of using cyclopentolate or tropicamide are minimal (Chapter 5). See also Chapter 14 for a further discussion of legal aspects with regard to consent to treatment.

If dilation has been attempted and an adequate view of the fundus not obtained, and when there is cause for concern regarding ocular health, the optometrist should refer to the family doctor, paediatrician or paediatric ophthalmologist for examination under sedation or general anaesthetic. This is most likely to be necessary in children with severe behavioural problems such as those with autism or other intellectual impairment.

INTRAOCULAR PRESSURE

There are few published data on the normal range of intraocular pressures (IOPs) in infants and children, mostly owing to the difficulties of measurement. Most of the data that are published pertain to pressures measured under general anaesthesia, using the Perkins hand-held tonometer, and are therefore not directly relevant to optometrists. Most general anaesthetic agents (CNS depressants) are reported to have the effect of lowering IOP and the amount of lowering is related to the depth of the anaesthesia. Other anaesthetics increase the IOP, while others have little or variable effects. Distress in the child before the onset of anaesthesia will also increase IOP. Referring a child for IOP measurement under anaesthesia is expensive due to the medical services involved, particularly when repeated measures over a period of time are required. There is also a time delay until results are known. Furthermore, there is always some risk in the use of general anaesthetics. For these reasons it is of benefit to all optometrists and ophthalmologists to be able to measure IOP in children without general anaesthesia. To do this we require an instrument which can take readings very quickly (so that fixation does not have to be maintained for any length of time), which can be used in free space (i.e. not attached to a major instrument such as the slit-lamp) and preferably with the child in any position. Obviously, the Perkins and the Goldmann do not fulfil these requirements and therefore cannot be used with a young child without general anaesthetic.

There are two currently available instruments which enable IOP measurement in young children, which are reasonably accurate and which fulfil the above requirements: the Tonopen and the Pulsair. Below, we review these two instruments, describe their use and present normal data that are available.

Pulsair

This is similar in principle to the AO Non Contact Tonometer (NCT), made by Keeler. For a description of the NCT see Henson (1983). The Pulsair is semi-portable and can be used with the child supine or upright. The other main advantage is that the instrument will automatically fire to take a reading when it is on axis and at the correct distance from the eye. For this reason it is a very useful instrument to use with infants and young children who cannot maintain steady fixation and also with older people who have difficulty with fixation, such as those with multiple challenges, nystagmus or low vision. As with the NCT, a reading is taken in a fraction of a second, unlike the Perkins or Goldmann applanation tonometer, where fixation has to be maintained for enough time for the practitioner to make adjustments in order to obtain a reading. Another advantage of the Pulsair over some other methods is that a topical anaesthetic is not required.

Procedure

To obtain a reading with the Pulsair, the room lights are dimmed and the child views a distance target. Young children can be asked to watch a video or toy as for ophthalmoscopy. The instrument is held in one hand while the other is used to balance against the child's forehead. It is possible to align the Pulsair by viewing through the instrument, but experience with children and adults with multiple challenges has shown that viewing from the side is easier. The instrument should be approximately one inch (about 2.5 cm) from the cornea. Two red targets (spots of light) are seen. When these are in focus and superimposed with each other on the corneal apex, the instrument is at the correct distance to take a reading. The practitioner must judge where the visual axis is and align the instrument with this. The instrument will fire when correctly positioned to take a reading. As with the NCT, four readings should be taken, if possible, on each eye. The new Pulsair 2000 takes multiple readings and averages them; it is still recommended to take four of these averaged readings per eye. If a reading is not taken within a short period of time, the reset button should be pressed.

Before attempting to take a reading the instrument should be demonstrated first on the child's hand, then on their forehead. Making a joke about the puff of air helps to allay the child's apprehension: for example, the instrument 'tickles' your eye, or 'blows a kiss' at it. As with the NCT, the demonstration button should always be pressed to prevent dust being blown onto the eye. Compliance may be improved by always having a parent present and letting them hold the child's hand, by turning the machine on beforehand (it does make a low rumbling) and by continuously talking to the child. In one British study (Evans and Wishart, 1992) some readings were obtained from 78% of children aged 6 months–9 years and four readings on each eye were obtained from 45%. Even in the youngest age group (0–2 years) some readings were obtained in 75% of cases and all readings were obtained in 35%.

Accuracy

Several studies have compared the Pulsair with the 'gold standard' of Goldmann (or Perkins) tonometry. Most of these studies show reasonable agreement and conclude that the Pulsair is clinically valid (Evans and Wishart, 1992; Moseley et al., 1993). Earlier studies of the original Pulsair demonstrated a tendency to underestimate at higher IOPs, but this does not seem to be the case with the new Pulsair 2000 (Pearce et al., 1992; Moseley et al., 1993) for which 79–90% of readings fall within 3 mmHg of Goldmann values. One must remember that the Goldmann itself involves a subjective judgement of alignment, whereas the Pulsair relies on digital results with less potential for interobserver error. When considering these comparisons between Pulsair and Goldmann one must keep in mind similar figures for test-retest repeatability of Goldmann: Phelps and Phelps (1976) found that 70% of the time inter-observer readings with the Goldmann were within 3 mmHg of each other and Motolko et al. (1982) found that 90% of the time Goldmann readings fell within 4.5 mmHg.

Readings from the original Pulsair tend to drift in time. The variability compared with Goldmann increases and the readings drift to lower values (Atkinson et al., 1992). It is therefore recommended that the Pulsair tonometers should be regularly recalibrated to maintain accuracy.

Tonopen

The Tonopen is an electronic hand-held tonometer, developed on the principle of the Mackay-Marg tonometer (Henson, 1996) and is about the size of a thick pen. It has a central steel probe which moves in and out of a steel sheath. The area of contact with the cornea is 1.5 mm, which is much smaller than for the Goldmann. The instrument contains a microchip which analyses the movement of the central probe with respect to the outer sheath, discards inaccurate readings and takes an average of four good readings, which is digitally displayed together with an indication of the variability of these readings. The Tonopen fulfils most of the requirements listed above as necessary for an instrument to use with children: the cornea simply has to be touched and a reading is taken in a fraction of a second, it can be used in either the seated or supine position and it is hand-held and small so that a child's apprehensiveness of large instruments is not a factor. Other advantages are that is is truly portable, makes use of a latex probe cover (thus eliminating the need for disinfection) and can be used without an anaesthetic, although it is more usual to use one. Note that the use of the latex probe cover means that allergy to latex must be ruled out before use.

Procedure

The technique is to hold the instrument like a pen, brace the hand on the patient's cheek and touch (not indent) the cornea on axis. The

Table 4.1 Intra-ocular pressure in children (only data not obtained under general anaesthetic are included)

Source	Premature (25–37 weeks gestation)	Newborn	1 mo–1 yr	1–2 yrs	2–3 yrs	3–4 yrs	4–5 yrs
Tonopen (Tucker et al., 1992)	10.2 ± 3.75						
Perkins (Goethals et al., 1983)		11.4 ± 2.4	8.4 ± 0.6				
Pulsair (Pensiero et al., 1992)		9.59 ± 2.3	10.61 ± 3.1	12.03 ± 3.1	12.58 ± 1.4	13.73 ± 2	13.56 ± 2
Pulsair (Kohn et al., 1989)				7.5			13.0

room lights do not need to be dimmed and the practitioner views from the side. Four readings are attempted on each eye and the average of these readings is digitally displayed.

Accuracy

The Mackay-Marg was considered an accurate instrument as compared with known manometric pressures (Henson, 1983; Christofferson et al., 1993). More recent clinical studies of the Tonopen have shown that 95% of readings are within 5 mmHg of Goldmann (Christoffersen et al., 1993) and that 64–74% of readings are within 3 mmHg of Goldmann (Kao et al., 1987). These compare favourably with the test-retest repeatability of Goldmann itself, mentioned above.

It is worth noting that there have been significant differences found between Tonopens (Kao et al., 1987) and that the Tonopen tends to underestimate readings above 20 mmHg as compared with the Goldmann.

Normal IOP in children

Although there is not a great deal of normal data for children, some idea of age-related norms can be gained from Table 4.1. It can be seen that infants tend to have lower pressures than adults. Normal adult values (range 10–22 mmHg, with a mean of 15; Henson, 1996) are reached by the approximate age of 10 years (Parssinen, 1990). When IOP is measured on young children it is therefore important to use these age-related norms and not those for adults when deciding if an individual pressure reading is normal. The cut-off for normality in adults is commonly taken as 21 or 22 mmHg, being the mean + 2 standard deviations. The equivalent criterion would mean that for infants in their first year, the normal/abnormal cut off would be 17 mmHg when using the Pulsair tonometer.

DISORDERS OF ANTERIOR EYE, LIDS AND LASHES

Epiphora

Reflex tearing begins at birth, but babies do not cry with tears until several weeks of age. Obstruction or impatency of the nasolacrimal canal causes epiphora (watery eyes) in 5% of babies, but the vast majority of cases resolve by 1 year of age. Other causes of epiphora must be excluded, namely, glaucoma, corneal abrasion, conjunctivitis, keratitis, allergy and foreign body. In the absence of any of these other causes, epiphora in the first year of life is treated with massage (to increase the patency of the nasolacrimal duct) and antibiotics (if secondary conjunctivitis occurs). Cases which do not resolve after 9 months, or when there is persistent infection, should be referred for probing of the duct.

Epicanthus

This is a skin fold which is frequently present in infants which runs from the upper to the lower eyelid, covering the medial canthus. Usually, as the bridge of the nose develops, this stretches the skin and the epicanthus decreases. Prominent epicanthal folds can give the impression of esotropia, since there is less nasal sclera visible. The cover test or Hirschberg test (Chapter 9) will distinguish true from pseudo-strabismus and gently pinching the bridge of the nose to pull the epicanthal folds away from the eyes is a useful way to check (and demonstrate to parents) that the eyes themselves are straight. Prominent epicanthus is typical in Down syndrome in which case it continues into adult life. It has no functional significance. Epiblepharon is a horizontal fold of skin across either the upper or lower lid margin which usually decreases during the first few years as the facial bones develop. Occasionally, the eyelashes can be turned inwards (entropion), scratching the cornea. This requires surgical correction.

Ptosis

This abnormal drooping of the upper lid is one of the commonest lid abnormalities in children. Congenital ptosis may be unilateral or bilateral and of varying severity. In mild ptosis the lid would cover an additional 2 mm, in moderate ptosis an additional 3 mm and in severe cases an additional 4 mm or more. Ptosis is due to a developmental dystrophy of the levator muscle and may be an isolated finding or occur in association with a superior rectus palsy. Innervational abnormalities are not usually referred to as congential ptosis. Congenital ptosis can also occur in association with other anomalies of the eyes and adnexa such as epicanthus, abnormal puncti, congenital cataracts or anisometropia. The main concern with congenital ptosis is its effect on developing vision and cosmesis. Usually parents are aware of its presence since birth but, if in doubt, ask them to bring in photographs of the child when younger. Typically, congenital ptosis worsens when the child is tired. Deprivation amblyopia from ptosis is rare (Hoyt and Lambert, 1990a; Catalano and Nelson, 1994), but visual acuity should be monitored and associated anisometropia, astigmatism or strabismus excluded. Except in cases where acuity is at risk or where the child develops a backwards head tilt in order to see, surgery is best left until the child is 2–4 years old, when accurate and repeatable assessment of levator function can be performed.

It is important to differentially diagnose between congenital and acquired ptosis, the latter being indicative of active neuropathy and requiring referral for neurological assessment. Acquired ptosis may have a number of causes: muscular disorders such as myasthenia gravis or progressive external ophthalmoplegia; neurogenic disorders such as third nerve palsy or Horner's syndrome; trauma; inflammation or tumours of the lid or orbit. Rapidly progressing ptosis is often the most prominent finding in rhabdomyosarcoma, a malignant tumour of striate muscles which is the most common orbital malignancy in children. All children with acquired ptosis should be referred for ophthalmological assessment, as should any child with proptosis (anterior displacement of the globe); this might result from rhabdomyosarcoma or from benign orbital haemangioma (Chapter 2).

Anterior eye infections and inflammations

Before entering this section, we need to offer a few words of explanation. There are many changes occurring in the scope of optometry in some countries such as the United States and Canada. In most US states the optometrist is allowed to use topical antibiotics, some steroids and even certain systemic medications. In other countries this is not the case, and optometry may not move in this direction. Optometrists (and other eye care professionals) must be aware of their legal and ethical responsibilities in the treatment or referral of eye diseases and must not go beyond what is legally allowed or in what they, individually, are adequately trained and experienced to handle. Therefore, in the following sections, we have listed the appropriate treatments without giving guidance regarding who should administer them.

Blepharitis

Chronic blepharitis (inflammation of the eyelid margin) is fairly common in children. The eyelids appear red, swollen and scaly. The aeteology is not always clear, but two components are common and can occur separately or, more commonly, together. These components are chronic infection and seborrhoea (oily skin or dandruff). The infection is usually bacterial, but in some cases can be with lice.

Staphylococcal blepharitis (infection with the bacterium *Staphylococcus aureus*) is the most common kind. As the disease progresses there is chronic irritation, burning, itching and photophobia. There are hard brittle scales which leave a small bleeding lesion when removed. In later stages there is madarosis (loss of lashes) and ulceration, scarring and notching of the eyelid margin. Conjunctivitis, styes (external hordeola) and internal hordeola are frequent secondary infections. Chalazion can be another sequela. Treatment consists of several components, as follows:

- Lid hygiene. Commercially available lid scrubs can be used or the lids cleaned with cotton wool using saline or a weak solution of baby shampoo. Special attention should be given to removing the crusts and to cleaning the eyelid margin.
- Antibiotic ointment. In severe cases these can be used in combination with steroids.
- Appropriate treatment for any attendant secondary infection or chalazion.

Seborrhoeic blepharitis is associated with dandruff of the hair, brows and behind the ears. In this case the scales are more greasy and do not bleed when removed. Conjunctivitis is not usually present, but Meibomian gland dysfunction may be a factor, in which case there may be droplets of oil at the orifices of the Meibomian glands. Excessive sebum in the tears can give rise to foaming and sometimes the Meibomian glands become blocked and wax can be seen when the eyelid is squeezed. Treatment consists of the following components:

- Lid hygiene as above.
- Treatment of any attendant dandruff (including the eyebrows) with medicated shampoo.
- Sulphacetamide can be used as it has antiseborrhoeic effects.
- Warm compresses followed by expression of Meibomian glands by squeezing or firm pressure in cases where Meibomian gland dysfunction causes blepharitis involving the posterior surface of the lids.
- Systemic antibiotics. In cases of Meibomian gland dysfunction which is unresponsive to the hot compresses and lid massage, the child can be referred for a course of systemic antibiotics (erythromycin). N.B. systemic tetracyclines, which are used in adults to treat this condition, should NOT be used in children (nor in pregnant or nursing women).

As mentioned above, blepharitis is commonly mixed, including components of both staphylococcus and seborrhoeic conditions, in which case treatment may consist of elements of treatment for both.

External hordeolum (stye)

This is an acute bacterial infection of a lash follicle and the associated gland of Moll or Zeis. Often it can be distinguished from other cysts and swellings in that there is a lash at the centre. It follows a natural course, with enlargement and finally rupture. Frequent styes indicate poor ocular hygiene or chronic infective blepharitis. Treatment consists of the following:

- Hot compresses applied four times daily.
- Removal of the lash to open a drainage channel.
- Topical antibiotic ointment.
- Systemic antibiotics.
- Excision to remove the purulent mucus is rarely neccessary.

Internal hordeolum

This is an acute staphylococcal infection of a Meibomian gland and often follows on from meibomitis and from chronic blepharitis as for external hordeolum. It appears as a red, tender swelling of the tarsal plate and it may resolve by discharging either posteriorly through the conjunctiva or anteriorly through the skin. In some cases it shrinks and leaves a small hard nodule. Treatment is the same as for a stye (except for lash removal).

Chalazion

This is a chronic inflammation of a Meibomian gland following on from Meibomian gland dysfunction and blockage of the duct. The end result is a lipogranuloma. Chalazia rarely resolve spontaneously. They are common in people with seborrhoeic blepharitis. Chalazia can cause pressure on the cornea, inducing irregular astigmatism. Glasses should therefore not be prescribed until the chalazion has been resolved. Treatment with hot compresses and topical antibiotics can be tried, as for internal hordeolum, but most will require incision. Direct injections of steroids can be effective prior to granuloma formation, but can cause depigmentation of the overlying skin.

Conjunctivitis

There are several types of conjunctivitis, but we will consider here the four types which most commonly affect children: bacterial, viral, chlamydial and allergic.

Bacterial conjunctivitis is usually associated with a purulent (festering) discharge. Two types require systemic antibiotics as soon as possible: *Gonococcal* conjunctivitis can lead to corneal ulceration and perforation if treatment is delayed; even more serious is *Neisseria meningococcus,* which if left untreated can lead to meningococcal meningitis (Lambert and Hoyt, 1990).

Other forms of bacterial conjunctivitis result from infections from *Staphylococcus aureus* or *Streptococcus pneumoniae.* These forms of bacterial conjunctivitis affect all age groups. The most common eye disorders caused by staphylococcal infection are marginal blepharitis and conjunctivitis. In addition, corneal complications may be present in these types of conjunctivitis. *Haemophilus influenzae* is a frequent cause of conjunctivitis in children aged 6–36 months in which conjunctivitis is associated with conjunctival chemosis, follicles, hyperaemia, and a mucopurulent discharge. It often occurs in winter and may be associated with respiratory tract infection. Corneal opacities, cellulitis and exudative uveitis may also occur (American Academy of Ophthalmology, 1994, p. 37). If a child develops cellulitis hospital treatment is required (American Academy of Ophthalmology, 1994, p. 38).

Conjunctivitis with mucopurulent discharge is serious in young children and mismanagement of childhood conjunctivitis has grave consequences including corneal ulcer, corneal opacification, possible perforation and cellulitis. Conjunctivitis can be treated in older children by topical administration of gentamycin, erythromycin or bacitracin.

Viral conjunctivitis, associated with a mucoserous (watery) discharge, is most commonly caused by the adenovirus infection (Lambert and Hoyt, 1990, p. 662). A very easily transmitted conjunctivitis from adenoviral infection is epidemic keratoconjunctivitis (EKC). The onset is usually unilateral. The initial complaints are of a foreign body sensation and periorbital pain (American Academy of Ophthalmology, 1994, p. 39). A diffuse superficial keratitis is followed by focal epithelial lesions. Infected children may need to be kept out of school or day care for up to 2 weeks. Topical steroids may ease symptoms, although they do not alter the course of the disease (American Academy of Ophthalmology, 1994, p. 39).

Pharyngeal conjunctival fever is a common adenovirus infection consisting of pharyngitis, fever and nonpurulent follicular conjunctivitis. Early signs of the infection include a foreign body sensation, hyperaemia and oedema of the conjunctiva with tearing and a mild sore throat. The infection resolves spontaneously after 2–3 weeks (American Academy of Ophthalmology, 1994, p. 39).

Herpes simplex conjunctivitis is usually associated with mucoserous discharge and vesicles on the eyelids. Dendritic keratitis may occur. Children with herpes simplex conjunctivitis should be treated with systemic acyclovir, and newborn infants need treatment with topical antiviral agents (Lambert and Hoyt, 1990).

Chlamydial trachomitis is the most common cause, in the United States, of ophthalmia neonatorum (a conjunctival inflammation occurring in the first few weeks of life). It is characterized by a mucopurulent conjunctivitis which manifests 5–14 days after birth. A correct diagnosis is important as it can give rise to superior corneal panus, conjunctival scarring and systemic complications such as otitis and pneumonitis. Treatment consists of oral erythromycin, with the addition of topical erythromycin and topical tetracyclines if necessary (Kanski, 1989; Lambert and Hoyt; 1990). Gonococcal conjunctivitis (see above) is still a common cause of ophthalmia neonatorum in some parts of the world and should be treated with systemic antibiotics.

Allergic conjunctivitis is characterized by epiphora, itching, and injection with slight chemosis. The allergy is typically to pollen or animals and often occurs in children with other atopic conditions such as hay fever, eczema or asthma. Treatment is with topical antihistamine and vasoconstrictors or sodium cromoglycate and, if possible, removing the allergen.

Acute allergic conjunctivitis can occur when there is a large exposure to an allergen. It is characterized by sudden severe chemosis and swelling of the eyelids. Usually it is necessary to simply reassure the parents and child, as the reaction often resolves in a few hours.

Vernal conjunctivitis, which is an allergic reaction which typically affects young males, is rare in infancy. It is a recurrent bilateral inflammation of the conjunctiva, associated with a thick, ropy, mucoserous discharge, photophobia and intense itching. It tends to occur during spring and summer and is most common in warm climates. Giant papillae can be seen under the upper eyelid or along the limbus. The tarsal conjunctiva of the upper lid is predominantly affected. Treatment involves sodium cromoglycate with the addition of topical steroids in more severe cases.

DISORDERS OF THE INTERNAL EYE AND RETINA

Cataracts

Slit lamp examination, ophthalmoscopy and retinoscopy will reveal the presence of cataracts. The course of treatment is very different for small anterior polar cataracts versus dense nuclear cataracts. The slit lamp examination will reveal if the cataract is on the anterior or posterior part of the lens. Small (1–2 mm) anterior cataracts are usually stable and may not interfere with vision. Children with this type of cataract need to be monitored, with regular checks of visual acuity and slit lamp examination to ensure that the cataract is not progressing.

Conversely, children with dense, nuclear, cataracts covering more than 3 mm of the central lens should be referred immediately to a paediatric ophthalmologist for surgery (extraction) in order to prevent profound amblyopia (Chapter 2). In symmetrical bilateral cases the interval between operations on the first and second eye should be no more than 1–2 weeks (American Academy of Ophthalmology, 1994, p. 262). After cataract removal the eye is highly hyperopic and requires a refractive correction (Chapter 5). Monocular cataracts require intensive patching after treatment to stimulate the previously deprived eye.

Traumatic cataracts result from injury to the eye. Severe traumatic cataracts in children under 8–10 years old should be removed within a few weeks of injury if possible (American Academy of Ophthalmology, 1994, p. 262).

Congenital (developmental or infantile) glaucoma

Glaucoma in children may be primary in nature or secondary, occurring in association with a number of syndromes. It is frequently hereditary and may be congenital (present from birth) or develop in the first few years of life (hence the suggestion that it should be called developmental glaucoma, or infantile glaucoma if it occurs in the first year). Primary glaucoma is very rare, affecting 1 in 10 000 births. Differing inheritance patterns have been suggested, either multifactorial (Hoyt and Lambert, 1990b) or autosomal recessive with incomplete penetrance, affecting more boys than girls (Kanski, 1989).

Glaucoma manifests differently in children than in adults. This is due to the fact that the tunics of the eye are more elastic in children under 3 years so that the eye will stretch when the pressure rises, rather than there being slow 'silent' neuronal loss as in primary open angle glaucoma in adults. The main clinical signs are buphthalmos (enlargement of the globe), corneal oedema, lacrimation, photophobia, and optic disc cupping. Buphthalmos is sometimes present at birth, in which case the IOP has been raised during the intrauterine period. In approximately 60% of cases the pressure elevates in the first year of life. Frequently, one eye is more affected than the other and inequality of eye size is easy to note and is strongly suggestive of glaucoma. Bilateral buphthalmos often goes undetected, the child being complimented for having attractive large eyes. Corneal diameters greater than 12 mm are suspect in the first year of life and 13 mm or more is suspect at any age. As the buphthalmos goes untreated, the anterior chamber increases in depth and corneal haze occurs due to endothelial oedema. There are breaks in Descemet's membrane and striae in the endothelium. These changes result in photophobia and lacrimation. Cupping in infants occurs early in the condition, but may regress if the pressure is successfully controlled.

Management of infantile glaucoma is usually surgical, involving goniotomy or trabeculotomy. Cryotherapy of the angle may be used in cases where previous surgery has been unsuccessful. Occasionally, surgery has to be supplemented with medical treatment and in cases of glaucoma secondary to inflammation, medical treatment would be the method of choice. In cases of pupil block, e.g. in ectopia lentis or persistent hyperplastic vitreous, lens extraction may be performed.

Even though the pressure may be eventually controlled, there is often a resultant loss of visual function. Visual acuity is frequently less than 6/15, as a result of optic nerve damage and corneal opacification. There is frequently strabismus, amblyopia in the more affected eye and anisometropia. In the case of amblyopia and anisometropia, occlusion therapy should be considered.

Glaucoma in children can be secondary to hyphaema as a result of trauma, retinopathy of prematurity (usually the more severe stages), retinoblastoma, ectopia lentis in Marfan's syndrome, persistent hyperplastic primary vitreous, chronic intraocular inflammation and complications of congenital cataract surgery. It occurs in association with a number of conditions and syndromes: rubella syndrome, aniridia, Rieger's anomaly, Peter's anomaly, Sturge–Weber syndrome and neurofibromatosis, to mention but a few. In the case of aniridia there are angle anomalies in association with the absent or vestigial iris. Glaucoma in rubella syndrome may be easily missed as it may occur in an eye which is already microphthalmic. When these angle anomalies give rise to IOP increases in later years (such as the teens), as can sometimes happen, the clinical manifestation is like that of primary open or closed angle glaucoma in adults, depending on how abruptly the pressure rises.

Retinoblastoma

Retinoblastoma, as its name suggests, is a retinal cancer that develops in infancy (Gallie, 1993). Its rarity means that primary care practitioners often fail to diagnose it, but early detection is essential to prevent severe loss of vision or even death (Simmons and Zabrycki, 1993). As retinoblastoma is often inherited, survivors' newborn children or siblings must receive genetic testing, where available, followed by regular eye examinations under anaesthesia if found to be at risk (such examinations must be done in any case if genetic testing is unavailable).

Parents usually do not report visual problems in the child, although occasionally nystagmus will be noted if the tumour is at the macula. Ninety percent of parents will make mention of a cat's eye pupil, an occasional strange white gleam in the child's eye. This is leukocoria (white pupil), caused by reflection of light from the tumour (it can be reproduced by shining a pen torch into the eye at an angle). The description of a cat's eye pupil is nearly universal in all cultures and is almost diagnostic of retinoblastoma; although other conditions can give rise to a white or grey pupil, it will not be described as having a cat's eye appearance. Parents will be very shocked by the news that cancer is suspected (see Chapter 14 on 'breaking bad news'), but can be reassured that the cure rate for the cancer is very high if the tumour is caught early. Immediate referral to an ophthalmologist is indicated for confirmation of the diagnosis and treatment, which may include enucleation, radiotherapy, cryotherapy or chemotherapy. As there are often bilateral tumours it is not uncommon for one eye to be removed and the other to have reduced vision. Recent results with chemotherapy have proved very successful, with 93% not only surviving, but keeping one eye and not requiring radiotherapy. Once the immediate crisis is over and the child's life has been saved, if vision is impaired there is an important need for low vision services.

Optic nerve anomalies

Optic nerve problems are varied, ranging from those associated with severe brain defects to those arising from benign developmental defects. Coloboma of the optic nerve results from a failure of normal embryonic development. The coloboma may appear as a notch or hole in the optic disc, which may be found also in the iris or choroid. The coloboma may be detected because of the misshapen iris, because of poor vision or, in unilateral cases, because of strabismus. In mild cases the defects resemble deep physiological cupping, and in severe cases there is a deep central excavation of the optic disc. The extent of impaired vision depends on the severity of the optic nerve coloboma.

An anomaly that may not be associated with any visual defect is the presence of myelinated optic nerve fibres in the retina. Normally, myelination of the optic nerve begins at the lateral geniculate nucleus, reaching the optic disc by birth and not extending anterior to the optic nerve. In about 1% of cases the myelination reaches some fibres of the retina in the first month of life (Taylor, 1990, p. 446). This can be seen as a white patch with frayed and feathered edges in a striate configuration coincident with retinal nerve fibres (American Academy of Ophthalmology, 1994, p. 138). This is usually adjacent to the optic disc. Vision is good unless the macula is involved, although there may be visual field defects corresponding to the area of myelination.

About 50% of cases of tilting of the optic disc are associated with myopia or astigmatism. The optic disc is D-shaped. There is a defect in the retinal nerve fibre layer adjacent to the flat arm of the D (Taylor, 1990, p. 454). Visual acuity may be mildly reduced and there will be visual field defects.

Optic nerve hypoplasia is a condition in which the optic disc is small and usually pale. An infant with bilateral severe optic nerve hypoplasia is usually legally blind with roving eye movements, strabismus and sluggish pupillary reactions. Lesser degrees of optic nerve hypoplasia result in fewer visual defects and/or strabismus. A child with unilateral optic nerve hypoplasia usually has strabismus, a relative afferent pupil defect and unsteady fixation in the affected eye (Taylor, 1990, p. 453). Optic nerve hypoplasia may be associated with a wide variety of central nervous system and systemic anomalies (American Academy of Ophthalmology, 1994, p. 139).

In a child with optic atrophy the optic disc is of normal size. Primary optic atrophy may be inherited as a dominant or a recessive defect. This type of optic atrophy is bilateral and usually results in some degree of visual impairment. There is no known treatment.

Acquired optic atrophy may be due to optic nerve and chiasmal tumours, retinal degenerative disease, glaucoma, hydrocephalus, neonatal anoxia, inflammatory vascular lesion near the optic nerve or craniopharyngioma. The degree of vision loss, the type of pupil defect and whether there is associated nystagmus or strabismus will depend on the specific cause of the optic atrophy. Unless already diagnosed, a child with optic atrophy should be referred for electrophysiological investigations and/or CT or MRI scans.

In children, optic neuritis is usually associated with widespread neurological or systemic illness. It may also be associated with childhood demyelinating diseases. The loss of vision in optic neuritis is sudden and often progressive (American Academy of Ophthalmology, 1994, p. 143).

Retinopathy of prematurity

As discussed in Chapter 3, the presence and degree of retinopathy of prematurity (ROP) are very dependent on the degree of prematurity and therefore on the birthweight. For example, ROP is rare in preterm infants with birthweights greater than 2000 g. On the other hand, preterm infants weighing less than 1500 g at birth are at risk of developing serious visual consequences of ROP and infants weighing less than 1250 g at birth, with a gestational age less than 28 weeks, are especially vulnerable. Infants born weighing less than 1500 g should have received ophthalmological assessments as part of their routine care. Children diagnosed as having ROP at birth should continue with regular eye examinations. In many cases the ROP regresses, but further complications may still arise in those who had severe ROP:

there may be further peripheral and posterior retinal changes; vitreoretinal traction may cause retinal detachment in the first or second decade; retinal folds and dragging of the macula may also occur (American Academy of Ophthalmology, 1994, p. 117).

CONCLUSION

Primary care practitioners have an important role to play in screening the ocular health of children under their care. In this chapter we have described the detection and management of those conditions which are of particular concern in infants and children and which are detectable through a primary care eye examination. Examining a child's ocular health can be a challenging process since standard instruments and methods of examination are not always appropriate for use with children, and we have outlined in this chapter some techniques which are conducive to success.

REFERENCES

American Academy of Ophthalmology (1994). *Basic and Clinical Science Course in Pediatric Ophthalmology and Strabismus.* 1994–1995. Section 6.

Atkinson, P.L., Wishart, P.K., James, J.N. et al. (1992). Deterioration in the accuracy of the Pulsair non-contact tonometer with use: need for regular calibration. *Eye*, **6**, 530–534.

Catalano, R.A. and Nelson, L.B. (1994). *Pediatric Ophthalmology, a Text Atlas.* Norwalk, Connecticut, Appleton & Lange.

Christoffersen, T. Fors, T., Ringberg, U. and Holtedehl, K. (1993). Tonometry in the general practice setting (1): Tono-Pen compared to Goldman applanation tonometry. *Acta Ophthalmologica*, **71**, 103–108.

Day, S. (1990). History, examination and further investigation. In D. Taylor (ed.), *Pediatric Ophthalmology.* Boston/London, Blackwell Scientific, pp. 7–10.

Evans, K. and Wishart, P.K. (1992). Intraocular pressure measurement in children using the Keeler Pulsair tonometer. *Ophthalmic & Physiological Optics*, **12**, 287–290.

Gallie, B.L. (1993). The misadventures of RB1. In I. Kirsch (ed.), *The Causes and Consequences of Chromosomal Aberrations.* Boca Raton, CRC Press, pp. 429–446.

Goethals, M. and Missotten, L. (1983). Intraocular pressure in children up to five years of age. *Journal of Pediatric Ophthalmology*, **20**, 49–51.

Henson, D.B. (1996). *Optometric Instrumentation*, 2nd edn. Oxford, Butterworth-Heinemann, p. 48.

Hoyt, C. and Lambert, S. (1990a) Lids. In D. Taylor (ed.), *Pediatric Ophthalmology.* Boston/London: Blackwell Scientific Publications, pp. 141–145.

Hoyt, C. and Lambert, S. (1990b). Childhood glaucoma. In D. Taylor (ed.), *Pediatric Ophthalmology.* Boston/London: Blackwell Scientific Publications, pp. 319–322.

Isenberg, S.J. (1994). Physical and refractive characteristics of the eye at birth and during infancy. In S.J. Isenberg (ed.), *The Eye in Infancy.* St. Louis/Baltimore/Boston, Mosby, pp. 31–47.

Isenberg, S.J., Molarte, A. and Vazquez, M. (1990). The fixed and dilated pupils of premature babies. *American Journal of Ophthalmology*, **110**, 168.

Kanski, J. (1989). *Clinical Ophthalmology*, 2nd edn. Oxford, Butterworth-Heinemann.

Kao, S.F., Lichter, P.R., Bergstrom, T.J. et al. (1987). Clinical comparison of the Oculab Tono-Pen to the Goldmann applanation tonometer. *Ophthalmology*, **94**, 1541–1545.

Kohl, P., Sabre, M. and Samek, B.M. (1989). Intraocular pressure measurements in children (birth–5 years of age) using the Keeler Pulsair non-contact tonometer. *Investigative Ophthalmology & Vision Science* (Suppl), **30**, 241.

Lambert, S. and Hoyt, C. (1990). Sticky eye in infancy. In D. Taylor (ed.), *Pediatric Ophthalmology.* Boston, Blackwell Scientific, pp. 662–663.

McCormack, A.Q. (1994). Transient phenomena of the newborn eye. In S.J. Isenberg (ed.), *The Eye in Infancy*. St Louis/Baltimore/Boston, Mosby.

Millodot, M. (1997). *Dictionary of Optometry*. 4th edn. Oxford, Butterworth-Heinemann.

Moore, A. (1990). Refraction of infants and young children. In D. Taylor (ed.), *Pediatric Ophthalmology*. Boston/Oxford, Blackwell Scientific, pp. 65–70.

Moseley, M.J., Thompson, J.R., Deutsch, J. et al. (1993). Comparison of the Keeler Pulsair 2000 non-contact tonometer with the Goldman applanation. *Eye*, 7, 127–130.

Motolko, M.A., Feldman, F., Hyde, M. and Hudy, D. (1982). Sources of variability in the results of applanation tonometry. *Canadian Journal of Ophthalmology*, **17**, 93–95.

Parsinnen, O. (1990). Intraocular pressure in school myopia. *Acta Ophthalmologica*, **68**, 559–563.

Pearce, C.D., Kohl, P. and Yolton, R.L (1992). Clinical evaluation of the Keeler Pulsair 2000 tonometer. *Journal of the American Optometric Association*, **63**, 106–110.

Pensiero, S., Da Pozzo, S., Perissutti, P. et al. (1992). Normal intraocular pressure in children. *Journal of Pediatric Ophthalmology*, **29**, 79–84.

Phelps, C.D. and Phelps, G.K. (1976). Measurement of intraocular pressure: a study of its reproducibility. *Albrecht von Graefes, Arch Klin Exp Ophthalmol.*, **198**, 39–43.

Robinson, J. and Fielder, A.R. (1990). Pupillary reaction and response to light in preterm neonates. *Archives of Diseases in Childhood*, **65**, 35.

Rosner, J. and Rosner, J. (1990). *Pediatric Optometry*, 2nd edn. Boston, Butterworths.

Simmons, J.N. and Zabrycki, M. (1993). Retinoblastoma: continuum of care. *Canadian Family Physician*, **39**, 1470–1471.

Taylor, D. (1990) (ed.). *Pediatric Ophthalmology*. Boston/Oxford, Blackwell Scientific Publications.

Tucker, S.M., Enzenauer, R.W., Levin, A.V. et al. (1992). Corneal diameter, axial length, and the intraocular pressure in premature infants. *Ophthalmology*, **99**, 1296.

5

Refraction

INTRODUCTION

This chapter is concerned with the development and measurement of refractive error in infants and children. A refractive error (ametropia) is said to occur when, although the eye is relaxed and not accommodating, light from infinity does not come to a focus on the retina. We begin this chapter with some basic explanations of the three types of refractive error and of anisometropia (differing refractive error in the two eyes). Knowledgeable eye professionals will wish to omit these brief introductory sections. We then discuss the effects of aphakia (missing lens) in children before describing in detail how refractive errors develop. The remainder of the chapter is devoted to a discussion of techniques for measuring refractive error and accommodation in children.

REFRACTIVE ERROR TYPES

Myopia and hyperopia

An eye which has no refractive error, in which light from infinity is brought to a correct focus on the retina, is termed emmetropic. Any eye which is not emmetropic is called ametropic. In the case of myopia (short-sight or near-sight), light from infinity (consisting of parallel rays) is brought to a focus in front of the retina. In practice, light from objects at 4 metres or more can be considered parallel. Light from progressively closer objects is focused gradually nearer to the retina so that there is a point for every myopic eye, the 'far point', which will give rise to a focused retinal image. Objects further than this are unfocused, but nearer objects may be focused by the accommodation system, which enables the eye to increase its dioptric power. There is, therefore, a finite range over which the eye can see clearly. The more myopic the eye, the closer this range is to the eye and the smaller the actual linear range becomes. Myopic eyes are corrected with negative (concave) lenses which have the 'side-effect' of making the retinal image smaller (but clearer). The degree of myopia is indicated in dioptres with a negative value, e.g. $-2.00\,\mathrm{D}$.

In hyperopia (long or far sight), light from infinity is brought to a focus behind the retina of the unaccommodating eye. Progressively closer objects give rise to gradually more defocused images. Thus, for the relaxed hyperopic eye, there is no real distance at which an object

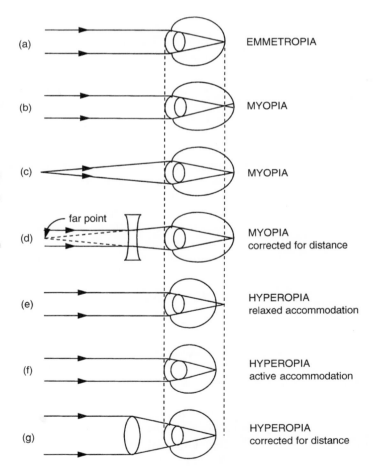

will give rise to a clear image. However when accommodation increases the dioptric power of the eye, it can bring into focus distant objects and then, by exerting more accommodation, near objects. The ability to focus objects at a range of distances depends, therefore on the relative amounts of hyperopia and accommodation. High amounts of hyperopia may prove too much for the accommodative system and the effort to maintain a clear image is abandoned, resulting in a defocused retinal image at any distance. Exerting accommodation for extended periods of time, although resulting in clear vision, may give rise to symptoms of accommodation stress such as headaches and tired eyes (asthenopia). Lapses of accommodation result in occasional blurred vision. Since more accommodation is required to focus a near object, these symptoms will be more pronounced when near objects are viewed for extended periods, as in reading. Therefore, the ability to simply read a letter chart successfully at the required distance does not prove the absence of a refractive error. Hyperopia is corrected with positive (convex) lenses which have the 'side-effect' of making

Fig. 5.1
Emmetropia and ametropia.
(a) Light from a distant object (parallel light) is focused on the retina of an emmetropic eye; (b) Light from a distant object is focused in front of the retina in an uncorrected myopic eye; (c) Light from a near object (divergent light) is focused on the retina in an uncorrected myopic eye; (d) A negative (concave) lens diverges parallel light and allows the myopic eye to see distance objects in focus; (e) Light from a distant object is focused behind the retina of an uncorrected, unaccommodating hyperopic eye; (f) An uncorrected hyperopic eye with sufficient accommodation can bring objects into focus by accommodating; (g) A positive (convex) lens converges parallel light and allows the unaccommodating, hyperopic eye to see distance objects in focus.

the retinal image size larger. The degree of hyperopia is indicated in dioptres with a positive value, e.g. +2.00 D.

Myopia and hyperopia are known as spherical refractive errors and are corrcted with spherical lenses. In general, people with myopia will be given their full refractive correction. Low myopes will only need to wear their distance prescription for occasional distance vision tasks while medium and high myopes will need to wear their prescription constantly. Those with hyperopia will sometimes be partially corrected. This is because the accommodation system of a hyperope who is unused to wearing the spectacle prescription is active and may not relax sufficiently to allow acceptance of the full prescription, resulting in blurred distance vision. In children and young adults the accommodation may not even relax fully during testing so that the measured hyperopia (manifest hyperopia) is less than the actual. Thus some amount (latent hyperopia) goes undetected unless cycloplegic drops are used which paralyse the accommodation. Throughout life the amplitude of accommodation decreases so that the latent hyperopia becomes manifest, symptoms of uncorrected hyperopia become more frequent and the full spectacle prescription becomes accepted. By the age of approximately 40 years all the latent hyperopia will have become manifest.

In cases of low and medium myopia and hyperopia, the refractive error is thought to stem from a miscorrelation of the optical elements of the eye. The dioptric power of the eye results from a number of elements within the eye (Chapter 1): the corneal curvature and refractive index, the refractive index of the aqueous humour, the lens curvatures (anterior and posterior surfaces), the lens refractive indices, and the positions of the surfaces relative to each other. If the total resultant dioptric power is too great relative to the axial length of the eye, or the axial length is too long for the dioptric power, myopia is the result, even if each element itself is within the normal range. This miscorrelation accounts for the majority of refractive errors. In some cases, however, one optical element is abnormal and usually a high refractive error is the result. Examples of this include high (progressive) myopia, where the axial length is abnormally great and continues to increase through life, and microphthalmos, where the axial length is abnormally small resulting in high hyperopia.

Astigmatism

Astigmatism occurs when the two meridians of the eye (e.g. the vertical as opposed to the horizontal) have different refractive errors. For example, the vertical meridian may be more hyperopic than the horizontal, or the vertical may be myopic while the horizontal is hyperopic. In regular astigmatism these two principal meridians are orthogonal (at right-angles) to each other. This is often due to the cornea not being spherical. In astigmatism the cornea can be pictured as being shaped like a rugby ball (or an American or 'Aussie Rules' football), while in the non-astigmatic eye it would be like a soccer ball. When a rugby ball is held vertically (i.e. pointed end up) the vertical meridian is flatter and the horizontal meridian steeper. These are equivalent to the principal meridians in an eye with astigmatism. Astigmatism may be present with either an overall hyperopia or myopia or can be 'mixed' when one meridian is myopic and the other hyperopic. A point object will result in an image with two focal lines which are perpendicular to each other, but at different distances from the retina. The result is that orthogonal lines or edges of any object will not be focused at the same distance from the retina and there is no distance at which an object gives rise to a clear retinal image. Since accommodation cannot occur differentially in two meridians, the eye cannot compensate for this refractive error by accommodating. The result of uncorrected astigmatism can be a meridional amblyopia (amblyopia along one orientation). Astigmatism is corrected by cylindrical lenses (toric lenses) which have a different power in each perpendicular meridian. The prescription is indicated by three components in the following order: the spherical refractive error, the cylindrical refractive error and the orientation of the cylinder axis, e.g. $-1.25/+0.50 \times 45$.

Astigmatism is of three types. In with-the-rule astigmatism, the vertical (or near vertical) meridian has the higher refracting power; in against-the-rule, the horizontal meridian has the most refracting power; in the oblique type an oblique meridian has higher refracting power. In some cases the two principal meridians are not orthogonal to each other, and this is known as irregular astigmatism. Such an eye cannot be completely corrected with a cylindrical lens. Eyes with irregular astigmatism are those with corneal or lenticular irregularities due to pathology such as keratoconus.

Anisometropia

Anisometropia is said to occur when there is a significantly different amount of refractive error in the two eyes. When uncorrected, it is impossible for there to be a clear retinal image in both eyes simultaneously (the eyes cannot exert different amounts of accommodation concurrently). The traditional theory states that since the image in one eye is blurred, there is a tendency for the image from that eye to be suppressed. Clinical experience shows that if both eyes are hyperopic, one more so than the other, the eye with higher hyperopia will be suppressed and may become amblyopic. In cases where one eye is hyperopic and the other myopic or where one is more myopic than the other, there is a tendency for one eye to be used for near tasks and the other for distance tasks. Since each eye is being used at least part of the time, amblyopia will be less likely, although the development of binocular vision may be compromised.

Since by definition a person with anisometropia will require a different power of corrective lens for each eye, each has a different effect on the retinal image size. This may give rise to a retinal image size difference between the two eyes, called aniseikonia. The visual cortex has difficulty fusing significantly different image sizes and the attempt can give rise to symptoms (asthenopia, photophobia, reading difficulty, space perception anomalies and nausea). With an extreme image size difference, binocular vision will break down, resulting in the suppression of one eye. Retinal image size differences may be minimized by the type of optical correction used. Spectacles will be the correction of choice if the anisometropia is due to different axial lengths in the two eyes (axial ametropia) but contact lenses are preferable if it is due to a different dioptric power in each eye (refractive ametropia). Spectacle lenses can be designed to reduce aniseikonia (size lenses) or eliminate it (iseikonic lenses).

Aphakia

An aphakic eye is one in which the crystalline lens is missing. This is usually due to surgical removal because of cataract. In rare cases the lens may be congenitally absent, but in these cases the remainder of the eye is also malformed resulting in low vision. Functional aphakia may occur with a dislocated lens (common in Marfan's syndrome) in which case light bypasses the lens.

Congenital cataracts are not uncommon and may be the result of intra-uterine infections or inherited with or without systemic disorders. The term 'congenital' is misleading as they may develop some weeks, months or even years after birth. There are frequently other malformations of the eye in association with the cataract, such as microphthalmos or microcornea and these eyes will have a worse prognosis. Cataracts in children may also be the result of trauma, in which case there may be other complications due to the trauma itself. Whatever the aetiology, dense cataracts will require surgery at the earliest possible date (in the first months of life) in order to prevent amblyopia. If surgery is delayed more than a year there is little chance of normal vision. Less dense cataracts may be left slightly longer and the decision about whether to remove the cataract will depend largely on the clarity of the view of the fundus, although forced choice preferential looking acuity and/or pattern visually evoked potentials may play some part in the decision.

Usually an extra-capsular operation is performed and frequently a secondary cataract (capsular thickening) occurs, in which case further surgery or YAG laser treatment is required. Intra-ocular lens implants are not generally used in infants and children as the long-term effect of these lenses and their effects on a growing eye are not known.

An aphakic eye will be highly hyperopic (unless it was highly myopic prior to surgery) and will have no accommodation. Since the lens removed has high power and the infant eye is small the resultant hyperopia is very large, often 20–30 D in neonates. An eye with a cataract is often smaller than its fellow eye. A full prescription for the hyperopia will be required with a bifocal correction for near. In babies a near prescription (preferably in contact lens form) with an add of 3 D is given since most of their world is in the intermediate and near zones. The add is gradually reduced to 1–1.5 D by the end of the first year. By the age of 2 the child can wear a distance prescription with bifocal correction.

Contact lenses have definite advantages over spectacles. High hyperopic prescriptions such as are required in aphakia give rise to a functional ring scotoma (visual field loss, due to the prismatic effect of the lens periphery) and the 'jack in the box' phenomonon whereby peripheral objects suddenly jump into view when the head is turned. In addition there is the problem of increased aberrations at the edge of a high plus lens, the weight of the glasses and the difficulties of getting a young child to wear them. These problems are eliminated with contact lenses which also have obvious cosmetic benefits.

In the case of a monocular congenital cataract (resulting in monocular aphakia) a contact lens in the aphakic eye is required for there to be any hope of binocular vision (monocular aphakia results in large refractive anisometropia). Even then there is likely to be a 5–10% size difference between the images of the two eyes (Bennett and Rabbetts, 1984), which is still enough to prevent binocular single vision. Occlusion therapy is always required, as the aphakic eye is invariably amblyopic to some degree. It was traditionally thought that due to the dense amblyopia and aniseikonia, the prognosis for monocularly aphakic eyes was poor. However, recent figures are more encouraging: Lewis, Maurer and Brent (1995) showed that if surgery and optical correction are done early (before 5 months) and if there is aggressive occlusion (3–8 hr per day) good acuity can be achieved. Birch's (1993) group has found similar results: if surgery is done before 1 month and patching is done 8 hr per day to the age of 5 years, normal acuity can be achieved without any ill effect on the other, phakic, eye.

DEVELOPMENT OF REFRACTIVE ERROR

Emmetropization

There is now a considerable body of evidence which suggests that in most eyes there is an active feedback mechanism, resulting in a co-ordinated growth of the optical components of the eye so that a state of near emmetropia is reached. This is known as emmetropization. Some of the evidence for this is as follows:

1. There are large changes in some optical components during the first few years of life, particularly the axial length, and yet there is relatively little change in refractive error. The total change in axial length quoted in Chapter 1 would, by itself, lead to 25 D of myopia! Therefore the changes in the other optical components must in some way compensate for this large change.
2. The distribution of refractive error at birth approximates a normal curve (as do most biological variables), but this becomes a narrower distribution at the age of 6 years, indicating that there is a co-ordinated growth of optical components towards emmetropia.
3. The distribution of each individual optical component is normally distributed. The exception to this is axial length, which has a tail towards longer axial length. If these elements were combined at

random (in each individual), the result would be a normal distribution of refractive error. However, in adults we find a distribution of refractive error which is steeper than normal, which indicates that the elements are combined not randomly, but in a co-ordinated fashion (Young and Leary, 1991).

4. We can look at the correlation of optical components and axial length in individuals. Sorsby, Benjamin and Davey (1957) showed evidence that, in emmetropic eyes, there is a correlation between corneal curvature and axial length: the cornea tends to be flatter when the axial length is greater. In all eyes there is a correlation between axial length and the lens curvature; this again indicates a co-ordinated growth process (Curtin, 1985), particularly for those eyes which do manage to achieve emmetropia or near emmetropia.

5. Animal studies show that visual experience affects refractive error. Eyes which are allowed to receive light, but no form, on the retina tend to become highly myopic. This is known as deprivation myopia and has been demonstrated in various species including monkeys, tree shrews, cats, and chickens (see Schaeffel, 1993, for a review). Once myopia has developed it can be reversed if normal viewing conditions are allowed as long as this occurs within a certain time period of development. Chicks can recover from both myopia and hyperopia. Additionally, chicks raised with lenses over an eye develop a refractive error in the same direction, e.g. an eye with a negative lens becomes myopic, as though the eye were trying to make the total combination of eye and lens emmetropic. These effects are also reversible (Irving, Sivak and Callender, 1992). Recent studies have shown similar changes in monkeys (Hung, Crawford and Smith, 1995). These findings indicate an active feedback process which is sensitive to the sign of optical blur, aiming towards emmetropia.

6. Observations in humans confirm the same process. Eyes which have not received a normal retinal image from birth, such as those with cataract, or those with low visual acuity (e.g. retinopathy of prematurity or optic atrophy) tend to be highly myopic and to have a much wider spread of refractive error (Young and Leary, 1991). Thus the reception of a reasonably clear retinal image is thought to have some controlling effect on refractive error.

Development of refraction: newborn to 3 years

When studying the development of refractive error and reviewing the studies mentioned below, we find some variation and apparent disagreement between studies. This may represent real differences between populations differing in ethnicity or socioeconomic status. Alternatively, it may be due to differences in exclusion or inclusion criteria, for example, in studies of neonates, all babies, or only those without complications, may have been included, and the exact time (days after birth) that the measurements were taken may vary. Differences in technique may also account for some of the variability, for example, method of measurement, whether cycloplegic drugs were used and the type of cycloplegic agent used. These factors must be kept in mind when comparing studies.

At birth (and even at age 6 years – Hirsch, 1963) it is generally found that there is a wider spread of refractive error than in the adult population and that the mean is more hyperopic. The mean varies somewhat between different studies (from +0.6–+2.6 D), but Banks (1980) amalgamated data from 11 other studies and found an overall mean of +2 D with a standard deviation (s.d.) of 2 D. Refraction in all these studies was performed under cycloplegia. This implies that 67% of newborns lie between 0 and +4 D, and 95% lie within −2 and +6 D. Therefore myopia is not uncommon in neonates.

At birth refractive error is normally distributed but at 6–8 years of age it is steeper than a normal curve (as it is in adults) with fewer myopes. Hirsch's data showed that in the first 8 years of life the mean decreased by 1 D from +2 to +1 D and the s.d. from 2.7 to 1.6 D.

Gwiazda et al. (1993) found that the mean uncycloplegic refraction changed from myopia to hyperopia during the first year of life and stayed hyperopic until 8 years of age. Refraction was measured with either distance or near fixation retinoscopy. They found as much variation as in studies with cycloplegia (i.e. an s.d. of approximately 2 D in neonates). By 6 years of age the s.d. was much smaller and the mean was hyperopic, as found in other studies. The myopia in the first 6 months is thought to be due to the child not fully relaxing accommodation during retinoscopy.

Figure 5.2 gives the distribution of data obtained by Cook and Glasscock (1951) who performed cycloplegic retinoscopy and found a slightly wider distribution than some studies (mean 1.8 ± 3.1 D), and data obtained by Gwiazda et al. (1993) (non-cycloplegic data at 0–3 months and at 6 years).

Other studies have shown a decrease in hyperopia in the first year to 15 months (Edwards, 1991; Saunders, Woodhouse and Westall,

Fig. 5.2
Distribution of non-cycloplegic refractive error (spherical equivalent) at 0–3 months (solid circles) and 6 years (open circles). Cycloplegic newborn data (☆) from Cook and Glasscock (1951). (From Gwiazda, J., Thorn, F., Bauer, J. and Held, R. (1993). Emmetropization and the progression of manifest refraction in children followed from infancy to puberty. *Clinical Vision Science*, **8**, 337–344. With kind permission of Elsevier Science Ltd.)

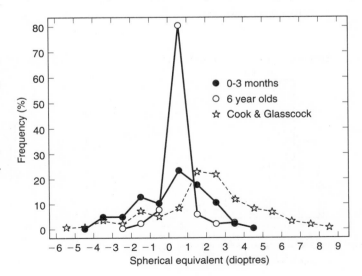

1995) (Figure 5.3). Saunders et al. used Mohindra retinoscopy (described later) and Edwards used retinoscopy under cycloplegia. The apparent difference between some studies and that of Gwiazda et al. (1993) may depend on the initial level of ametropia. Saunders, Woodhouse and Westall (1995) showed that the rate of emmetropization depends on the initial amount of ametropia; that is, the further the eye has to go to reach emmetropia, the faster it changes (Figure 5.4). This seems to apply to moderate amounts of ametropia, but not to extreme refractive errors which are less likely to emmetropize during the first few years of life. When Gwiazda's population was separated into those children who were initially myopic and hyperopic, it became evident that both groups moved towards emmetropia. Similarly, Atkinson and Braddick (1988) and Ehrlech et al. (1995) found that hyperopes and myopes, respectively, progressed towards emmetropia or low hyperopia, while the emmetropes, as a group, remained unchanged. The apparent movement of the *mean* will thus depend on relative proportions of infants with myopia and hyperopia in the initial sample.

Fig. 5.3
Distribution of cycloplegic spherical equivalent refractive error at approximately 10 weeks (1st visit), 20 weeks (2nd visit), 30 weeks (3rd visit) and 40 weeks (4th visit) of age. (From Edwards (1991) The refractive status of Hong Kong Chinese infants. *Ophthalmic and Physiological Optics,* **11,** 297–303. With kind permission of Elsevier Science Ltd.)

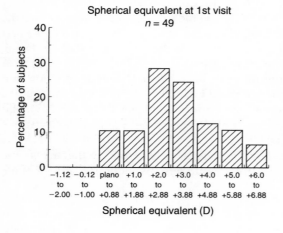

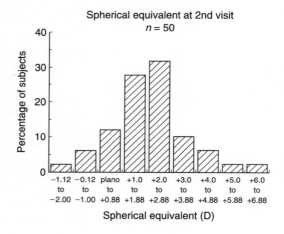

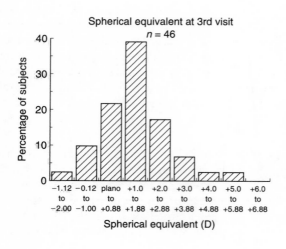

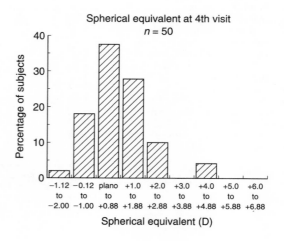

Fig. 5.4
Rate of change of ametropia
with respect to initial ametropia.
(From Saunders, K., Woodhouse,
J.M. and Westall, C.A. (1995)
Emmetropization in human
infancy: Rate of change is related
to initial refractive error. *Vision
Research,* **35,** 1325–1328. With kind
permission of Elsevier Science
Ltd.)

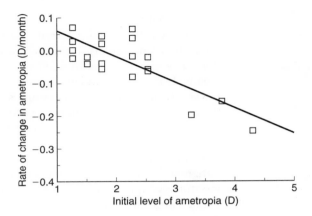

To conclude, most studies which use cycloplegic agents find that newborns are hyperopic and that there is a decrease in hyperopia in the first few years of life. Some earlier studies show an increase of hyperopia during this time, but these are usually much earlier studies, some of which used ophthalmoscopy rather than retinoscopy to measure refractive error.

Preterm babies

Low birthweight infants are less hyperopic at birth than normal weight babies and the distribution is not normal. Banks (1980) found an overall mean from four cycloplegic studies of +0.87 D and a range of means of − 1.3 to +1.1 D so it appears that the whole curve is simply shifted towards myopia. The s.d. is very similar to that of full-term babies (between 1.6 and 3.2 D). Scharf, Zonis and Zelter (1975) found 45% to be myopic. Amongst preterm babies with retinopathy of prematurity there is even more myopia and of higher degree (Fletcher and Brandon, 1955).

There is also evidence that the amount and prevalence of astigmatism increases as gestational age decreases (Dobson et al., 1981), that there is a higher prevalence (83–90%) of against-the-rule astigmatism (Dobson et al., 1981; Abrahamson, Fabian and Sjostrand, 1988) and a higher prevalence of anisometropia.

Preterm babies also show some emmetropization. Most preterm babies with myopia show a shift towards emmetropia by 6 months. However, some studies show that this may not be as complete as in full-term babies: children who were preterm are 0.5 D more myopic (mean value) than those that were full-term.

Small eye error

In most studies of refractive error in infants, measurements are undertaken by retinoscopy, during which light reflects from the vitreo-retinal border rather than the photoreceptors. Since the vitreo-retinal border is anterior to the photoreceptors by a finite distance, there is a small intrinsic error in retinoscopy. Since the finite distance between the two surfaces remains constant while the eye grows, this distance, proportional to the size of the eye, is greater in smaller eyes. This has been termed the small eye error. However, when calculated (Banks, 1980; Howland, 1983) this error is about 0.5–0.8 D in newborns and 0.37 D in adults. This difference is not enough to account for the greater hyperopia found in infants, as has been suggested by some. However, some eye care practitioners will reduce their prescription by 0.5 D in newborns to compensate for this error.

Astigmatism

Astigmatism is more common in newborns and until the age of 12–18 months (Mohindra et al., 1978; Atkinson, Braddick and French, 1980; Gwiazda et al., 1984; Edwards, 1991, Ehrlech et al., 1995). Mohindra found that 45% of infants (in the first year of life) had clinically significant amounts of astigmatism which is almost 10 times that found in children and 5 times that found in adults. In the adult population approximately 6.5% have astigmatism of 1 D or more (Kragha, 1987). In the cross-sectional study of Mohindra et al., astigmatism was greatest at 11–20 weeks (50–60% had 2 D or more between 1 and 31 weeks) and had declined by 5–6 months. Ninety per cent of these infants with high astigmatism will lose it over the following two years of life (Mohindra et al., 1978; Atkinson et al., 1980; Abrahamson, 1990a). Thus both the amount and prevalence of astigmatism decline with age. Atkinson et al. found that by 18 months most infants have no more than the average astigmatism in adults (0.75 D), while Gwiazda (1993) found that approximately 45% still had 1 D or more at age 2 years which dropped to 20% at 4 years of age (Figure 5.5). Edwards found fewer high astigmats and that the astigmatism decreased more rapidly (Figure 5.6).

Although there is, then, some disagreement between studies about rate of decline, most show that it does decline over the first few years, the rate of decrease varying between individuals.

Examination of various studies shows that no single type of astigmatism predominates. Most studies show more against-the-rule in newborns, which either decreases during the first year or is maximum at about half to one year (Mohindra et al., 1978; Fulton, Dobson and Salem, 1980; Dobson et al., 1984; Howland and Sayles, 1984; Atkinson, 1993). Two studies showed fairly equal prevalence of with-the-rule and against-the-rule (Mohindra et al., 1978; Gwiazda et al., 1984) while Edwards (1991) found that most astigmatism was with-the-rule in the first year of life. Oblique astigmatism also has a high prevalence (Howland and Sayles, 1984). The differences between studies may indicate genuine differences between populations.

Atkinson et al. (1980) and Atkinson (1993) in Britain found roughly equal percentages of with-the-rule, against-the-rule and oblique astigmatism amongst children with hyperopia and that with-the-rule astigmatism decreased more rapidly than against-the-rule. This resulted in a higher predominance of against-the-rule in hyperopic 1.5–3 year olds. Hyperopic infants with significant astigmatism

Fig. 5.5
Distribution of astigmatism with respect to age in a longitudinal study. (From Gwiazda, J., Thorn, F., Bauer, J. and Held, R. (1993) Emmetropization and the progression of manifest refraction in children followed from infancy to puberty. *Clinical Vision Science,* **8,** 337–344. With kind permission of Elsevier Science Ltd.)

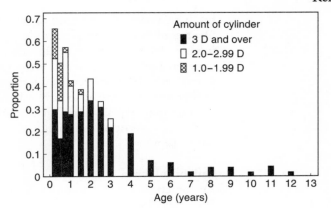

Fig. 5.6
Distribution of astigmatism at approximately 10 weeks (1st visit), 20 weeks (2nd visit), 30 weeks (3rd visit) and 40 weeks (4th visit) of age. (From Edwards (1991). The refractive status of Hong Kong Chinese infants. *Ophthalmic and Physiological Optics,* **11,** 297–303. With kind permission of Elsevier Science Ltd.)

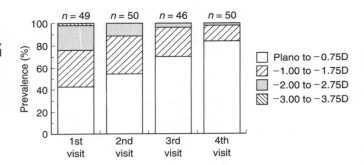

tended to retain their hyperopia, while those without astigmatism tended to emmetropize.

The conclusion is that the prevalence of all types of astigmatism is high in the first few years of life and decreases during that time. Most children will show some decrease of their astigmatism in the first year, but approximately 10% do not lose it or have increasing astigmatism which remains into adulthood. Unfortunately, at present, there does not seem to be any way of predicting which children will maintain and which will lose their astigmatism (apart from the fact that children with very high amounts are less likely to show a decrease or lose all their astigmatism). For medium amounts of astigmatism, we are left with the alternative of tracking astigmatism over a period of time in an individual before prescribing.

This infantile astigmatism (first year) does not appear to affect meridional grating acuity significantly, i.e. acuity will come into the normal range with correction and visual acuity in adulthood is essentially normal. However, Gwiazda et al. (1986) found that, if sensitive tests such as vernier acuity are used, meridional amblyopia can be demonstrated in the meridian which was most blurred in the 6–24-month period. From her data it seems that astigmatism in the first 6 months does not affect acuity. This may be because the poor resolving power of the young visual system makes it insensitive to blur. She found that the age of maximum sensitivity to astigmatic blur is 15 months falling sharply at 24 months. She found no correlation between the adult refractive error (or even the refractive error at 3 years) and the presence of meridional losses of acuity. The high proportion of infants who have astigmatism between the ages of 6–15 months may explain some of the differences in resolution between horizontal, vertical and oblique meridians found in most adults (anisotropy).

Anisometropia

Anisometropia is more common in young children up to the age of 3.5 years than in adults. Zonis and Miller (1974) found 17% of neonates had anisometropia greater than 1 D. Between the ages of 1 and 3.5 years, prevalence is between 7 and 11% (Ingram and Barr, 1979; Abrahamson et al., 1990b). Abrahamson et al. found a 10% prevalence of anisometropia greater than or equal to 1 D between the ages of 1 and 4 years and a 2% prevalence of anisometropia greater than or equal to 2 D. The prevalence of anisometropia 1 D or greater in the adult population is in the region of 4% (Hirsch, 1967; Kragha, 1987).

However, recent longitudinal studies have shown that there is an almost zero rate of persistent anisometropia. Over the first 3.5 years of life, some children lose their anisometropia, while others temporarily gain it. In a study which stretched through birth to 10 years, of the children who returned for subsequent visits, no children were anisometropic throughout (Almeder, Peck and Harland 1990). It has been suggested that the rates of progression towards emmetropia can be different in each eye resulting in temporary anisometropia which lasts for a short duration giving no increased risk of amblyopia. Persistent anisometropia throughout these years gives a 30% risk of amblyopia. Almeder et al. (1990) suggest the theory that anisometropia may be the result rather than the cause of amblyopia.

Refractive risk factors for amblyopia

Abrahamson et al. (1990a,b) and Ingram et al. (1986) found that there was an increased chance of amblyopia (monocular or binocular) in the following conditions:

- One year old with $\geq 3.5\,D$ in one meridian.
- Four years old with the most hyperopic meridian $\geq 2\,D$.
- Four years old with with-the-rule or oblique astigmatism.
- Increasing or unchanged high refractive error between 1 and 4 years.
- Persisting anisometropia.

Atkinson (1993) showed that partial correction of medium to high hyperopia (3.5 D or more in one meridian) reduced the incidence of strabismus and allowed acuity to develop normally. Without correction the children with medium to high hyperopia had poorer acuity on average than those with low hyperopia. Aurell and Norrsell (1990) showed that it was the infants with more than 4 D of hyperopia which did not decrease towards emmetropia, who went on to develop esotropia. In Chapter 14 we have suggested guidelines for when to correct ametropia in children, and it will be seen that they are closely related to these amblyopia risk factors.

Development of refractive error: 3–20 year olds

As noted above, between 1 year and 6–8 years there is a trend towards less hyperopia and there is less variation between individuals. At 6–8 years of age there is a mean hyperopia of 1 D with an s.d. = 1.6 D (Hirsch, 1963). Most of this change occurs in the first 3 years so that there is little change from 3–7 in either spherical correction or astigmatism. The cycloplegic and non-cycloplegic findings are within 0.75 D from age 5 upwards. Hyperopia which is much greater under cycloplegia is more likely to regress.

It has been shown that a high refractive error at 1 year old is predictive of a high refractive error later in life, that is, the higher refractive errors change little and fail to emmetropize fully (both hyperopia and myopia). Gwiazda et al. (1993), in a longitudinal study, found that refraction at 1 year was predictive of refraction from 7 years upwards. The smallest s.d. of the population was found at 6 years. Infants who were myopic at 6 months became hyperopic or emmetropic at 1 year, but not as hyperopic as those who were hyperopic at 6 months (Figure 5.7). There appeared to be a convergence towards emmetropia at 6 years, followed by an increase in spread again as those destined for myopia progress that way.

In the study of Gwiazda et al. (1993), hyperopic infants who had against-the-rule astigmatism at 6 months remained hyperopic, while myopes with against-the-rule became myopic later in life, that is, although the astigmatism reduced, the spherical error tended to remain. Infants with with-the-rule astigmatism, whether hyperopic or myopic in infancy, remained emmetropic later in life and also lost their astigmatism.

There is a gradual change in mean refraction from hyperopia through emmetropia to myopia in school years, progressing until the age of 15. It has been suggested that this is due to a few children becoming myopic while most remain emmetropic or progress very slowly to myopia (at the rate of 0.07–0.21 D per year – Goss, 1991). Myopia which begins during these years is called early onset, or juvenile, myopia. The incidence of myopia (number of new cases) is greatest between the ages 8–13 for girls and 10–13 for boys (Goss, 1991).

Since it is usual for a child to be slightly hyperopic, if this is not the case, there is increased risk that myopia, rather than emmetropia will be the final result. If a child enters school with hyperopia of 1.5 D or more, he or she is likely to be still hyperopic by the age of 13–14 while those who are between 0–0.5 D are likely to be myopic by then (Goss, 1991). The earlier a child shifts over to myopia, the more myopic they are likely to become. For those children who become myopic, the

Fig. 5.7
Mean spherical equivalent refraction (non-cycloplegic) from 31 children with negative spherical equivalents in the first 6 months (solid squares) and from 20 children who had positive spherical equivalents (≥0.5 D) in the first 6 months (solid circles). (From Gwiazda, J., Thorn, F., Bauer, J. and Held, R. (1993). Emmetropization and the progression of manifest refraction in children followed from infancy to puberty. *Clinical Vision Science*, **8**, 337–344.)

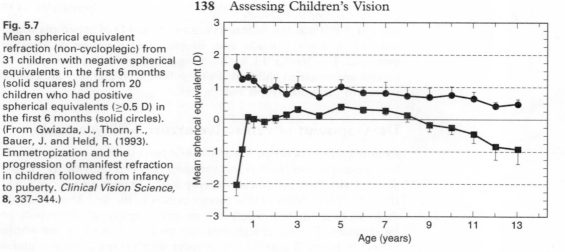

progression tends to be constant, about 0.5 D per year, slowing or stopping at the age of 15 (Goss, 1991).

Most adolescents are relatively emmetropic, but there is a tail towards myopia (Sorsby et al., 1957). Another group becomes myopic from 20 onwards (late onset, or young adult, myopia).

Sex differences

There are only slight differences of refractive error according to sex. Females have a slightly higher prevalence of high myopia in infancy (congenital or early acquired myopia) while males have a slightly higher incidence of early and late onset myopia. As a result, the total prevalence of myopia is the same in both sexes. Girls develop early onset myopia slightly earlier, but the progression ceases earlier. Girls and women have a higher prevalence of high astigmatism. No sex differences in hyperopia have been found.

MEASUREMENT OF REFRACTIVE ERROR

When testing young children and non-comunicative people, objective measures are necessary. Refractive error can be measured with relatively inexpensive equipment – the retinoscope. Although cycloplegic retinoscopy is the 'baseline' technique, against which others are measured, it is not always desirable or necessary to undertake cycloplegia. Instilling drops will always upset a child to some degree, may remind the child of previous unpleasant examinations and result in a reduction of co-operation, not only on that visit but on future visits also.

Retinoscopy

Static retinoscopy

Retinoscopy involves the observation of shadows within the pupil area while a moving beam of light from the retinoscope is shone into the eye from a distance of 50–66 cm; the direction of movement of the shadows, either in the same direction or in the opposite direction as the incident beam, indicates whether the eye is myopic or hyperopic relative to the position of the retinoscope and lenses are held in front of the eye to 'neutralize the movement'. For a full explanation of the theory and technique of retinoscopy see Bennett and Rabbetts (1984).

Traditional static retinoscopy involves the person regarding a distant object, preferably red in colour (to relax accommodation further) and without detail which would stimulate accommodation. Once the working distance lenses of +1.5 or +2 D are in place, the detail of the target should be unresolvable. Alternatively, a spot light can be utilized. However, the colour of the target probably has little effect on the final result. If a child is old enough and co-operative enough this can be undertaken as for an adult. A child of this ability will usually accept wearing a trial frame if it is shown to the child first (with a joke) before attempting to place it on the face. It is important to accustom the child to the idea slowly rather than abruptly placing the frame on the face.

Creativity is required when devising distance fixation targets for younger children. The child's attention can be attracted to the distance target by a number of methods, such as by giving the child the controls of the test chart and asking him or her to attempt to extinguish all the panels without looking at the control box (this applies to British internally illuminated charts). Alternatively, a specially purchased stimulus can be used such as an illuminated musical box, or flashing lights or simply a translucent toy which fits over a penlight. This would be held at the other end of the room by a co-worker or parent. A video-player showing a child's cartoon film also makes a good distance target which will gain the attention of children down to the age of 3.

Until the age of approximately 7 years, trial frames should be used rather than the phoropter, which is too intimidating for most children and results in a loss of contact with the child as it is harder to see how the child is reacting behind it. Several trial frames have been specially designed for children. The authors find that a drop cell frame is more acceptable to children than the more common clip or Oculus type, being lighter and less cumbersome and intimidating. Alternatively, a child's spectacle frame can be glazed with +2 D lenses and the lens holders from Halberg clips permanently stuck to the front of the lenses. Halberg clips are useful for children, allowing an 'over-refraction' to be undertaken over their own spectacles.

For infants and toddlers, although it may be possible to use a trial frame, especially if it is introduced gradually and playfully, hand-held trial lenses may be more acceptable. Lens bars can also be used for speed (Figure 5.8). However, it must be remembered that most infants will be hyperopic, in order to relax accommodation, it is important to have a fogging lens over the fixing eye, while performing retinoscopy on the other eye. While using spheres it is possible to achieve this with hand-held trial lenses, holding two lenses in one hand (Figure 5.9). To measure astigmatism, spheres can be used for each meridian separately (streak retinoscopy) or, after the main spherical portion of the prescription in each eye has been determined by hand-held lenses, the sphere-cylinder combination can be checked using the trial frame. This latter method can work for infants who only have a short tolerance period for a trial frame or $+2\,D$ fogging glasses. The method of using the sphere-cylinder combination is probably preferable as accommodation may change between the measurement of each meridian, resulting in a wrong estimation of the amount of astigmatism.

Fogging of the fixing eye is very important. If, while undertaking retinoscopy on the first eye, a considerable amount of hyperopia is found, the fogging lens for the other eye should be increased accordingly, under the assumption that both eyes will have a similar degree of hyperopia.

During this time the retinoscopist should be watching the child's pupil. When constricted it indicates that accommodation is active, and the results should be ignored. Use the results during dilation of the pupil when accommodation is more relaxed. Additionally, always look for the most 'with' movement, ignoring occasional 'against' movements.

Given the limited attention span of a child it is always important to work fast and obtain the maximum amount of information in the minimum time. For example, gaining some idea of the refractive error

Fig. 5.8
Distance fixation (static) retinoscopy being performed on a child using lens bars.

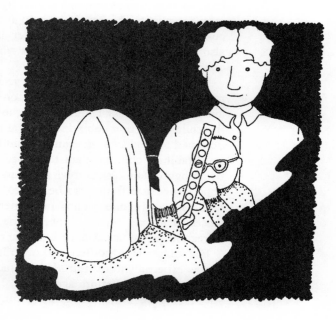

Fig. 5.9
Distance fixation (static)
retinoscopy using hand-held trial
lenses.

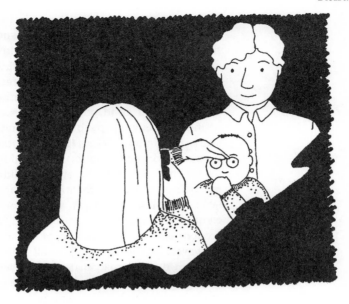

of each eye is more important than refining the axis of a small cylinder in the first eye. Therefore, obtain a rough retinoscope result on each eye and then return to each eye (if the child is still co-operating) to refine the result.

Near fixation retinoscopy (Mohindra Technique)

For a child who will not consistently fixate on the distant target, and for younger infants, the Mohindra technique can be used. All the room lights are extinguished (slowly, not suddenly) and the child encouraged to fixate the retinoscope light by calling her or his name and talking reassuringly. This is a good time for an infant to be allowed to bottle feed as accommodation then relaxes and the child will fixate well on the light. Since Mohindra advocates occluding the eye not being measured, the technique works well with hand-held lenses. A sphere and cylinder lens can be held before the eye being tested, while the palm of the hand occludes the other eye. Alternatively, lens bars can be employed. A working distance of 50 cm is used and a correction of 1.25 D is subtracted to allow for tonic accommodation and working distance. Some authors have suggested that occluding the unmeasured eye makes little difference to the retinoscopy result (Griffin, 1982; Wesson, Mann and Bray, 1990).

The near fixation technique makes two assumptions: that the retinoscope light is not a stimulus to accommodation and that therefore the eye assumes its tonic (resting) accommodative level. Owens, Mohindra and Held (1988) showed that these assumptions are essentially correct. The main theoretical objection to near retinoscopy therefore appears to be the range of tonic accommodation between individuals, from 0 to 4 D. Tonic accommodation may also be refractive-error dependent, those with hyperopia having a closer dark focus than those with myopia (Maddock et al., 1981; McBrien and Millodot, 1987; Rosner and Rosner, 1989). If tonic accommodation is greater in hyperopia, this would lead to an underestimate of the degree of hyperopia in these individuals.

The results from Mohindra retinoscopy must therefore be interpreted with caution. Mohindra and Molinari (1979) concluded that there is a good correlation between cycloplegic refraction and Mohindra retinoscopy but their study was on older children, 3–7 years. Borghi and Rouse (1985) concur that there is good agreement between Mohindra and cycloplegic retinoscopy. However, other studies have shed doubt on the validity of the technique, especially for infants (the group for which the technique will be primarily used) (Wesson, Mann and Bray, 1990), for children with higher refractive errors (Maino, Cibis and Cress, 1984) and for the spherical component of the correction (Wesson, Mann and Bray, 1990). However, Saunders and Westall (1992) found no better agreement between two retinoscopists doing cycloplegic than near retinoscopy. On children and infants they found that most of the variability was due to poor confidence ratings (when there was poor co-operation from the child, poor fixation or variable pupil size indicating active accommodation). They agreed that near retinoscopy may tend to underestimate hyperopia. They found that a correction factor of 1.25 D was appropriate for adults, but suggested 1 D for children older than 2 years and 0.75 D for those under 2.

Choice of distance or near fixation retinoscopy
Our recommendations are as follows:

- Use distance fixation for retinoscopy when possible, i.e. when the child is old enough and co-operative enough to fixate a distance target.
- With infants or older children who cannot co-operate for distance fixation, use near fixation retinoscopy.
- If confidence is poor (poor fixation or variable pupil size) or if high hyperopia is detected with near fixation retinoscopy, use a cycloplegic. There are other, additional indications for using cycloplegia (see below).
- In the case of aphakia or functional aphakia, let the child observe the retinoscope beam (accommodation is absent) and subtract the normal working distance.

Cycloplegic refraction

Some eye professionals feel that cycloplegic refraction is necessary almost routinely. Our experience in Cardiff was that a number of children had a history of bad experiences with 'drops' (and clinicians in white coats); this was particularly true for children with low vision or those who had had major illnesses and hospitalizations. We therefore try to avoid the use of drugs in order to instil confidence in the child. With the majority of infants, when routine examinations are undertaken, sufficiently reliable results can be obtained using Mohindra or distance fixation.

However, cyclopegia should be used when:

1. High hyperopia is detected in a child < 2 years, particularly if measured with near fixation retinoscopy.
2. A high refractive error of any type is detected so that spectacles are likely to be prescribed and a poor result is obtained using Mohindra or distance fixation, i.e. the retinoscope reflex constantly changes, the pupil is small (indicating active accommodation) or the child does not maintain reasonably constant fixation.
3. A strabismus is detected, especially esotropia.
4. Anisometropia of greater than 1 D is detected.

Cyclopentolate is the cycloplegic of choice, using 0.5 (two drops separated by 5 minutes) or 1% in most cases. If maximum pupil dilation is required for a dilated fundus examination as well, then cyclopentolate together with 2.5% phenylephrine can be used. For children under 3 months of age, 1% cyclopentolate should NOT be used, but two drops of 0.5% cyclopentolate (Moore, 1990).

Tropicamide does not reduce accommodation sufficiently to be used as a cycloplegic in normally pigmented eyes. There is still 40–60% of accommodation remaining in brown eyes and 20–40% in blue eyes. Atropine is rarely, if ever, necessary and may serve to break an intermittent convergent strabismus to a constant strabismus due to its long duration of action (10 days). It also is inconvenient and potentially injurious as it has to be prescribed in advance, inserted by a parent for 3 days prior to the visit and has a number of potentially harmful systemic effects (thirst, fever, urinary retention, restlessness and tachycardia). Allergic reactions of the lids and cornea are also known (North and Kelly, 1987).

The only adverse reactions to cyclopentolate are the systemic effects of incoherent speech, disorientation, restlessness, visual hallucinations and drowsiness, lasting 1–5 hours. Usually these are reported in darkly pigmented children who require more doses of the drug for adequate cycloplegia or on occasions when cyclopentolate 2% is used. No permanent consequences have been found (Jones and Hodes, 1991). Allergic reactions to cyclopentolate are very rare (Jones and Hodes), but take the form of a local skin rash and some breathlessness. In these cases, cyclopentolate should not be administered at a future date and parents should be warned of potential allergic reactions to other anticholinergic agents, some of which can be bought over the counter, e.g. travel sickness preparations.

Methods
Cycloplegic refraction is performed at the end of the examination. With the exception of the fundus examination, other procedures (such as binocularity tests, assessing the effect of increased plus on esotropia or esophoria, low vision assessment, stereopsis tests) are performed before the cyclopentolate is instilled.

There are several methods for instilling drops in children.

1. Attempt to get one drop in each eye as quickly as possible.
2. Use a local anaesthetic before instilling the cycloplegic in order to reduce the substantial discomfort that cyclopentolate causes. Proparacaine hydrochloride 0.5% is the anaesthetic of choice as it causes a minimal stinging sensation itself. It has very little effect on the time course of cyclopentolate or the depth of the cycloplegia (Lovasic, 1986).
3. With the head back or the child lying supine, place drops at the inner canthus while the child has his or her eyes closed. On opening the eyes, sufficient quantities of the drops will enter.
4. Spray drops using a sterilized perfume atomizer. These can be applied to the open or closed eyes and are sprayed at a distance of 5–10 cm. The child does not have to be supine as with conventional drops. The use of a spray is said to decrease discomfort.

Minims are the preferable form in which to obtain drugs. They may appear more expensive, but certainly compare well in price if a whole bottle of cyclopentolate has to be discarded when it accidentally comes into contact with an eyelid, a frequent occurrence when dealing with children. Also, they do not contain preservative, thus reducing the chance of an allergic reaction. When instilling drops into an infant's eye, let her or him lie on the parent's lap with the head towards the parent's knees (see Figure 4.4). Let toddlers and preschoolers sit or lie on the parent's lap. After instillation, the punctae should be occluded for 1–2 minutes (the child or parents can do this) in order to reduce the rate of absorption of the drug into the blood system. Closing the eyes will also reduce systemic absorption and will increase the uptake through the cornea.

The authors' experience is that the use of Proparacaine makes the instillation of cyclopentolate far less traumatic. However, the disadvantage of using a topical anaesthetic is that co-operation in getting the subsequent drops of cycloplegic into the eyes may be reduced. Therefore, if the child has received drops before, it is usually easier to instil the cyclopentolate as quickly as possible (method 1 or 3 above). If the child has never had drops, then the prior use of a local anaesthetic is the best route. The usual precaution about not rubbing the eyes after use of an anaesthetic must be explained to the parent.

With older children the use of the local anaesthetic is not warranted but, as we have said before, we must be honest about the fact that there will be some stinging sensation.

Refraction is performed 30 minutes after instillation of cyclopentolate. Cyclopentolate does not completely eliminate accommodation: as much as 1 D may remain. Therefore, the use of a distance fixation target is still preferable during cycloplegic retinoscopy, although fixation of the retinoscope light is possible. In the latter case a 2 D, rather than a 1.25 D, correction for working distance should be used as tonic accommodation will be substantially reduced. As there may still be some residual accommodation, the retinoscope reflex may be seen to fluctuate from with to against. The retinoscopist should follow the 'with' movement, ignoring occasional 'against' movements. Since the pupil will be dilated, the retinoscopist should also concentrate on the movement of the reflex at the centre of the pupil.

Cycloplegia in special populations

Cycloplegics (and mydriatics) can be used in special populations as long as the usual precautions are taken. In Down syndrome there is some evidence of increased sensitivity to cholinergic drugs which may result in an extended period of dilation and cycloplegia (Doughty and Lyle, 1992). However, there is no evidence that there is any increased risk from cycloplegia itself. People with cerebral palsy may also show prolonged effects. Children and adults who are intellectually challenged may show unpredictable responses and therefore their carers should be warned appropriately. Psychosomatic responses may be more common. Persons with multiple sclerosis may also show unpredictable reactions. Those with a history of epilepsy should be questioned regarding the possible triggering effect of bright lights (once the pupils are dilated, there will be more retinal illumination and therefore any light will be effectively brighter). This seems a sensible precaution even though light-induced seizures are usually triggered by a regular pulsing or strobe light rather than a constant light such as a retinoscope. The frequency of seizures should also be considered. If a seizure seems likely, cycloplegia would only be undertaken if there were a clear advantage to this, and then only after advantages and disadvantages have been discussed with the parent or other carer. The alternative which can be offered in the case of hyperopia is that glasses may have to be changed more frequently, as more of the hyperopia becomes manifest.

Amongst visually impaired people there is no contraindication to the use of cyclopentolate except in the case of obvious anterior segment anomalies (e.g. dislocated lenses, aniridia, congenital glaucoma, microphthalmos) which may predispose to an attack of closed angle glaucoma. If an optometrist deems that cycloplegia is necessary in such cases, he or she should make contact with the child's ophthalmologist first. Although it is not documented specifically (Doughty and Lyle, 1992), it may be assumed that children with albinism may show a different time course to the drug due to reduced pigmentation.

Advantages of cycloplegic refraction

1. A more accurate measurement of the full refractive error is determined. This is essential in some cases.
2. Latent hyperopia is revealed.
3. A dilated fundus examination can be performed.

Disadvantages of cycloplegic refraction

1. The child is upset to a greater or lesser extent and made wary of eye professionals.
2. There is a very small risk of CNS effects.

3. Cycloplegia does not guarantee an accurate refraction. Lack of co-operation may result in more drug being instilled into one eye than the other, resulting in unequal cycloplegia. Alternatively, if a child will not allow any view of the retinoscope reflex, no advantage is gained from cycloplegia; in this case, referral for examination and refraction under general anaesthetic or sedation can be considered.

Autorefraction

Autorefraction may be an alternative for some children and has been undertaken on infants as young as 1.5 months, although children of 4–18 months may be too active and unable to respond to simple instructions (Aslin, Shea and Metz, 1990). A large proportion of individual measurements will have to be discarded and the need for cycloplegia is not eliminated. Aslin et al. showed that the astigmatic error is frequently overestimated compared with the retinoscopy result, although the spherical error is more in agreement. It seems likely that if the child will not maintain fixation during retinoscopy, she or he will not maintain fixation and relax accommodation during autorefraction, which requires in the region of 500 ms steady fixation without a blink. Autorefractors have more difficulty with abnormal eyes, such as aphakic and pseudoaphakic eyes and those with cataract. In these groups Wesemann and Rassow (1987) found that only 67–80% of adult eyes could be measured and amongst these there was frequent disagreement of up to 6 D in the spherical component and 3 D in the astigmatism compared with subjective techniques. These results indicate that autorefraction is unlikely to replace retinoscopy for the routine measurement of refraction.

Photorefraction

Photorefraction has been advocated as an additional technique. Flash photographs of the child's eyes are taken with the camera at 1.5 or 0.75 m while the child is encouraged to fixate an object at the same distance. The pattern and size of the reflected light from the retina indicate whether the child is hyperopic or myopic relative to the distance of the fixated object. Since photorefraction results in a measure at a single instant in time, the child only having to look at a target momentarily, little co-operation is required. There is little to upset or scare a child: there is no unusual stimulus or unknown person getting close to the child, no lenses are held up to the eyes and most children are familiar with having their photograph taken.

Several 'generations' of photorefraction exist. The original technique has become known as orthogonal photorefraction. The fibre-optic light source is centred at the front of the camera lens and four segments of a cylindrical lens are used to defocus the returning light. If the retina is conjugate (in focus) with the lens no reflected light is observed (the reflected point of light falling on the fibre optic, not the camera lens). If the retina is not conjugate, then the returning light extends over the cylindrical lens and a four-pointed star is seen, the length of its 'rays' depending on the degree of defocus of the eye (Braddick, Atkinson and French, 1979). Using this technique significant astigmatism and anisometropia can be detected, but not the sign of spherical refractive errors. Also, the cylindrical segments are at predetermined axes so that astigmatism at other axes cannot be measured or might go undetected.

Because of these limitations, isotropic photorefraction was developed (Howland, Dobson and Sayles, 1987). In this technique the camera is defocused (no cylindrical lenses being used) first beyond, and secondly closer than, the plane of the pupil, thus allowing the sign of any spherical refractive error to be determined. Astigmatism manifests as a blur ellipse rather than a blur circle. Isotropic photorefraction has been developed into videorefraction (for immediate results) and eccentric photorefraction (which gives more accurate results). In videorefraction a video camera and frame grabber are used to record an image onto a computer screen for immediate or subsequent analysis involving image processing techniques. Eccentric photorefraction involves placing the flash source at some angle to (usually above) the visual axis and results in a crescent of light. The crescent is the same side of the light source in the case of myopia and the opposite side in hyperopia.

Isotropic photorefraction, including eccentric photorefraction can only measure a limited range of refractive errors; large refractive errors can be detected, but not measured, and very small errors (to about 0.8 D) cannot be detected (Bobier and Braddick, 1985). Both of these techniques, especially the former, involve expensive equipment and are therefore unlikely to be used in optometric practice.

Photorefraction does not eliminate the need for cycloplegia in cases of significant refractive error (as active accommodation will still influence the results) and it is not recommended that the results should be used for the prescription of glasses. It may have some use in specialized children's clinics, in screening (Chapter 2) and in research, but it is unlikely to replace the use of a retinoscope in experienced hands. It may occasionally be useful for the very uncooperative child who will not consistently fixate for retinoscopy and for some mentally-challenged people (Bobier et al., 1992). However, there are very few children for whom some measure of refractive error cannot be obtained with retinoscopy, particularly if a cycloplegic is used.

Subjective techniques

With older children (even some as young as 4) subjective techniques are possible using a shortened form of the usual routine. Questioning should be more careful than with adults as children will be more easily led to give the answer they think the examiner wishes to hear (Chapter 3).

If the child accepts more minus during the subjective, check that this results in an increase of acuity. Similarly, if there is a significant change in cylinder power or axis, expect an increase in acuity. In other words, use acuity as an arbiter and check for the accuracy of the child's responses. Children with uncorrected high hyperopia will have very active accommodation and may well not accept the full retinoscopy result. This can be seen during the subjective as acuity with the retinoscope result is initially good and then worsens during the subjective examination. Accommodation should be allowed to be active during crossed-cylinder technique but more plus should be 'pushed' in rechecking the spherical component. More plus may well be accepted binocularly. Binocular balancing may be difficult as accommodation is constantly variable. The duochrome method with polaroid dissociation can be successful. In many cases with these children, the original retinoscopy result or dynamic retinoscopy can be used to give the balance point.

ACCOMMODATION

Traditionally it has been assumed that children have the expected amplitudes of accommodation for their age. The routine measurement of accommodation involves bringing a target with fine detail closer to the person (moved along an amplitude rule) until she or he reports that the target begins to blur. This technique is clearly inappropriate with infants and those with communication difficulties who may not be able to comprehend or communicate about the blur point. It is also inappropriate for children with visual impairment, to whom the idea of the moment of blur will be foreign or, at least, less specific. Nevertheless, there is an increased likelihood of reduced accommodation in these groups: children with Down syndrome, cerebral palsy and low vision have been shown to suffer frequently from reduced accommodation (Lindstedt, 1983; Duckman, 1984; Lindstedt, 1986; Woodhouse et al., 1993; Leat, 1996). There are two possible clinical techniques for assessing accommodation in these cases depending on the child's communication ability: dynamic retinoscopy and measurement of distance and near acuity.

Normal accommodative response

The normal stimulus for accommodation is the maintenance of a clear retinal image (Cuiffreda, 1991). Reflex accommodation is the automatic adjustment of accommodation to maintain this image. Blur will give information regarding the magnitude of accommodation change required but not the direction. There are a number of cues to accommodation (which give information about the direction of accommodation shift required): these include chromatic aberration, spherical aberration, asymmetry of astigmatism in the eye and disparity vergence, size and proximity of the target and other monocular cues regarding the relative depth of objects such as overlap.

Objective measures of accommodation in adults generally show that for a stimulus at a distance of 0.66 m or closer (1.5 D or greater) there is a lag (the eye under-accommodates) which tends to increase as the demand increases, i.e. as the stimulus becomes closer. For a target at a distance greater than 0.66 m, there is a lead – the eye does not completely relax its accommodation or there is over-accommodation.

Accommodation in infants has been measured objectively with dynamic retinoscopy and with photorefraction. It is thought that neonates have a larger depth of focus of the eyes than do adults. The pupil diameter is smaller until the age of 2 months and the visual acuity is poorer, both these factors increasing the depth of focus. Early data seemed to show that a baby's accommodational response is 'locked' into the accommodated position (that they cannot relax their accommodation). Subsequent studies showed that they can make accommodational changes and that occasionally their accommodation is accurate (Brookman, 1983; Howland et al., 1987; Cuiffreda, 1991). That is, they have the physical ability to change their accommodation, but they do not use it consistently or accurately. Their accommodation is more consistent and accurate to near, rather than distance, stimuli.

Accommodation accuracy improves until by 5–6 months accommodative responses are essentially adult-like (Braddick, Atkinson and French, 1979; Brookman, 1983; Bobier, 1990). The stimulus-response curves for accommodation have a slope of 0.5 at 1 month, 0.75 at 2 months and 0.8 (which is similar to the adult) at 6 months. Perfect accommodative response would give rise to a slope of unity.

Dynamic retinoscopy for measurement of accommodation

As early as 1952 Pascal recommended the use of dynamic retinoscopy to measure accommodation in cases where subjective measurements would not be reliable. However, the technique does not seem to have gained wide acceptance. Various techniques for dynamic retinoscopy have been advocated. Those that will be mentioned here are designed to be simple measures of the lag (or lead) of accommodation while a near target is viewed (Locke and Somers, 1989). Bell retinoscopy makes use of a bell to gain the child's attention and the bell is moved to find the neutral position. In MEM retinoscopy (monocular estimation method) the accommodative lag (or lead) is estimated and trial lenses held very briefly in front of one eye with the assumption that this will not influence the accommodation. During Nott retinoscopy the child reads a near point card while retinoscopy is performed through a hole in the card. The observer moves away from the card until neutrality is found (Locke and Somers, 1989). Haynes, White and Held (1965) and Brookman (1983) used a dynamic retinoscopy technique to measure accommodation and we have recently adapted that technique. We use a variation of Nott dynamic retinoscopy in which the target is held closer to the eye than the retinoscope (Woodhouse et al., 1993; Leat and Gargon, 1996).

Fig. 5.10
Dynamic retinoscopy technique
(Woodhouse et al., 1993).

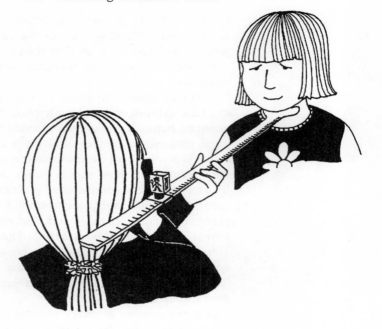

We use an internally illuminated target with pictures made up of detail that can be detected by eyes with various acuities, including fine detail to stimulate accurate accommodation (Figure 5.10). Dynamic retinoscopy is performed after the distance refraction has been determined and with the distance refractive correction in place. The target is placed at certain dioptric distances from the eyes. The child is encouraged to watch the target and the retinoscopist moves until the neutral position is found. Using this technique trial lenses do not have to be used, which many infants find disturbing and which may have some influence on the state of accommodation even if introduced quickly, as in MEM retinoscopy. If the child is accommodating accurately for the target distance, neutral will be at the same distance as the target. In fact, most normally sighted children tend to under-accommodate by 0.35 D. A lead is found if the neutral is closer than the stimulus. The data of Rousse et al. (1984) indicate that 95% of school age children from the general population will lie between having a lag of 1 D to a lead of 0.35 D. The lag increases slightly with age.

The normal range for each dioptric distance and for different age groups is shown in Figure 5.11 and in Table 5:1. The results using a 4 D stimulus to accommodation (25 cm distance, which is a common working distance for children) are very similar between age groups. For ages above 6 years there is a 0.5 D lag with a 95% confidence limit of 0.9 D. This means that the normal range can be said to be from a lead of 0.4 D to a lag of 1.4 D. From the age of 11 years, the lag increases with accommodational demand. In all age groups, the s.d. of responses increases with increasing accommodational demand.

The amplitude of accommodation can be estimated by dynamic retinoscopy by noting the maximum accommodational response obtained whatever the target distance.

Dynamic retinoscopy can also be used to estimate the required reading addition in children who show a reduced accommodative response and who may require a reading addition (see below). The target is placed at the child's habitual distance for near tasks and the neutral position is found. If this is outside the normal range, plus lenses can be added binocularly in 0.5 D steps until the neutral position is brought within the normal range. Clinical experience currently indicates that the minimum positive lens to bring the neutral into the normal range should be prescribed as a reading addition, either in bifocal or single vision reading glasses form. Children with multiple challenges frequently benefit from single vision reading glasses as they may not comprehend the concept of using bifocals (see below for the populations commonly affected with reduced accommodation) and it limits their attention to the near task in hand.

Distance and near acuity for measurement of accommodation

If the same measure of acuity is used at distance and near (for example, single isolated letters), the same result should be obtained,

Fig. 5.11
Mean accommodative response with respect to accommodative demand for four age groups, measured with dynamic retinoscopy. The 95% confidence limits are given ($\pm 1.96 \times$ the standard deviation). The dashed line gives response equal to stimulus. (From Leat, S.J. and Gargon, J.L. (1996). Accommodative response in children and young adults using dynamic retinoscopy. *Ophthalmic and Physiological Optics,* **16**, 375–384. With kind permission of Elsevier Science Ltd.)

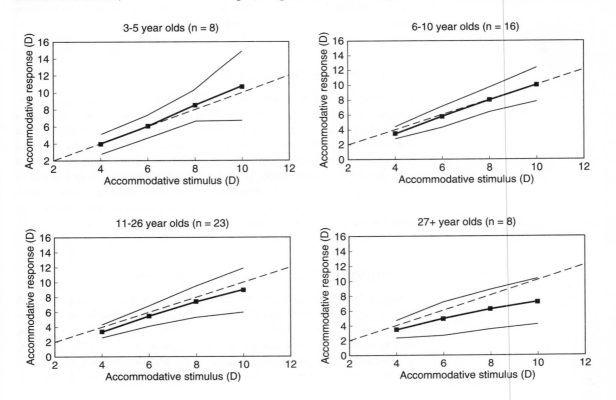

Table 5.1 Normal range of accommodative response. Position of neutral with dynamic retinoscopy

| Age | Accommodative response | |
	Target Distance = 25 cm (4D)	Target distance = 16.7 cm (6D)
3–5 years	19.6–35.7 cm (5.1–2.8D)	13.5–21.3 cm (7.4–4.7D)
6–10 years	23–37 cm (4.3–2.7D)	14–23.5 cm (7.1–4.3D)
11–26 years	23–40 cm (4.3–2.5D)	14.4–24 cm (6.95–4.15D)
27+ years	45.6–21.6 cm (4.6–2.2D)	14–39 cm (7–2.6D)

as the resolution of the eye is not distance dependent. Differing results indicate that the eye is not correctly focused (either the distance refractive correction is not correct or the accommodative response is not accurate). Thus by measuring the acuity using a test which is identical at distance and near (such as Snellen letters or illiterate Es, as appropriate for the child – see Chapter 7), we can determine if the eye is accommodating accurately (assuming the distance prescription is correct). Any deficit of near in comparison with distance acuity indicates insufficient accommodation. A reason for reduced accommodation should be sought or a reading addition determined (Chapter 12). It must be emphasized that the visual task must be the same at distance and near; using isolated letters at distance and lines of letters for near, or a Snellen chart at distance and continuous text at near, are NOT equivalent tests of acuity.

Eccentric photorefraction

Eccentric photorefraction can also be used for measuring accommodation in infants (Bobier, 1990), although at present this is a research rather than a clinical tool. Using this technique, the accommodative responses of infants 6 month and older with minimal refractive errors were found to be similar to adults, that is, a lag of accommodation over most of the range. Children with uncorrected high hyperopia (+3.5 D or greater in at least one meridian) show more variability of accommodative response both between individuals and for an individual person.

Accommodation in special populations

Using dynamic retinoscopy we have found that 50% of children with Down syndrome have significantly reduced accommodation (4 D or less) and 80% have some reduction of accommodation, being outside the normal range for their age (Woodhouse et al., 1993). These children must be considered for reading additions or their education, reading and attention span for near work will be compromised.

Reduction of accommodation may explain why some of these children will not gladly accept their full prescription for myopia.

Another group with a high frequency of reduced accommodation is children and young adults with cerebral palsy. Duckman (1984) comments that children with cerebral palsy almost demonstrate 'paralysis' of accommodation, being unable (subjectively) to make shifts of even 0.25 D. In fact, 100% of children with cerebral palsy were unable to 'clear' their vision through -2 D lenses. He suggests that accommodation can be trained by the use of accommodative facility flippers ($+2$ D lenses presented binocularly and alternated with -2 D lenses). Our data measuring accommodative response objectively with dynamic retinoscopy indicate that approximately 46% of children and pre-presbyopic adults with cerebral palsy have reduced accommodation for their age and 38% have less than 4 D of accommodation (Leat, 1996). They also frequently show a limited ability to maintain accommodation: they may accommodate accurately for a few seconds before accommodation relaxes and an obvious 'with' movement is seen with the retinoscope. These children will often benefit from a near reading addition. This may be confirmed either by a loaned pair of glasses of the approximate prescription, by subjective questioning (some children may be able to indicate a clear preference for the reading lenses) or by dynamic retinoscopy itself (see above).

Lindstedt (1986) found reduced near acuity compared with distance acuity in a group of children with low vision. Near acuity was frequently a factor of two to three worse than distance acuity even in children with only a moderate visual impairment (6/9–6/18). We have also found that that children with albinism may have reduced accommodation. Figure 5.12 shows some examples of the accommodative response in albinism and it can be seen that many have virtually no accommodation while the response of others gives an abnormal slope to the accommodative response curve. Ong, Cuiffreda and Tannen (1993) found similar variability of results in people with both ideopathic nystagmus and albinism.

A number of factors may lead to reduced accommodative accuracy in children with low vision. The accuracy of accommodation has been shown to be affected by the spatial frequency content of the image, low frequencies being used as a coarse guide for accommodation and the high frequencies for fine tuning (Cuiffreda, 1991). Therefore, we may expect those with low vision for whom the high frequencies are not detected to have decreased accuracy of accommodation. Indeed, if visual acuity is artificially reduced, accommodative response is rendered progressively less accurate. On the other hand, accommodation seems to be relatively robust to changes in the contrast of the image (being essentially unaffected until contrast drops from 63 to 2.6%). Retinal eccentricity also affects the accommodative response, which is thought to be driven by the cones. As a target is positioned more eccentrically (e.g. out to 10–15 degrees) the accommodative

Fig. 5.12
Accommodative response for four
people with albinism (solid
circles), superimposed on the
normal response and 95%
confidence limits for their age. (a)
Subject aged 9; (b) Subject aged 8;
(c) Subject aged 17; (d) Subject
aged 6.

response decreases; this is also relevant to people with low vision who
use eccentric fixation. During retinal image motion the accommodative response slips towards the tonic position and this has obvious
relevance for children with nystagmus. Many of the cues to the
required direction of an accommodative shift (described earlier) may
be abnormal, absent or go undetected in an eye with low vision.

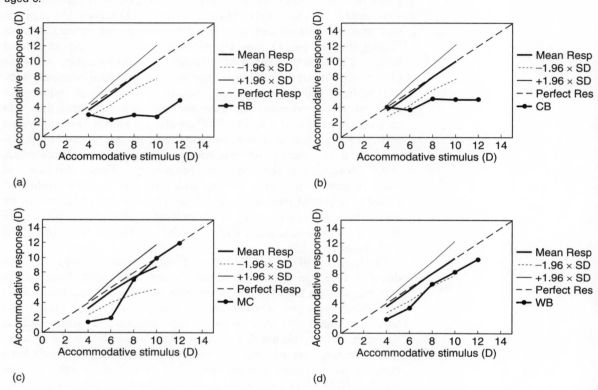

(a)   (b)

(c)   (d)

In amblyopia, subjective measures of accommodation are higher
than objective measures. Hokoda and Cuiffreda (1982) found that
objective measures of accommodation using dynamic retinoscopy
were lower in the amblyopic than the dominant eye while subjective
amplitudes using the conventional 'push-up' technique were higher.
Detection of defocus during the subjective measurement is rendered
less specific due to lower visual acuity and perceptual fading of the
target together with eccentric fixation. Accommodation is also less
well sustained in the amblyopic eye (Hokoda and Cuiffreda, 1982).
An objective technique therefore gives the better estimate. Interestingly, when the accommodation is driven consensually (i.e. stimulus
to dominant eye while objectively measuring accommodation in the
amblyopic eye) the amplitude in the amblyopic eye is approximately
equal to that in the dominant eye. This indicates that the lower
accommodation in the amblyopic eye is the result of the poorer
afferent rather than efferent pathways; that is, poorer acuity gives rise
to poorer stimulus for accurate accommodation.

CONCLUSION

In refracting infants and children, it is important to appreciate the changes in refractive error that occur with age and to be aware of errors which are indicative of a risk of amblyopia. In this chapter we have presented a summary of the available evidence. We have also described and evaluated various objective techniques for refracting infants and young children, concluding that in most routine examinations reliable results can be obtained using the Mohindra technique or distance fixation, although cycloplegia is indicated under some circumstances. Autorefraction and photorefraction have limited value, while subjective techniques are possible with older children. Although accommodation is not traditionally assessed in children, we believe that it is of importance, especially in children with special needs, and we have described some techniques which may be used.

REFERENCES

Abrahamson, M., Fabian, G., Anderson, A.K. and Sjostrand, J. (1990a). A longitudinal study of a population based sample of children. I Refraction and amblyopia. *Acta Ophthalmologica*, **68**, 428–434.

Abrahamson, M., Fabian, G., Andersson, A.K. and Sjostrand, J. (1990b). A longitudinal study of a population based sample of children. II The changeability of anisometropia. *Acta Ophthalmologica*, **68**, 435–440.

Abrahamson, M., Fabian, G. and Sjostrand, J. (1988). Changes in astigmatism between the years 1 and 4 years: a longitudinal study. *British Journal of Ophthalmology*, **72**, 145–149.

Almeder, L., Peck, L. and Howland, H. (1990). Prevalence of anisometropia in volunteer laboratory and school screening populations. *Investigative Ophthalmology & Vision Science*, **31**, 2448–2455.

Aslin, R.N., Shea, S.L. and Metz, H.S. (1990). Use of the Canon R-I autorefractor to measure refractive errors and accommodative responses in infants. *Clinical Vision Science*, **5**, 61–70.

Atkinson, J. (1993). Infant vision screening: Prediction and prevention of strabismus and amblyopia from refractive screening in the Cambridge photorefraction program. In K. Simons (ed.), *Early Visual Development, Normal and Abnormal*. New York/Oxford, Oxford University Press.

Atkinson, J. and Braddick, O.J. (1988). Infant precursors of later visual disorders: correlation or causality? *20th Symposium on Child Psychology*, **20**, 35–65.

Atkinson, J., Braddick, O.J. and French, J. (1980). Infant astigmatism: Its disappearance with age. *Vision Research*, **20**, 893–894.

Aurell, E. and Norrsell, K. (1990). A longitudinal study of children with a family history of strabismus: factors determining the incidence of strabismus. *British Journal of Ophthalmology*, **74**, 589–594.

Banks, M. (1980). Infant refraction and accommodation *Int. Ophthal. Clin.* **20**(1), 205–232.

Bennett, A.G. and Rabbetts, R.B. (1984). *Clinical Visual Optics*. London, Butterworths.

Birch, E.E., Swanson, W.H., Stager, D. et al. (1993). Outcome after very early treatment of dense congenital unilateral cataract. *Investigative Ophthalmology & Vision Science*, **34**, 3687–3699.

Bobier, W.R. (1990). Eccentric photorefraction: A method to measure accommodation of highly hypermetropic infants. *Clinical Vision Science*, **5**, 45–60.

Bobier, W.R. and Braddick, O.J. (1985). Eccentric photorefraction: optical analysis and empirical measures. *American Journal of Optometry & Physiological Optics*, **62**, 614–620.

Bobier, W.R., Schmitz, P., Strong, G. et al. (1992). Comparison of three photorefractive methods in a study of a developmentally handicapped population. *Clinical Vision Science*, **7**, 225–235.

Borghi, R.A. and Rouse, M.W. (1985). Comparison of refraction obtained by "near retinoscopy" and retinoscopy under cycloplegia. *American Journal of Optometry & Physiological Optics*, **62**, 169–172.

Braddick, O., Atkinson, J. and French, J. (1979). A photorefractive study of infant accommodation. *Vision Research*, **19**, 1319–1330.

Brookman, K.E. (1983). Ocular accommodation in human infants. *American Journal of Optometry & Physiological Optics*, **60**, 91–99.

Cuiffreda, K.J. (1991). Accommodation and its anomalies. In W.N. Charman (ed.), *Visual Optics and Instrumentation, Vision and Visual Dysfunction*. Boca Raton, CRC Press.

Cook, R.C. and Glasscock, R.E. (1951). Refractive and ocular findings in the newborn. *American Journal of Ophthalmology*, **34**, 1407–1413.

Curtin, B.J. (1985). *The Myopias; Basic Science and Clinical Management*. Philadelphia, Harper & Row.

Dobson, V., Fulton, A. and Sebris, S. (1984). Cycloplegic refraction of infants and young children: The axis of astigmatism. *Investigative Ophthalmology & Vision Science*, **25**, 83.

Dobson, V., Fulton, A., Manning, K. et al. (1981). Cycloplegic refractions of premature infants. *American Journal of Ophthalmology*, **91**, 490–495.

Doughty, M.J. and Lyle, W.M. (1992). Ocular pharmacogenetics. In Fatt, H.V., Griffin, J.R. and Lyle, W.M. (eds), *Genetics for Primary Eye Care Practitioners*. Boston, Butterworth-Heinemann.

Duckman, R. (1984). Accommodation in cerebral palsy, Function and remediation. *Journal of the American Optometric Association*, **55**, 281–283.

Edwards, M. (1991). The refractive status of Hong Kong Chinese infants. *Ophthalmic & Physiological Optics*, **11**, 297–303.

Erhlech, D.L. Atkinson, J., Braddick, O., Bobier, W. and Durden, K. (1995). Reduction of infant myopia: a longitudinal study. *Vision Research*, **35**, 1313–1324.

Fletcher, M.C. and Brandon, S. (1995). Myopia of prematurity. *American Journal of Ophthalmology*, **40**, 474.

Fulton, A.B., Dobson, V. and Salem, D. (1980). Cycloplegic refractions in infants and young children. *American Journal of Ophthalmology*, **90**, 239–247.

Goss, D.A. (1991). Childhood myopia. In T. Grosvenor and M.C. Flom (eds), *Refractive Anomalies*. Boston, Butterworth-Heinemann.

Gwiazda, J., Bauer, F., Thorn, F. and Held, R. (1986). Meridional amblyopia does result from astigmatism in early childhood. *Clinical Vision Science*, **1**, 145–152.

Gwiazda, J., Scheiman, M., Mohindra, I. and Held, R. (1984). Astigmatism in children: changes in axis and amount from birth to six years. *Investigative Ophthalmology & Vision Science*, **25**, 88–92.

Gwiazda, J., Thorn, F., Bauer, J. and Held, R. (1993). Emmetropization and the progression of manifest refraction in children followed from infancy to puberty. *Clinical Vision Science*, **8**, 337–344.

Griffin, J.R. (1982). *Binocular Anomalies: Procedures for Vision Therapy*. Chicago, Professional Press.

Haynes, H., White, B.L. and Held, R. (1965). Visual accommodation in human infants. *Science*, **148**, 528–530.

Hirsch, M.J. (1963). The refraction of children. In Hirsch, M.J. and Wicks, J.E. (eds), *Vision of Children*. Philadelphia, Chilton.

Hirsch, M.J. (1967). Anisometropia: A preliminary report of the Ojai longitudinal study. *American Journal of Optometry*, **44**, 581–585.

Hokoda, S.C. and Cuiffreda, K.J. (1982). Measurement of accommodative amplitude in amblyopia. *Ophthalmic & Physiological Optics*, **2**, 205–212.

Howland, H.C. (1983). Infant eyes. Optics and accommodation. *Current Eye Research*, **2**, 217.

Howland, H.C., Dobson, V. and Sayles, N. (1987). Accommodation in infants as measured by photorefraction. *Vision Research*, **19**, 1319–1330.

Howland, H.C, and Sayles, N. (1983). Photokeratometric and photorefractive measurements of astigmatism in infants and young children. *Vision Research*, **25**, 73.

Howland, H.C. and Sayles, N. (1984). Photorefractive measurements of astigmatism in infants and young children. *Investigative Ophthalmology & Vision Science*, **25**, 93.

Hung, L.F., Crawford, M.L.J. and Smith, E.L. (1995). Spectacle lenses alter eye growth and the refractive status of young monkeys. *Nature Medicine*, **1**, 761–765.

Ingram, R.M. and Barr, A. (1979). Changes in refraction between the ages of 1 and $3\frac{1}{2}$ years. *British Journal of Ophthalmology*, **63**, 339.

Ingram, R.M., Walker, C., Wilson, J.M. et al. (1986). Prediction of amblyopia and squint by means of refraction at age 1 year. *British Journal of Ophthalmology*, **69**, 851–853.

Irving, E.L., Sivak, J.G. and Callender, M.G. (1992). Refractive plasticity of the developing chick eye. *Ophthalmic & Physiological Optics*, **12**, 448–456.

Jones, L.W.J. and Hodes, D.T. (1991). Possible allergic reactions to cyclopentolate hydrochloride: case reports with literature review of uses and adverse reactions. *Ophthalmic & Physiological Optics*, **11**, 16–21.

Kragha, I.K.O.K. (1987). The distribution of refractive errors in Nigeria. *Ophthalmic & Physiological Optics*, 7, 241–244.

Leat, S.J. (1996). Reduced accommodation in children with cerebral palsy. *Ophthalmic and Physiological Optics*, **16**, 385–390.

Leat, S.J. and Gargon, J.L. (1996). Accommodative response in children and young adults using dynamic retinoscopy. *Ophthalmic & Physiological Optics*, **16**, 375–384.

Lewis, T.L., Maurer, D. and Brent, H.P. (1995). Development of grating acuity in children treated for unilateral or bilateral congenital cataract. *Investigative Ophthalmology & Vision Science*, **76**, 2080–2095.

Lindstedt E. (1986). Accommodation in the visually-impaired child. In G.C. Woo (ed.), *Low Vision: Principles and Applications*. New York, Springer-Verlag.

Lindstedt, E. (1983). Failing accommodation in cases of Down's syndrome. *Ophthal Paediatr Genet.*, *3*, 191.

Locke, L.C. and Somers, W. (1989). A comparison study of dynamic retinoscopy techniques. *Optometry and Vision Science*, **66**, 540–544.

Lovasic, J. (1986). Pharmacokinetics of topically applied cyclopentolate HCL and Torpicamide. *American Journal of Optometry & Physiological Optics*, **63**, 787–803.

McBrien, N.A. and Millodot, M. (1987). The relationship between tonic accommodation and refractive error. *Investigative Ophthalmology & Vision Science*, **28**, 997–1004.

Maddock, R.J., Millodot, M., Leat, S. and Johnson, C.A. (1981). Accommodative responses and refractive error. *Investigative Ophthalmology & Vision Science*, **20**, 387–391.

Maino, J.H., Cibis, G.W. and Cress, P. (1984). Non-cycloplegic vs. cycloplegic retinoscopy in pre-school children. *Annals of Ophthalmology*, **16**, 880–882.

Mohindra, I., Held, R., Gwiazda, J. and Brill, S. (1978). Astigmatism in infants. *Science*, **202**, 329–330.

Mohindra, I. and Molinari, J.F. (1979). Near retinoscopy and cycloplegic refraction in early primary grade schoolchildren. *American Journal of Optometry & Physiological Optics*, **56**, 34–38.

Moore, A. (1990). Refraction in infants and young children. In D. Taylor (ed.), *Pediatric Ophthalmology*. Boston/London, Blackwell Scientific Publications.

North, R.V. and Kelly, M.E. (1987). A review of the uses and adverse effects of topical administration of atropine. *Ophthalmic & Physiological Optics*, 7, 109–114.

Ong, E., Cuiffreda K.J. and Tannen, B. (1993). Static accommodation in congential nystagmus. *Investigative Ophthalmology & Vision Science*, **34**, 194–204.

Owens, D.A., Mohindra, I. and Held, R.H. (1986). The effectiveness of a retinoscope beam as an accommodation target. *Investigative Ophthalmology & Vision Science*, **19**, 942–949.

Pascal, J.I. (1952). *Selected Studies in Visual Optics*. St. Louis, C.V. Mosby.

Rosner, J. and Rosner, J. (1989). Relation between clinically measured tonic accommodation and refractive status in 6- to 14-year-old children. *Optometry and Vision Science*, **66**, 436–439.

Rousse, M.W., Hutter, R.F. & Shiftlett, R. (1984). A normative study of the accommodative lag in elementary school children. *American Journal of Optometry & Physiological Optics*, **61**, 693–697.

Saunders, K. and Westall, C. (1992). Comparison between near retinoscopy and cycloplegic retinoscopy in the refraction of infants and children. *Optometry and Vision Science*, **69**, 615–622.

Saunders, K., Woodhouse, J.M. and Westall, C.A. (1995). Emmetropisation in human infancy: Rate of change is related to initial refractive error. *Vision Research*, **35**, 1325–1328.

Schaeffel, F. (1993). Visually guided control of refractive error: results from animal models. In K. Simons (ed.), *Early Visual Development, Normal and Abnormal*. New York/Oxford, Oxford University Press.

Scharf, J., Zonis, S. and Zelter, M. (1975). Refraction in Israeli premature babies. *Journal of Pediature Ophthalmology* **12**, 193.

Sorsby, A., Benjamin, B., Davey, J.B. et al. (1957). *Emmetropia and its Aberrations*. London, Medical Research Council Special Report No. 293.

Wesemann, W. and Rassow, B. (1987). Automatic infrared refractors – A comparative study. *American Journal of Optometry & Physiological Optics*, **64**, 627–638.

Wesson, M.D., Mann, K.R. and Bray, N.W. (1990). A comparison of cycloplegic refraction to the near retinoscopy technique for refractive error determination. *Journal of the American Optometric Association*, **61**, 681–684.

Woodhouse, J.M., Meades, J.S., Leat, S.J. and Saunders, K.J. (1993). Reduced accommodation in children with Down syndrome. *Investigative Ophthalmology & Vision Science*, **34**, 2382–2387.

Young, F.A. and Leary, C.A. (1991). Refractive error in relation to the development of the eye. In W.N. Charman (ed.), *Visual Optics and Instrumentation*. Boca Raton/Ann Arbor/Boston, CRC Press.

Zonis, S. and Miller, B. (1974). Refraction in the Israeli newborn. *Journal of Pediatric Ophthalmology*, **2**, 77.

6

Psychophysical testing of infants and children

INTRODUCTION

The purpose of this chapter is to examine general issues concerning
the psychophysical testing of visual functions, especially the problems
of doing so when the testee is very young or has a disability. The
principles outlined here are relevant for the various behavioural
methods of assessing visual function described elsewhere in the book.
Many familiar vision tests, such as the Snellen letter chart, are
unsuitable for young children and those with disabilities. New tests
and techniques have been developed in recent years which widen the
range of individuals who can be tested and the nature of visual
functions which can be assessed, and there has been a steady flow of
new children's tests onto the market. We have given emphasis in this
chapter to the technique of preferential looking, which has been
especially influential in encouraging visual assessment at an early age.
Most acuity tests mentioned here are discussed further in the
following chapter.

SPECIAL CONSIDERATIONS IN TESTING CHILDREN

The most obvious reason why the familiar Snellen chart is unsuitable
for use with young children is the requirement to recognize and name
letters of the alphabet. Another problem is that each letter to be
identified is embedded within the whole chart, and it can be difficult
for a small child to attend to a stimulus within such a confusing
context. To overcome this, letter tests for children have been
developed in which the letters are presented one at a time (for
example, the Sheridan–Gardiner). However, this is itself a drawback
on occasions when it is important to discover whether a child's acuity
is reduced in context, a phenomenon known as crowding (e.g.
Atkinson and Braddick, 1982); for this reason the Cambridge test
includes not only individual letters but also cards where the target
letter is embedded in a row of other letters. Still another reason why
the Snellen chart is not suitable for young children is that it has been

devised for use at a distance (6 m) that is too far away to enable a young child's attention to be maintained (Sheridan, 1976). Furthermore, because many consulting rooms are not 6 m long the chart may be situated above the head but viewed through a mirror placed 3 m away (the letters on the chart are reversed so that they appear in the correct orientation when viewed in the mirror). While this is practical and straightforward for adults, the use of a mirror often confuses young children. Tests devised specially for use with children are designed to be used at a shorter viewing distance.

Although picture symbol charts and special letter-based tests maintain young children's interest, their design presents some technical difficulties and they depend upon the child having the ability to understand the instructions, to be willing to co-operate with the tester, to be able to give verbal answers (or, in some cases, to point at a target) and to maintain concentration. Even apparently simple tests require a range of cognitive abilities in relation to attention, learning, memory, symbolic understanding and communication, and perhaps understanding of concepts such as same/different (such as when the task requires a symbol to be matched with a sample) (Lindstedt, 1986). They will not be useful, therefore, if the child has limited cognitive abilities because of being very young or developmentally delayed (nor if the tester puts across the task in an unacceptable way).

One way of simplifying the task is to remove the symbolic component by making use of real objects such as the sweets (candies) hundreds and thousands (Bock, 1960) or balls and toys of various sizes (Sheridan, 1969, 1973), which can also help to maintain a child's interest. However, the acuity calculations are very rough and ready, measure a different type of visual acuity (Chapter 7) and the youngest infants cannot be tested by these methods. As we shall see later, preferential looking makes minimal demands on a child's cognitive and motor capacities, enabling even newborns to be assessed.

The emphasis of this chapter on measurement should not lead us to overlook the human context within which such measurement occurs. Good measurements are only possible if the tester is responsive to the child's needs. This was discussed in detail in Chapter 3, and a quote from Garbarino and Stott's (1989) book serves as a brief reminder here: 'In eliciting perceptual information from young children, it is important to use familiar materials and to structure tasks and situations that make human sense' (p. 50). A parent will be able to assist in choosing suitable tests, for example, by saying whether a child knows the letters of the alphabet (some children know lower-case letters, but not the upper-case letters typically used in vision tests). In the event that a child proves unable to cope with a task, it is important not to give any sense of failure, but to praise the child and say, 'Now let's try something else.' Similarly, once the end-point of a task has been reached, return to a target to which the child was able to respond correctly so that he or she experiences success on the final trial.

PSYCHOPHYSICAL TESTING

As the word suggests, psychophysics (at least as it was originally conceptualized in the mid-19th century) is concerned with the relationship between the mind and the physical world. Traditionally, researchers were concerned with trying to determine the nature of 'the psychophysical law'. This concerns the relationship between the magnitude of a stimulus and the sensory experiences to which it gives rise. For example, by how much must a light or a sound be increased for an observer to report that it is twice as bright/loud? Research efforts later expanded into investigating the neural correlates of sensation (Stevens, 1975).

One offshoot of traditional psychophysics has been the development of techniques for measuring visual abilities within a clinical context. Snellen acuity is just one example, but others include the measurement of visual fields, colour vision, stereopsis and sensitivity to contrast. Such tests measure the functioning of the visual system as a whole (i.e. optics, retina, and higher centres of the nervous system), and have the advantage of being non-invasive and permitting quantitative investigation of visual functions (Fitzke, 1988).

The early psychophysicists found that translating adults' visual sensations into something quantifiable was a challenging task and, until the preferential looking technique was developed, it was regarded as impossible for a clinician to know how well a baby could see. It is not easy to devise tasks that may be regarded as 'pure' tests of visual capacity given that factors such as memory, learning, attention and understanding may be involved. Bruce and Green (1989) have argued convincingly that almost everything we perceive visually involves the processing of information from sources other than the incoming light. They maintain that most visual perception necessitates some element of higher, cognitive, processing, which involves internal 'representations' of the world.

Some of the complexities of perception were apparent from the earliest psychophysical studies, which set out to try and measure the limits of sensory abilities. The notion of a 'threshold' was introduced by Herbart in 1824, and indicates the point at which a faint stimulus becomes detectable (absolute threshold) or the point at which two similar stimuli become just noticeably different from one another (discrimination threshold). Studies soon demonstrated that even a so-called absolute threshold is not, in reality, a fixed point. An observer responds to presented stimuli with some variability, influenced by factors such as external distractors, anxiety, boredom and a wish to please the experimenter, as well as by random fluctuations in nervous system activity, or 'noise'. This variability means that thresholds have to be estimated through multiple stimulus presentations and probability estimates: for example, a particular stimulus may be detected by the observer on, say, 50% or 75% of occasions, and conventions are established by which a particular level of response probability is taken as the threshold estimate.

Assessment of visual function frequently involves the estimation of thresholds, with acuity being a prime example. Various methods of estimating acuity have been developed over the years, all based, in essence, on the task of discriminating a black stimulus from a white background (Coren, Porac and Ward, 1979). The need to present multiple stimuli may be dealt with in a number of different ways. In some instances (as with the Snellen chart) all the stimuli (in this case, letters of various sizes) are presented at once and the observer has to respond to each in turn. In other tests, single stimuli are presented successively and repeatedly, either in steadily increasing or decreasing order, or randomly: towards the end of the 19th century Kraepelin devised the 'method of limits', whereby stimulus intensity is increased and decreased on alternate trials to determine the point at which the observer respectively begins to detect and can no longer detect the stimulus. An alternative to the traditional method of limits is the 'staircase method', in which the stimulus value is decreased until responding ceases, then increased until the response recurs. Further reversals are made, so that the stimuli presented are in the region of the threshold value; this is clinically valuable, especially with infants, as it reduces the number of presentations, and therefore the time, needed. Another method for estimating threshold is to use 'bracketing' – establishing the upper and lower boundaries of a bracket within which the endpoint lies and gradually reducing its size until the viewer can no longer make a choice, the middle of this bracket being taken as the threshold value.

It is important to note that vision test results depend very much upon the precise nature of the task. For example, acuity may be measured by assessing whether the person can detect the presence of a stimulus, as in the Catford Drum test (Catford and Oliver, 1971) or the STYCAR rolling balls test (Sheridan, 1973). Such tests yield a higher acuity level in comparison with tests which require the person to recognize a stimulus, such as a particular letter on a Snellen chart (this is termed the detection-recognition hierarchy). In recognition tasks, task difficulty is dependent on the number of alternative responses from which the observer has to choose (Coren et al., 1979). On a Snellen chart, therefore, although not all letters of the alphabet are used, a testee is unlikely to know this and therefore decides which of 26 alternatives is being presented. With so many alternatives, guessing is not really a problem, and a single reading of the chart is all that is needed to establish the acuity level. If, however, the test is one with fewer alternatives (such as the Tumbling E, which has four alternatives), then more presentations are needed to eliminate the effect of chance responding.

Yet another form of acuity is resolution acuity, measured using black and white stripes, or gratings (the notation used for these was explained in Chapter 1). It forms the basis of what is perhaps the most important infant visual assessment method, preferential looking, which is discussed below. Since vision test results are so dependent upon the exact method used, it is vital that appropriate norms are used. For example, it must be realized that infant (resolution) acuity is not interchangeable with adult (recognition) acuity, and that acuity obtained using psychophysical methods will be different from that using electrophysiological techniques.

Teller (1981) noted a number of necessary features for a psychophysical test to be of value in a clinical setting. First, efficiency is necessary: given that infants have a shorter attention span than adults, the prolonged testing required by standard psychophysical procedures is unsuitable and in need of streamlining. It was with this in mind that staircase procedures were developed, limiting the number of presentations needed. The test should also be valid. For example, it should be demonstrable that infants with reduced acuity due to binocular cataracts will fail the acuity screening. What Teller refers to as 'on-line utility' is also needed; the test results must be of value to the client, perhaps by suggesting treatment options or by promoting parental acceptance of diagnoses. We should also add to this that the test should be reliable, that is, it should give similar results when used by different testers and/or on different occasions.

PREFERENTIAL LOOKING

In 1981, Teller noted 'a tendency to imagine that psychophysical testing of organisms as irresponsible and impulsive as human infants must be impossible'. At the time she wrote this, psychophysical studies of infant vision were only about five years old.

These studies owed their existence to the pioneering work of Fantz (1958), who originated the preferential looking technique. Fantz noted that infants prefer to look at a patterned surface rather than a plain one. Fantz originally used visual targets such as schematic faces, scrambled faces and bullseyes but, for the purposes of assessing visual acuity, gratings are used, presented on cards or sometimes, in laboratory experiments, by computer. An infant will visually fixate a striped target in preference to a plain grey one of equal luminance presented simultaneously. If, however, the stripes are decreased in width, there comes a point at which the infant's visual system reaches the limit of its ability to differentiate, or resolve, the stripes (an adult reaching this threshold will report that both targets appear plain grey). This point is considered to have been reached when the infant shows no preference for one target over the other.

Clinically, the usual way of determining preference is to present stripes of a given width several times, the side of presentation being varied randomly. An adult observer who cannot see which side the stripes are on makes a judgement about this by observing the infant's eye movements. If the observer performs better than chance, it is assumed that the infant can resolve the stripes. A 75% correct value is used to derive the acuity level. Care must be taken to ensure that the child has been given sufficient time to respond: the younger the child, the slower the response, so that the examiner may need to wait several seconds for a tiny infant's eyes to move.

Norms have been established by testing infants of different ages with presumably normal vision, so that an individual infant's acuity can be compared with such norms to determine whether acuity is in the expected range for their age. Heersema and van Hof-van Duin (1990) have noted consistency of results across various laboratories, with the most rapid development of acuity occurring over the first 6 months. As measured by behavioural methods, infant acuity continues to improve over several years, the age at which adult values are reached depending on the exact stimuli and methods used (McDonald, 1986). It is important that norms are selected appropriately (Heersema and van Hof-van Duin, 1990), i.e. one should not apply norms from one test to a different test.

The original procedure devised for testing acuity in the way described above forces the observer to choose on each trial which target the infant is fixating, so the method is sometimes referred to as forced-choice preferential looking, or FPL. As originally devised, the method has limitations. FPL has been found to be most successful with infants aged 6 months and under; older infants and toddlers become bored and restless (e.g. Atkinson and Braddick, 1982). However, modifications have been found to expand the age range (Chapter 7). McDonald et al. (1985, 1986) developed the quick and simple 'acuity card procedure', for use with infants up to 36 months of age, while Heersema and van Hof-van Duin (1990) developed modifications which permitted the acuity cards to be used up to the age of 4 years. Another variation, which was also incorporated into McDonald's acuity card procedure when used with older infants, is operant preferential looking or OPL (e.g. Mayer and Dobson, 1980). Here, the infant receives a reward, or reinforcement, for responding appropriately to the task. Simple social reinforcement may be sufficient, such as saying 'Good', 'Well done' 'That's right', and smiling and nodding, or applause, toys, glove puppets or even a small piece of food (with parental permission) may be used. They found this method extended the usefulness of preferential looking up to 3 years of age.

Another way of increasing infants' attention to testing is to use a screen to mask all other objects in the room, thus reducing distractions. A screen may be supplied with the test or made by any handyperson. It may be free-standing or table-mounted and should be painted matt grey, as close as possible to the shade of the test cards. These are presented through an opening in the screen, as are any puppets used as reinforcement (hence the description of this arrangement in the Cardiff clinic as the 'Punch and Judy' or in Waterloo as the puppet show).

Although preferential looking has been mainly used for measuring acuity, the technique is also applicable to other visual functions, including contrast sensitivity, colour vision and stereopsis. Clinically appropriate tests, as well as those suitable mainly for experimental purposes, continue to be developed.

PSYCHOPHYSICS WITH PRESCHOOLERS

We have already seen that it is possible to modify preferential looking procedures in such a way as to extend acuity testing up to the age of 4 years. However, preschoolers also become increasingly capable of undertaking some of the other types of task referred to earlier, such as matching or naming letters or pictures. In fact, for children who are capable of such tests, preferential looking may be inappropriate, giving a lower acuity assessment because the task is boring for them (Shute et al., 1990). However, it is important to ensure that any alternative task selected is not too difficult for the child.

Hill (1984) attempted to classify tasks according to their difficulty for children, ranging from simple detection tasks through to those involving problem-solving. Overall, his review demonstrated that even though a test may have been specially designed for use with children that in itself is not evidence that it is suitable for its intended purpose. For example, if a test is intended as a screening device, yet many children have difficulty with the nature of the task, then the test will produce many false positives (children who fail the test, but in fact have normal vision).

In selecting a test to use with a young child, it is important to have adequate information about procedures, success rates with the age group in question and established norms. In reviewing acuity tests for preschoolers Fern and Manny (1986) noted that available tests often fall short on such issues: criteria for determining acuity, such as number of presentations needed and the percentage of correct responses used to establish threshold, differ among authors and are often not stated at all. These authors note a couple of points made earlier in this chapter, that measured acuity is affected by whether symbols are presented singly or in an array, and that testability is affected by distances. In addition, there is a ceiling effect in some tests, where the best possible score is below adult levels.

A common way of attempting to produce tests which will be interesting for a small child, but which do not assume a knowledge of letters, has been to use picture symbols, and these have now been devised for assessing a wide range of visual functions. Their design presents technical problems, however, and performance will be influenced by the abstractness of the figures, the child's familiarity with the object depicted, verbal ability and cultural changes over time (Fern and Manny, 1986).

In assessing acuity charts for children, Blakey (1988) concluded that those tests which are based on a matching task seem to be usable over the widest age range. Tests such as the Sheridan–Gardiner (which uses letters) and Ffooks symbols (which consist of outline shapes such as squares) have the advantage that results can be related to the established standard of Snellen acuity. Blakey also makes a point which may seem obvious, but which is all too easily overlooked: if a test is being repeated (for example, so that monocular acuities can be assessed) care must be taken that the chart has not been remembered from the first occasion (charts should not be left on show and, preferably, there should be alternative versions).

Although they are not yet widely used outside the research context, electronic methods are potentially of benefit in psychophysical testing in children. In the mid-1980s, Abramov et al. (1984) responded to the fact that the growing body of data on infant vision was not being matched by progress in measuring the sensory capacities of preschool and early school age children. They developed methods designed to overcome the repetitive, boring nature of adult psychophysical tests by disguising the procedures as electronic space games. The young 'space cadets' had to identify and shoot down such things as 'dangerous cloud bands' (with appropriate sound effects) in return for (fictitious) scores, space stamps and space rations. A forced-choice paradigm was used, whereby the child was forced to choose between two alternative screens (as in the case of preferential looking with infants). To avoid frustration near threshold when discrimination becomes difficult, the method of descending limits was used, whereby the stimulus was presented well above threshold and reduced until an error was made; this was repeated several times and the mean taken to calculate the threshold.

By maintaining the children's attention with this attractive format it proved possible to measure several aspects of visual function, under both normal and dark-adapted conditions, something that would be impossible with normal testing methods. The method proved reliable, in that re-testing weeks or months later gave similar results. In all tests, the children proved to be less sensitive than adults, and the authors believed this was primarily due to non-visual factors, particularly performance near threshold, when the children tended to adopt a guessing strategy. It is noteworthy here that adults' contrast sensitivity functions can be apparently reduced to that of children if they are instructed to pay less attention to the task (Bradley and Freeman, 1982). This demonstrates both the importance of using age-matched norms and of carrying out tests in accordance with standardized procedures.

CHILDREN WITH SPECIAL NEEDS

In this chapter so far, we have discussed some basic psychophysical principles and seen how procedures used for assessing adult vision may be unsuitable for use with children. There may be additional considerations if the child has a disability.

First, it is important to be aware of any communication problems the child may have and to adapt accordingly. In Chapter 1, ways of communicating with children with hearing impairments in particular were discussed. Some children with disabilities may use a communication board, or sign language, or they may be able to indicate yes and no nonverbally. It is essential to have any necessary information and assistance from carers in this respect, so that it can be ensured that the child understands test instructions.

Some children with an intellectual impairment may be quite capable of understanding what is happening during vision testing if simple explanations are given, and be able to co-operate with normal procedures. Some are perfectly able to respond to a Snellen chart or to children's tests such as the Sheridan–Gardiner.

If understanding seems to be a problem, or if a child's disabilities prevent verbal or pointing responses, acuity cards provide a useful alternative. Duckman and Selenow (1983) examined the proposition that FPL would remain suitable at a later age than usual for children who are developmentally delayed, and obtained clear preferential looking responses in 11 of 12 children tested, aged between 6 months and $3\frac{1}{2}$ years.

Hertz (1987) tested children with Down syndrome with acuity cards and obtained results which seemed to be valid, in that they compared well with those obtained using a children's picture chart. The majority of children responded well, by speech, gesture or fixation, but they became frustrated near threshold, and a third alternative response, that there were 'no stripes', had to be given to them to solve this. The number of presentations also had to be kept to a minimum.

Hertz (1987) also used the acuity cards to test intellectually impaired children with cerebral palsy, but obtained rather unreliable results. She noted that carers report that these children appear to see better on some days than others, so the variability noted on different occasions may have represented genuine fluctuations. In another report, Hertz (1988) examined children with intellectual impairment, and found reliable measurements in those with acuity better than 2/60. Successful use of acuity cards with children with cerebral palsy was reported by Hertz and Rosenberg (1988); although the most severely affected children had greater test-retest variabilities, the majority showed an acceptable agreement.

Our experience is in accordance with that of other workers, who have noted the short attention span of those with intellectual impairments. The Cardiff Acuity Test (Chapter 7), a preferential-looking type of test which uses pictures rather than stripes, has been developed with the aim of improving attention to testing. Motivation may also sometimes be increased by supplying small quantities of food (with a carer's permission), meted out in small quantities contingent on correct responding, for example, one potato crisp per correct response. Protecting costly equipment such as acuity cards from sticky fingers is also advisable; presenting them behind perspex sheets is suitable, provided care is taken to avoid reflections from room lights.

Oculomotor problems can cause difficulty with acuity card testing if a child has severe and multiple impairments: if strabismus is present, or there is difficulty in controlling eye movements, it is not always easy to determine where the child is looking. A simple arrangement of two light bulbs spaced about 15 inches apart, which can be switched on and off alternately (known as the 'Leat lights' after one of the present authors, who devised them) is helpful. This simple arrangement enables the tester to determine whether the child can reliably move the eyes from one target to another, and to determine any idiosyncracy which the child has; for example, some require a considerable time, perhaps as long as 10 seconds, to change fixation. The knowledge gained from this procedure can then be applied to the acuity cards.

Another method is the 'en face' method for children who cannot make right and/or left eye movements (Rodier, Raye and Mayer, 1993). The card is presented so that first one then the other side is directly ahead of the child. The observer is naive regarding the position of the stripes and watches for evidence of more visual attention or preference when one side of the card is presented than when the other side is presented, e.g. more staring or eye widening, or stopping fidgeting or sucking.

Shentall and Hosking (1986) found that some children with disabilities respond less well to symbolic picture charts than to non-symbolic tests (such as being able to see 'hundreds of thousands', indicating an acuity of at least 6/60). Similarly, the present authors once saw a boy with multiple impairments who would not attend to any test, including the acuity cards, but paced around the room; he was tested by rolling the STYCAR balls along the floor and estimating acuity using the distance of his eyes from the carpet which, fortunately, provided good contrast. Sometimes, rough and ready calculations such as these are all that is possible: they may be somewhat lacking in reliability and validity, but are often better than gaining no information at all. In this case it was at least established that the boy responded to moving stimuli of a certain size.

It is especially important to maintain a game-like quality to the testing, and the value of this even for children without disabilities was shown by the 'space psychophysics' example given earlier. A game format is also used in a combined test of acuity and visual form perception for use with children with visual and/or intellectual impairments developed by Lindstedt (1986). The test consists of a set of playing cards, the BUST-LH cards, which display symbols of different sizes. The tester can use the cards flexibly, playing games with the child, to gain an indication of functional acuity.

In some cases, if equipment is available, electrophysiological techniques may useful. For example, Orel-Bixler and associates (1989), in measuring the vision of multiply-challenged clients, were able to measure acuities in 95% of cases using a spatial frequency sweep VEP technique in comparison with 70% using acuity cards. Similarly, Saunders, McCulloch and Kerr (1995) found that they were unable to use preferential looking successfully with girls with Rett syndrome, but they were able to use VEPs with checkerboard targets, establishing acuities of at least 24 seconds of arc in all the girls.

CONCLUSION

In this chapter we have outlined the special considerations which apply when using psychophysical procedures with infants and young children. Factors of importance include choosing a valid and reliable test (with appropriate norms) which is within the child's capabilities and interesting enough to maintain attention; it should also have clinical utility. Emphasis has been given to the method of preferential looking, used initially for acuity measurement but being increasingly applied to other visual functions. It has been enormously valuable in facilitating the early visual assessment of infants, toddlers and children with disabilities and is an indispensable tool for today's child vision care practitioner.

REFERENCES

Abramov, I., Hainline, L., Turkel, J. et al. S. (1984). Rocket-ship psychophysics. Assessing visual functioning in young children. *Investigative Ophthalmology and Vision Science*, **25**, 1307–1315.

Atkinson, J. and Braddick, O. (1982). Assessment of visual acuity in infancy and early childhood. *Acta Ophthalmologica (Copenh)* Suppl 157, 18–26.

Blakey, J. (1988). A review of children's test charts. *Optician, June 24*, 17–25.

Bock, R.H. (1960). Amblyopia detection in the practice of pediatrics. *Archives of Pediatrics* 77, 335–339.

Bradley, A. and Freeman, R.D. (1982). Contrast sensitivity in children. *Vision Research*, **22**, 953.

Bruce, V. and Green, P. (1989). *Visual Perception: Physiology, Psychology and Ecology*. Hove, Lawrence Erlbaum.

Catford, G.V. and Oliver, A. (1971). A method of visual acuity detection. In *Proceedings of Second International Orthoptics Congress*. Amsterdam: Excerpta Medica, pp. 183–187.

Coren, S., Porac, C. and Ward, L.M. (1979). *Sensation and Perception*. New York, Academic Press.

Duckman, R.H. and Selenow, A. (1983). Use of forced preferential looking for measurement of visual acuity in a population of neurologically impaired children. *American Journal of Optometry and Physiological Optics*, **60**, 817–821.

Fantz, R.L. (1958). Pattern vision in young infants. *Psychological Records*, **8**, 43–47.

Fern, K.D. and Manny, R.E. (1986). Visual acuity of the preschool child: A review. *American Journal of Optometry and Physiological Optics*, **63**, 5, 319–345.

Fitzke, F.W. (1988). Clinical psychophysics. *Eye*, **2**, Suppl S223–S241.

Garbarino, J., Stott, F.M. and Faculty of the Erikson Institute (1989). *What children can tell us*. San Francisco, Jossey Bass.

Heersema, D.J. and van Hof-van Duin, J. (1990). Age norms for visual acuity in toddlers using the acuity card procedure. *Clinical Vision Science*, **5**, 2, 167–174.

Hertz, B.G. (1987). Acuity card testing of retarded children. *Behav, Brain Res.*, **24**, 85–92.

Hertz, B.G. (1988). Use of the acuity card method to test retarded children in special schools. *Child: Care, Health Dev* 14, 189–198.

Hertz, B.G. and Rosenberg, J. (1988). Acuity card testing of spastic children: preliminary results. *Journal of Pediatric Ophthalmology and Strabismus*, **25**, 139–144.

Hill, A.R. (1984). Defective colour vision in children. In A. Macfarlane (ed.), *Progress in Child Health, vol.1*. Edinburgh, Churchill Livingstone.

Lindstedt, E. (1986). Early vision assessment in visually impaired children at the TRC, Sweden. *British Journal of Visual Impairment*, **IV**, 49–51.

Mayer, D.L and Dobson, V. (1980). Assessment of vision in young children: A new operant approach yields estimates of acuity. *Investigative Ophthalmology and Vision Science*, **19**, 566–570.

McDonald, M.A. (1986). Assessment of visual acuity in toddlers. *Survey of Ophthalmology*, **31**, 3, 189–210.

McDonald, M., Ankrum, C., Preston, K. et al. (1986). Monocular and binocular acuity estimation in 18- to 36-month-olds: Acuity Card Results. *American Journal of Optometry and Physiological Optics*, **63**, 3, 181–186.

McDonald, M.A., Dobson, V., Sebris, S.L. et al. (1985). The acuity card procedure: A rapid test of infant acuity. *Investigative Ophthalmology and Vision Science*, **26**, 1158–1162.

Orel-Bixler, D., Haegerstrom-Portnoy, G. and Hall, A. (1989). Visual assessment of the multiply handicapped patient. *Optometry and Vision Science*, **66**, 530–536.

Rodier, D., Raye, K. and Mayer, D. (1993). Unconventional acuity card testing: tester reliability and notable cases. *Investigative Ophthalmology and Visual Science*, **34**, S1422.

Saunders, K.J., McCulloch, D.L. and Kerr, A.M. (1995). Visual function in Rett syndrome. *Developmental Medicine and Child Neurology*, **37**, 496–504.

Shentall, G.A. and Hosking, G. (1986). A study of the visual defects detected in children with cerebral palsy and Down's syndrome. *British Orthoptic Journal*, **43**, 22–25.

Sheridan, M.D. (1969). Vision screening procedures for very young or handicapped children. In P. Gardiner, K. MacKeith and V. Smith (eds.), *Aspects of Developmental and Pediatric Ophthalmology. Clinics in Developmental Medicine No. 32*. London, Spastics International Medical Publications.

Sheridan, M.D. (1973). The STYCAR graded balls vision test. *Developmental Medicine and Child Neurology*, **15**, 423–432.

Sheridan, M.D. (1976). *Manual for Stycar Vision Tests*. Slough, National Foundation for Educational Research.

Shute. R., Candy, R., Westall, C. and Woodhouse, J.M. (1990). Success rates in testing monocular acuity and stereopsis in infants and young children. *Ophthalmic and Physiological Optics*, **10**, 133–136.

Stevens, S.S. (1975). *Psychophysics. Introduction to its Perceptual, Neural, and Social Prospects*. New York, Wiley.

Teller, D.Y. (1981). Infant psychophysics: the laboratory and the clinic. In L.M. Proenza, J.M. Enoch and A. Jampolsky (eds), *Clinical Applications of Visual Psychophysics*, Cambridge, Cambridge University Press, pp. 111–120.

7

Visual acuity

Kathryn Saunders

INTRODUCTION

As indicated in previous chapters, visual acuity (VA) refers to the spatial limit of visual discrimination: it is a description of the finest detail (or smallest object) which a person can perceive. It is measured in high levels of illumination and at high contrast and although it reflects only a small part of a person's visual performance it is traditionally the measure most widely used to describe the functional capability of the visual system. In this chapter the various types of visual acuity are defined and a range of acuity tests for children described. Age norms are also provided for several tests.

TYPES OF VISUAL ACUITY

Within the general definition of visual acuity, some obvious subdivisions can be recognized:

1. Detection (minimum visible): this refers to the smallest test object which can just be detected. Hecht and Mintz (1939) demonstrated that under ideal conditions a dark line of width just 0.5 second of arc could be detected.
2. Resolution (minimum resolvable): this refers to the smallest angular separation between neighbouring targets that can be resolved. Resolution acuity is usually in the region of 30 seconds to 1 minute of arc. This value is very close to that predicted by the optical limitations of the eye and the retinal photoreceptor spacing. Preferential looking tests (described below) provide a measure of resolution acuity.
3. Identification (minimum recognizable): this refers to the capacity to identify a form or its orientation and is the type of acuity measured by the Snellen acuity chart and letter/picture naming and matching tests. Recognition acuity differs from resolution acuity in several ways. The targets used to assess recognition acuity are more localized, threshold recognition stimuli are usually much smaller than resolution stimuli which may contain equally fine detail, but tend to cover a larger area. Recognition stimuli are affected by contour interaction from nearby stimuli whereas resolution stimuli are not. Contour interaction reveals the

'crowding' phenomenon, in which acuity thresholds increase when contour interaction is present. Typically the amblyopic eye's performance is reduced under such conditions, making recognition acuity the more sensitive measure in detecting amblyopia. Finally, resolution acuities are less degraded in the normal and pathologic peripheral retina than recognition acuities (Loshin and White, 1984). This results in strabismic amblyopes demonstrating falsely high acuities with resolution tests whose larger targets stimulate extra-foveal areas. It is clear that recognition acuities are more sensitive to pathological and physiological degradation than resolution acuities.

4. Hyperacuity (minimum discriminable): this refers to the ability to determine the differences between 2 stimuli, e.g. the presence of offsets. The visual system is capable of making much finer spatial discriminations than the minimum recognizable acuity. For example, relative position, size and orientation can be judged with an accuracy of 3–6 seconds of arc or better (Klein and Levi, 1985). Foveal inter-cone spacing is at best 30 seconds of arc and the smearing of a point of light caused by the optics of the eye spreads the image over several cones. Therefore, hyperacuity cannot be explained in terms of retinal or optical limitations and, whilst it is not fully understood, hyperacuity is believed to reflect cortical processing. Resolution acuity and hyperacuity demonstrate different developmental time-courses in infants, further suggesting that they reflect different underlying mechanisms (Shimojo and Held, 1987). Stereoacuity, which can have thresholds of a few seconds of arc, may also be considered a type of hyperacuity, but its processing probably differs somewhat from that in ordinary hyperacuity.

Because different types of acuity are unequally affected by pathology, the disparity between detection, resolution and recognition acuity increases with low vision and amblyopia. Children with low

Fig. 7.1
Different levels of visual acuity. (a) Detection task (minimally visible); (b) Resolution task (minimum visible); (c) Isolated identification task (minimum recognizable); (d) 'Crowded' identification task (minimum recognizable with horizontal contour interaction); (e) Hyperacuity task.

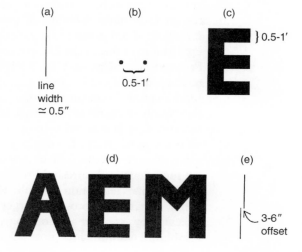

Table 7.1 Acuities achieved by grating and recognition acuity tasks for normal eyes and for amblyopes or those with macular problems (from Mayer, D.L., Fulton, A.B. and Rodier, D. (1984). Grating and recognition acuities of pediatric patients. *Ophthalmology*, **91**, 947. Reprinted with permission of Lippencott-Raven Publishers)

Grating acuity	Recognition acuity	
	Amblyopes and foveal or macular abnormalities	Normal eyes and other non-ocular visual abnormalities
6/15 (20/50)	6/30 (20/100)	6/21 (20/70)
6/30 (20/100)	6/120 (20/400)	6/45 (20/150)
6/60 (20/200)	6/420 (20/1400)	6/120 (20/400)
6/120 (20/400)	6/960 (20/3200)	6/240 (20/800)

vision may be noted to detect small specks on the floor or stars in the sky. Such a detection task is often less impaired by low vision than resolution or recognition tasks. Mayer, Fulton and Rodier (1984) describe acuities achieved by grating and recognition acuity tasks for normal eyes and for amblyopes or those with macular problems. Their data, adapted in Table 7.1, illustrate the increasing disparity between resolution and recognition measures with low vision.

SNELLEN ACUITY

Adult visual acuity is most often recorded in Snellen notation. This was explained earlier in the book, but a brief reminder is in order here. A Snellen acuity chart (named after its designer) consists of black letters on a white, brightly-lit background (some are internally illuminated). The letters decrease in size down the chart and the testee is asked to read the letters aloud, while the examiner records the lowest line that is accurately read. The usual testing distance is 6 m (20 ft), at which distance the eye's accommodation system is considered to be fully relaxed, so that the chart is considered a true 'distant' target. The chart is designed such that the width of the limbs making up each letter is 1/5th of the overall size of the letter. A normally-sighted adult would be expected to be able to discriminate the limbs and therefore identify the letter when the limbs subtend one minute of arc (see Figure 1.4). Each line of the chart is therefore described by the distance at which a normally-sighted observer could identify the size of letters on that line. The topmost letter on the chart is usually large enough that a normally-sighted observer could identify it at 60 m. A person able to identify only this letter on the chart when viewed at 6 m is said to have an acuity of 6/60. A person able to read letters that the normally-sighted observer could identify at 24 m would have an acuity of 6/24 and so on. Snellen acuity in a visually normal adult is usually regarded as at least 6/6 (1 minute of arc). As mentioned in the previous chapter, the required distance is often obtained through the use of a chart reflected in a mirror, which is sometimes problematic when working with children.

The traditional Snellen chart is the most commonly used form of acuity measure and is used with children by many clinicians, including some school nurses, with a home-made key card (see section below on Letter Matching Tasks). However, the Snellen chart has come under criticism for the following reasons. As can be seen in Figure 7.2a the number of letters on each line of the chart is unequal and the spacing between the letters on the lower lines is greater, making each line a different acuity task. In addition, the decrease in letter size from line to line is not uniform. These criticisms have been redressed in the Bailey–Lovie acuity chart (Figure 7.2b), which provides a more sensitive and repeatable measure of acuity (Lovie-Kitchin, 1988). It can be used at any distance and the values obtained directly compare with those at other distances, making it very useful for assessing those with low vision, who may be unable to recognize any of the letters at the usual 6 m distance.

THE BAILEY–LOVIE ACUITY CHART

The Bailey–Lovie acuity chart does not record acuity as a Snellen fraction, but uses logMAR notation (Bailey and Lovie, 1976). This notation describes acuity in terms of the logarithm of the minimum angle of resolution (MAR). An acuity of 6/60 is represented by 1.0 and 6/6 by 0.0. Acuities better than 6/6 have a negative value. Each line on the Bailey–Lovie chart represents a change in acuity by 0.1 logMAR and acuity doubles every third line. This system allows each letter to be valued individually as 0.02 logMAR such that acuity can be scored per letter rather than per line. The poorest acuity which can be recorded with this type of chart is 0.5/60 (with the chart at 0.5 m from the testee's eye), equivalent to 6/720.

Both the Snellen and Bailey–Lovie acuity charts rely on the literacy of the testee, requiring the detection, resolution and recognition of the letters and the relaying of this information to the examiner. Clearly neither test is suitable for infants, young children or those with neurological impairment who are unable to perform such a task. For this reason alternative acuity tests have been devised and are described below.

LETTER MATCHING TESTS

Letter matching tests relate most closely to the Snellen and Bailey–Lovie tests. They provide the child with a key card on which all the letters used in the test are reproduced. The key card is either held by the child or the parent and the child's task is to point to the letter on the key card which matches that shown at a fixed distance by the examiner. There are several versions of the letter matching test available, most of which have chosen letters which are symmetrical about their vertical axes (H, O, T, V, X, Y, A, U) in order to avoid right-left confusion and maintain approximately equal legibility between letters. Some of the most useful letter matching tests are described below.

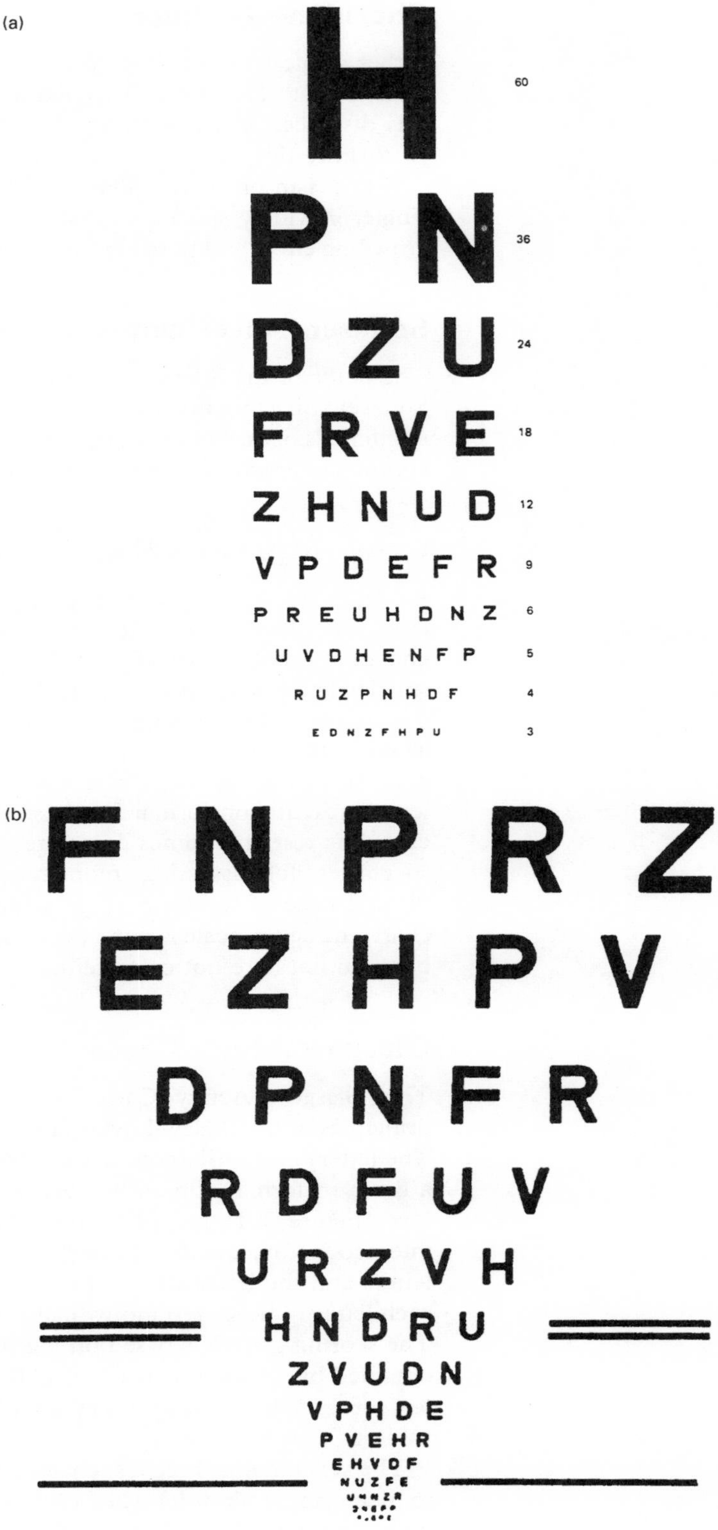

Fig. 7.2
(a) A complete Snellen letter acuity chart for use at 6 m. (b) A Bailey–Lovie letter acuity chart. (From Rabbetts, R.B. (1998). *Bennett and Rabbetts' Clinical Visual Optics*, 3rd edn. Oxford, Butterworth-Heinemann, pp. 28 and 30.)

(a)

H	60
P N	36
D Z U	24
F R V E	18
Z H N U D	12
V P D E F R	9
P R E U H D N Z	6
U V D H E N F P	5
R U Z P N H D F	4
E D N Z F H P U	3

(b)

F N P R Z
E Z H P V
D P N F R
R D F U V
U R Z V H
H N D R U
Z V U D N
V P H D E
P V E H R
E H V D F
N U Z F E
U H N Z R
P V H P V

Sheridan–Gardiner

Either single letter or linear presentations can be used, both in a flip card format. The test is designed for use at 6 m. Rather than using this distance, or achieving it with a mirror, it may be preferable to perform testing at 3 m and convert the acuities obtained.

A criticism of the Sheridan–Gardiner test is that it presents either single or widely spaced letters, thus not allowing evaluation of the crowding effect and possibly over-estimating acuity in amblyopic eyes.

Sonksen–Silver acuity system

The faults of the Sheridan–Gardiner test have been addressed in the Sonksen–Silver acuity test. The letters are presented in a row, spaced at intervals of one letter width. This spacing allows the introduction of contour interaction, although only in the horizontal direction.

Cambridge Crowding Cards

As its name suggests, the Cambridge test also introduces the crowding phenomenon. It improves on the Sonksen–Silver test by containing both vertical and horizontal contour interaction and smaller letter spacing of one half letter width. The child's task is to match the central letter with the identical one on the key card. To avoid confusion the letters surrounding the central letter are not present on the key card. The Cambridge test also contains a single letter presentation format for those children too young to perform a crowding test and comes complete with brightly coloured occluding spectacles for assessing monocular acuities (Figure. 7.3). One disadvantage of the Cambridge acuity cards is that, like the Snellen chart, the acuity scale is not a log scale such that the changes in acuity between lines are not consistent.

Glasgow Acuity Cards

The Glasgow Acuity Cards (GAC) were devised to reflect the principles of the Bailey–Lovie acuity test (McGraw and Winn, 1993). The letters in the Glasgow test are designed for presentation at 3 m in a flip card format. On each page, four letters are contained within a box (Figure 7.4) providing both horizontal and vertical contour interaction for each letter. Each line contains the same number of letters and the letter size decreases in a logarithmic fashion allowing each letter to be scored individually. Every letter has a score of 0.025. The scoring system is based on logMAR, although the GAC score is obtained by subtracting the logMAR score from unity. Therefore the test scores 6/6 as 1.0, 6/60 as 0.0 and acuities below 6/60 as negative values.

The set contains three test charts in order that children are not able to memorize letter order when testing monocular acuities or on repeat visits. An additional feature of the Glasgow Acuity Cards is the

Fig. 7.3
(a) The Cambridge Crowding Cards can be used either in single letter or crowded presentation form and the child matches the test letter to the identical one on their key card. (b) The Cambridge Crowding Cards require the child to match the test letter to the appropriate one on the key card. Occluding spectacles are useful for obtaining monocular acuity estimates.

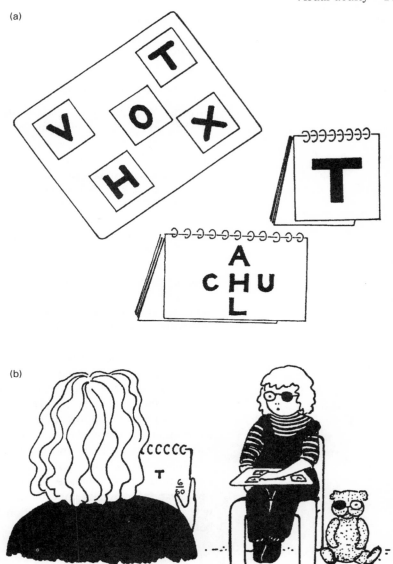

(a)

(b)

Fig. 7.4
The Glasgow Acuity Cards present four letters at each size surrounded by a box to maintain vertical and horizontal contour interaction.

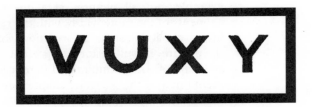

provision of a time saving screening sequence at the start of each test which allows testing proper to commence close to the acuity threshold.

The letter matching procedure

In order to gain useful results with either single or multiple letter presentation in the above tests the child must first be shown what is expected of him or her. The examiner should hand the key card to the child and initially stand close to the child and indicate the letter on the test chart. The child should be instructed to show the examiner a letter on their key card which is the same as the one the examiner is pointing to. The parent may need to help the child with the first response, but testing at 3 or 6 m should not continue until the examiner is confident that the child is able to correctly match letters and understands what is required. All correct responses should be praised to encourage the child to continue with testing and maintain co-operation. Testing at 3 or 6 m should commence with a large letter and the size should be decreased until the letters are no longer correctly matched. Once this point has been reached the examiner should increase the letter size again to ensure that correct responses are once more achieved. It is important to know whether failure to match is due to lack of interest or acuity limitations. Once a binocular acuity is achieved, monocular measures can be made. Slightly more encouragement for co-operation may be needed during monocular acuity measurement as occlusion can be distracting. An occluding sticky patch is useful for infants but not ideal for toddlers and older children. Occluding glasses, converted from children's sunglasses, can encourage toddlers and older children to participate.

Whilst it is preferable to assess crowded letter acuity, the presence of multiple letters increases the complexity of the task. Single letter presentation matching may be attempted from 2–2.5 years of age, whereas multiple letter presentation tests are not normally successful before 3 years of age.

PICTURE NAMING AND MATCHING

Some acuity tests designed for younger children use pictures or familiar shapes as targets rather than letters. While early versions of these tests failed to conform to standard Snellen principles recent tests are more satisfactory, although a problem still remains with these charts because recognition is not uniform for all pictures. For example, not all pictures at a given acuity level are made up of elements of the same width, with the result that some pictures contain lower spatial frequency information which could be utilized to identify the picture. Despite efforts to present objects drawn in a standardized style and of equal familiarity differences remain (Osterberg, 1936). As mentioned in the previous chapter, cultural differences also exist. In addition, as with single letter optotype tests, many picture optotype tests suffer from the disadvantage of not inducing the crowding phenomenon.

The Kay Picture test

The Kay Picture test, designed around Snellen principles and aimed at the age group 2–3 years, presents a series of 25 isolated pictures in a flip card format (Kay, 1983). Testing can be done at either 3 or 6 m. The child is asked to name the pictures shown to him or her by the examiner. Whilst the use of 25 different optotypes aims to maintain the child's interest and prevent guessing, it is a reasonably demanding task for a child. An alternative is to use the Kay Picture key card which uses only eight different pictures and allows picture matching, rather than naming. A useful addition to the test is a booklet containing the Kay Picture symbols which can be made available to the parent prior to testing and allows the child to practise naming the optotypes. Acuity estimates may be successfully achieved from children as young as 2 years of age with this test (Kay, 1983). Kay measured Kay Picture test acuities in older children with a range of Snellen acuities and found a close correlation (0.9) between the two measures of acuity, although the Kay Pictures tended to slightly underestimate acuity.

Allen cards

These are picture symbols of a constant size, and visual acuity is measured by varying the viewing distance. They were calibrated using adult subjects whose vision was degraded by blurring lenses. The distance cards are seldom used, but similar symbols are used in the American Optical projection slide and a near card, which do have symbols of varying sizes.

Ffooks symbols

The Ffooks test presents three shapes, a square, circle and triangle, either singly on a cube or in a linear fashion on a flip chart. The child is required to name each symbol presented or match it with one of three equivalent cut-outs in front of him or her. With only three symbols to choose from the child has a one-in-three chance of guessing the answer correctly and older children may soon become bored with the test.

Illiterate/tumbling E test

This test uses Snellen letter Es presented either singly on a cube, or linearly on a chart. The Es are positioned with the prongs of the E pointing either up, down, left or right and the child is required to match its orientation with a cut-out E or describe its orientation using his or her fingers to represent the prongs of the E. Because right and left orientations are frequently confused acuity estimates should be made largely on the responses to vertical orientation of the prongs. Children often find this test tedious because of its repetitive nature.

Landolt C and the broken wheel test

A similar test to the tumbling E is the Landolt C test which requires the child to identify where the break in the C is positioned. It is also the basis of the broken wheel test which shows pictures of cars, one with a 'broken' wheel which the child is required to identify.

Lighthouse test

The three symbols utilized by the Lighthouse test and which the child must name are a house, an umbrella and an apple. This test suffers from the flaw that at the acuity threshold the shapes do not blur equally, the umbrella still being distinguishable when the others are not.

LH symbols

There are four LH symbols, a circle, square, heart (or apple) and house. Unlike the Lighthouse symbols they do blur equally at the acuity limit. They are available in a variety of charts, including a logMAR version similar to the Bailey–Lovie chart, and single and crowded symbols on flip over cards. They come with a matching card for children who cannot verbalize the shapes.

Sjögren's hand test

This test is similar to the tumbling E test, but uses a hand positioned in various orientations instead of an E. It suffers from the same limitations as the tumbling E and, in addition, its design does not conform to Snellen principles.

Because of the difficulty in interpreting verbal answers and the difficulty in adhering to Snellen principles in designing picture and symbol tests, where possible letter matching tests are the preferred test of optotype acuity.

PREFERENTIAL LOOKING

The Teller and Keeler Acuity Cards

As discussed in the previous chapter, preferential looking is a way of estimating visual acuity in infants and others who are non-verbal and unable to complete a letter/picture matching test. It is based on the observation that infants would rather look at a pattern than a blank stimulus (Fantz, Ordy and Udelf, 1962). Much early work utilizing this observation involved the use of computer-generated stimuli to assess preferential looking acuities and limited the access of clinicians to preferential looking techniques. However, commercially available, portable and clinically useful versions of the preferential looking test have since been developed. The Teller Acuity Cards and the Keeler Acuity Cards consist of a series of large grey cards with a central peephole. On one side of each card is a black and white grating of a specific spatial frequency (as explained in Chapter 1). Each full set of Keeler and Teller cards contains cards covering a range of spatial frequencies in 1/2 octave steps. Acuity results are usually recorded in cycles per degree although both tests provide a Snellen conversion which can help the clinician relate the acuity measured to more familiar Snellen fractions. However, it should be recalled that these preferential looking techniques provide a measure of resolution acuity which does not strictly equate to a Snellen (recognition) acuity and such conversions have limited meaning.

The Keeler cards (Figure 7.5) were developed in response to criticisms regarding an artefact in the Teller acuity cards (Robinson, Moseley and Fielder, 1988). This artefact is a consequence of the absence of a border surrounding the grating on the Teller cards which results in an edge artefact for gratings with spatial frequencies greater than 6 cycles per degree. Although adult observers report this artefact, it is not clear whether infants utilize it to determine grating position. In order to prevent an edge artefact the Keeler cards contain a circular white border on both sides of the card: one contains the grating and the other contains the isoluminant (equal average luminance as the stripes) grey background.

Fig. 7.5
The Keeler Acuity Cards can be used to estimate resolution acuity.

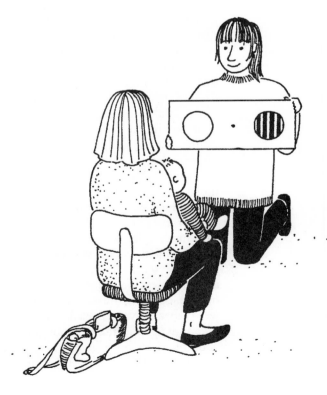

Obtaining an acuity estimate using preferential looking

The principle of the test is as explained in the previous chapter. If the spatial frequency is above the child's acuity threshold it provides an interesting target and he or she will look towards it. Each card is presented four times, the examiner randomly alternating the position of the grating at each presentation. The observer must correctly identify the position of the grating on at least three of the four presentations for that particular size of grating to be judged above the infant's resolution acuity threshold. Increasingly fine gratings are presented, from well above threshold to the point where it is not possible for the examiner to judge the grating's position from the infant's eye movements. At this point the spatial frequency is decreased again in 1/2 octave steps until a correct judgement is once again made. The finest grating that is correctly identified on two consecutive occasions is regarded as the acuity threshold. Testing with the Keeler and Teller acuity cards is normally performed at 38 cm.

A more rapid method of assessing acuity thresholds was introduced by McDonald et al. (1985). The 'acuity card procedure' has been shown to provide fast and accurate estimates of acuity and increase success rates (Lewis et al., 1993). One tester makes a selection of nine acuity cards centring on the expected acuity of the infant; the other tester only sees the backs of these, numbered from low to high, but does not know the absolute values of each card. This tester, the observer, is free to vary the order and orientation of the cards and to make as many presentations as judged necessary to make a decision on whether the child can see the stripes, using additional information which is disregarded in more traditional preferential looking techniques such as that described above. The examiner not only makes judgements on the basis of the infant's eye movements, but on the quality of their fixation, utilizing the fact that fixation preference is likely to be slight at or just above threshold and strong when coarse, low spatial frequency gratings well above threshold are presented. This additional information allows the examiner to reach threshold more quickly and not 'waste' valuable attention time assessing intermediate spatial frequencies. This freer method produces results that prove reliable on retesting, and which give acuity values close to those expected using FPL, for both binocular and monocular testing (McDonald et al., 1986).

Heersema and van Hof-van Duin (1990) also devised a rapid acuity card method for use up to the age of 4 years. They began with a large stripewidth the child was expected to resolve easily, then presented narrower widths in rapid succession in large steps until the child appeared less confident. Smaller steps between gratings were then used, each being presented at least twice. Near threshold, stripewidths were repeatedly decreased or increased until the observer could make a confident judgement about the finest grating the child could see. This required on average three reversals with at least 12–15 trials around threshold. Acceptable reliability between observers was found on repeat testing. Monocular acuity was tested successfully in 50% of 1 year olds and 100% of 4 year olds, failure always being due to unwillingness of the child to patch one eye. The age norms based on this procedure were slightly higher than those in previous studies, again demonstrating the importance of standardization of procedures, in terms of stimuli, methods and response patterns.

Another 'shortcut' method (for which no norms are available but which is really a variant of the above rapid method) can be used early in the testing sequence, as follows. The examiner presents the card 'blind' to the position of the stripes and judges their position based on the child's response. Then, still without looking at the card, the examiner turns it through 180 degrees. If the child is judged to look at the opposite side this time, the examiner checks the expected location of the stripes and, if correct, moves on to the next card. As soon as the examiner makes a mistake or cannot make a judgement, he or she returns to the last 'correct' card in the sequence and uses the fuller procedure from then on.

The use of operant methods to increase the age range of preferential looking tests was described in Chapter 6.

The Cardiff Acuity Test

As discussed in the previous chapter, success rates with simple grating acuity tests fall after 12 months of age, and it is increasingly difficult to obtain acuity estimates for children of toddler age (Shute et al., 1990). The Cardiff Acuity Test was developed in response to this problem. It is based on similar principles to the grating tests, but utilizes pictures constructed of black and white lines as the stimulus. As with the grating tests, these 'vanishing optotypes' disappear into the grey background when the lines are beyond the resolution limit of the infant. The stimuli are presented in a vertical format allowing an easier assessment of subjects with nystagmus whose own horizontal eye movements make discrimination of horizontal preferential look-ing eye movements more difficult (Figure 7.6). Children can be encouraged to point to or name the pictures, but decisions regarding the position of the target should only be made on the basis of the child's more reliable eye movements. Each size of target in the Cardiff Acuity Test is represented on three cards with either two targets at the top of the card and one at the bottom or vice versa. As with the grating tests, testing usually commences with a gross target expected to be well above threshold in order to demonstrate the test to the child and determine the child's eye movement patterns when presented with a visible stimulus. The designers of the Cardiff Acuity Test suggest that the smallest size of target at which two of the three cards elicit the correct response be regarded as the acuity threshold. However, practical experience with the Cardiff Acuity Test indicates that a more reliable threshold may be obtained by presenting four cards at each acuity level. This can be achieved by shuffling the three cards available at each acuity level for the fourth presentation. The acuity threshold is then regarded as the smallest target size at which three of four

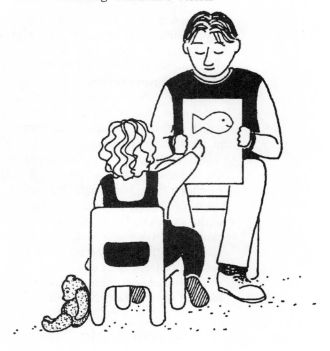

presentations are correctly judged. The Cardiff Acuity Test presents stimuli in 1/3 octave steps and can be used at either 50 cm or 1 m, although when testing at 50 cm a ceiling acuity of 0.3 logMAR (6/12) is present.

Preferential looking provides an *estimate* of acuity, influenced by both the examiner's ability and the infant's attention and behaviour. However, such tests have been shown to be repeatable, suggesting that the estimates obtained accurately reflect the resolution acuity present (Heersema and van Hof-van Duin, 1990). Whilst resolution acuity is the only acuity measure available when testing infants and young children unable to perform letter or picture matching tasks, the limitations of resolution acuity outlined above must be recognized. Once a child is able to perform a matching task, recognition acuities should be attempted.

An alternative method to preferential looking which is used when testing children whose ability to interact with the examiner is limited is the visual evoked potential. This method also provides an estimate of resolution acuity and will be discussed in Chapter 13.

OPTOKINETIC NYSTAGMUS

The presence or absence of optokinetic nystagmus (Chapter 12) in response to moving targets of different spatial frequencies has been used as an indicator of visual acuity (Fantz, Ordy and Udelf, 1962; Enoch and Rabinowicz, 1976). The basis of optokinetic nystagmus (OKN) as an indicator of visual acuity is that contours moving across

Fig. 7.7
The OKN drum.

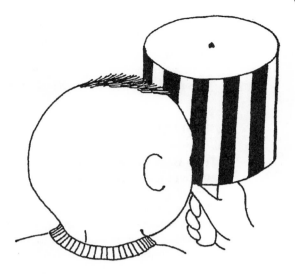

a subject's visual field will produce OKN if resolved. Although OKN is not mature at birth, it is present and OKN tests may be utilized from birth. Clinical OKN tests of acuity are traditionally performed using an OKN drum on which a grating of fixed spatial frequency is presented (Figure 7.7). In order to present different spatial frequencies and hence obtain an acuity estimate the drum must be used at a variety of distances. The criticism of this technique is that the size of the overall stimulus will vary with presentation distance, making it a less compelling target at the farthest test distances. A more recent, commercially available, test is the Catford drum which presents an oscillating black dot on a white background. Various dot sizes are available in order that a threshold size can be obtained. Unfortunately, the choice of target results in an estimation of detection rather than resolution acuity and is likely to overestimate visual acuity (Atkinson et al., 1981).

The use of OKN as a measure of acuity has several limitations. First, it is a measure made in response to a moving stimulus rather than the more standard static acuity measures. Second, it can be elicited in cortically blind children apparently reflecting a subcortical contribution to the OKN pathway (van Hof-van Duin and Mohn, 1983; Westall, 1991) and third, failure to detect OKN may reflect inattention rather than an inability to perceive the stimulus. Finally, when testing infants and children with neurological impairment it is the author's experience that the abnormal ocular posture and eye movements which are relatively common in this group make OKN more difficult to detect and assess.

A modification to the Catford drum apparatus has been described by Hopkisson et al. (1991). This applies a series of vernier offset targets to the Catford drum apparatus. These offsets are designed to correspond to Snellen letter sizes from 6/6 to 2/60 when presented at 50 cm. The offsets are viewed by the child through a narrow window placed in front of the oscillating drum and, if detected, elicit smooth pursuit movements as the offsets move across the visible field and disappear, then reappear again moving in the opposite direction. Hopkisson et al. note that the acuities they measure are not true hyperacuities but report a good correlation between the acuities recorded with their procedure and Snellen.

EQUIPMENT FOR ACUITY TESTING

In order to provide acuity assessment for infants and children over a wide range of ages it is not practical for the practitioner to use only a single acuity test. A useful set of tests might include a preferential looking test such as the Cardiff Acuity Test or the Teller or Keeler cards which can be used from birth to 2 years and a single and crowded letter matching acuity test such as the Sheridan–Gardiner single letter acuity test and the Glasgow Acuity Cards or the Cambridge Crowding Cards.

EXPECTED NORMS FOR AGE

Visual acuity at birth is relatively poor and shows a rapid improvement from birth through the first 6 months of life, when estimates improve from about 1 cycle per degree (20/600) to about 25 cycles per degree (20/24). Subsequently, visual acuity refines more slowly to adult levels during childhood (Mayer and Dobson, 1982; McDonald et al., 1985). Much of this improvement can be explained by changes in the optics of the eye and the size, shape and distribution of retinal photoreceptors (Banks and Bennett, 1988; see also Chapter 1). However, ocular development cannot fully explain the increase in acuity seen during this period. Significant maturation also occurs at a post-receptoral level, with the pruning of synaptic connections and the introduction of cortical inhibitory responses which improve the sensitivity of the visual system and hence increase visual performance (Wilson, 1988).

Figure 7.8 illustrates the improvement in acuity demonstrated through infancy and early childhood (Saunders, Westall and Wood-house, 1996). These measures were obtained using a preferential looking technique. Acuity development measured using sweep visual evoked potentials (Chapter 13) shows a more rapid increase in acuity reaching close to adult levels by 12 months of age (Norcia and Tyler, 1985). The reasons for the disparity demonstrated between VEP and preferential looking measures of acuity are not fully resolved. They may originate from different threshold criteria, the use of a temporally modulating stimulus in many VEP studies or the difference may arise from the level of response required by the two different techniques. Whilst the VEP assesses response produced up to the level of the primary visual cortex, the preferential looking response is also likely to involve the association and motor cortices. Although VEP and preferential looking estimates of acuity differ, when preferential

Fig. 7.8
Monocular grating acuity versus age (replotted from Saunders et al., 1996). Each data point represents an acuity estimate for a single child. The central solid line denotes mean acuity and the outer lines illustrate 95% confidence intervals for monocular acuity development. (Replotted from Sauders, K.J. et al. (1996). Longitudinal assesment of monocular grating acuity: predictive value of estimates in infancy. *Neuro-ophthalmology*, **16**, 15–25. © Aeolus Press.)

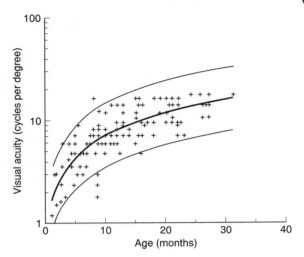

looking or VEP data are compared between different laboratories and authors, there is remarkable agreement, indicating that the data accurately reflect the maturation of visual acuity.

Interpretation of the significance of acuity findings is aided if clinicians have access to age norms for the particular test they are using. Results falling outside age norms or failing to reach the expected level for age warrant repeat testing or further investigation. Preferential looking techniques, which originated from laboratory-based tests, have been far more rigorously validated than more traditional clinical techniques such as optotype-matching tests which have frequently been produced without accompanying normative data. There is, in many cases, a lack of published literature from which to gain age-appropriate norms for these tests. Age norms for a variety of acuity tests are described below. In general, data have been quoted for the age groups for which the test is most appropriate. The normal ranges are described in the units used by the individual tests. Conversion of resolution acuities to Snellen equivalents has been avoided given that such conversions can be misleading.

Table 7.2   Teller Acuity Cards

Age (months)	Acuity range (cycles per degree*)	
	Binocular[†]	Monocular[‡]
Newborn	1.1–0.4	
1	1.7–0.4	1.66–0.60
2	3.3–0.9	3.13–1.11
4	6.8–1.7	4.70–1.66
6	9.1–2.2	9.60–3.13
9	9.1–2.2	9.60–4.70
12	9.1–2.2	9.60–4.70
18	13.0–4.7	13.00–6.36
24	19.0–6.4	13.00–6.36

*Higher scores indicate better visual acuity
[†]Teller Acuity Card Manual (reproduced with permission from Vistech Consultants Inc.)
[‡]Derived from Mayer et al., 1995

Age norms for preferential looking tests

Age norms for both grating acuity tests and the Cardiff Acuity Test have been produced and are given in Tables 7.2, 7.3a and 7.3b. These allow the clinician to compare his/her results with those expected from published norms. Infants with lower than normal values for their age require more detailed investigation.

Table 7.3   Cardiff acuity test

(a) Based on data from Deves et al., 1996

Age (months)	Binocular acuity range (logMAR*)
12	0.21–0.73
18	0.01–0.45
25	0.00–0.21

*Higher logMAR scores indicate poorer vision

(b) Based on Adoh and Woodhouse, 1994

Age (months)	Monocular acuity range (logMAR*)
12–< 18	0.40–0.80
18–< 24	0.10–0.70
24–< 30	0.10–0.50
30–36	0.00–0.30

*Higher logMAR scores indicate poorer vision

Age norms for optotype naming tests

Table 7.4   Kay Picture Test (isolated optotypes) (based on data from Deves et al., 1996)

Age (months)	Binocular acuity range (logMAR*)
25	− 0.24–0.28
31	− 0.18–0.10

*Higher logMAR scores indicate poorer visual acuity

Age norms for optotype matching tests

Table 7.5   Sjögren's hand test (isolated optotypes) (derived from Fern and Manny, 1986)

Age (years)	Mean binocular acuity value (Snellen fraction)
3	6/18
4	6/12
5	6/11
6	6/10

Table 7.6 Sonksen–Silver (3 m linear test) (Salt et al., 1995)

Age (years)	Acuity achieved by 90% of children (Snellen fraction)	
	binocular	monocular
2.5– < 3.5	3/6	3/6
3.5– < 5.0	3/4.5	3/6
5.0– < 6.0	3/4.5	3/4.5
6.0 and over	3/3	3/4.5

Acuities of 3/3 were only achieved by 85% of children aged between 8 and 9 years, the oldest age group tested in this study

Table 7.7 Cambridge Crowding Cards (crowded letter-matching test) (Cambridge Crowding Cards manual)

Age range (years)	Expected binocular acuity Snellen equivalent
3.5–4.5	6/9
5.0–6.0	6/6

REPEATABILITY OF ACUITY TESTS

When making clinical decisions about the significance of acuity estimates several factors need to be considered. The importance of understanding the limitations of measurements of resolution rather than recognition acuity and single rather than crowded acuities has already been discussed. In addition, when making clinical judgements it is important that information is available regarding the repeatability of acuity tests. Repeatability reflects the amount of inherent variability within a technique and hence its precision or lack of scatter. Once the level of repeatability is established for a given technique, the clinician can assess the significance of differences in acuity between the two eyes and between visits. When testing adult subjects Lovie–Kitchin (1988) demonstrated that for a change or difference in acuities to be significant, acuity must differ by at least eight letters on the Bailey–Lovie chart and by approximately two lines on the Snellen chart. Her results show that the minimum visual angle measured by the Snellen chart has to double before a difference can be said to be significant, i.e. from 6/6 to 6/12. Because of the improved design and scoring criteria of the Bailey–Lovie chart it is a more sensitive test for detecting significant differences in acuity, requiring a difference of only 0.16 logMAR (eight letters).

Despite the importance of repeatability measures they are remarkably scarce in instructions accompanying commercially available acuity tests.

Several studies have examined the repeatability of preferential looking grating acuity tests (McDonald et. al., 1986; Birch and Hale,

1988; Heersema and van Hof-van Duin, 1990). In general, they conclude that repeatability remains constant with age and the test-retest differences are limited to within one octave in more than 90% of cases. The acuity cards present spatial frequencies in 1/2 octave steps, making one card the limit of repeatability. Using the Teller acuity cards McDonald et al. (1986) report that a difference in acuities, either between eyes or between visits, of two or more cards can be regarded as a significant difference.

Adoh and Woodhouse (1994) investigated the repeatability of the Cardiff Acuity Test which presents stimuli in 1/3 octave steps. Their results suggest that an *increase* in acuity from one occasion to the next of more than three cards (more than one octave) or a *decrease* in acuity of more than two cards (one octave) could be regarded as significant. Therefore, when measured in octaves, the repeatability of the Cardiff cards is similar to the Teller cards.

There are fewer published data regarding repeatability of letter and picture matching acuity techniques than for preferential looking tests. Unpublished data from the Department of Vision Sciences, Glasgow Caledonian University, demonstrate that the repeatability of the Glasgow Acuity Card Test is limited to four letters. As each letter has a score of 0.025 logMAR a difference on repeat testing or between eyes of more than 0.1 logMAR is regarded as significant.

INTEROCULAR ACUITY DIFFERENCES

Brief examination of the age norms described in Tables 7.2 and 7.3 and those illustrated in Figure 7.8 reveals a wide normal range for resolution acuity tests, such that infants at both 4 and 18 months of age could have the same level of acuity and still be considered within normal limits. This wide normal range during infancy limits the use of binocular resolution acuity measures to excluding binocular visual impairment. A more sensitive and useful measure is that of interocular acuity difference. Significant interocular acuity differences

Table 7.8   Significant interocular acuity differences with different acuity tests

• Teller/Keeler Acuity Cards (preferential looking test)	2 cards
• Cardiff Acuity Test (preferential looking test)	2 cards
• Kay Picture Test (isolated picture naming/matching test)	2 lines
• Sheridan–Gardiner Singles (single letter matching acuity test)	2 lines
• Sonksen–Silver Acuity System (linear letter matching acuity)	2 lines
• Cambridge Crowding Cards (crowded letter matching acuity)	2 lines
• Glasgow Acuity Cards (crowded letter matching acuity)	4 letters

may be common during the first few months of life (Thompson, 1987), but are not normal outside this time and should be thoroughly investigated for underlying cause, such as amblyopia, pathology or anisometropia. But what constitutes a significant interocular acuity difference? As discussed above, the answer depends on the repeatability of the acuity test. Some acuity tests which are used in practice are listed in Table 7.8 and the level of significant interocular acuity difference given. These valuable figures have been obtained by testing large populations of visually normal children and should ideally be provided with every commercially available test. However, when unavailable they can be calculated by individual practitioners collecting their own normative data from visually normal subjects of a range of ages.

NEAR VISION TESTING

Near vision testing is an important aspect of testing children with low vision. Near vision assessment can provide educators and carers with information regarding the size of educational material that a particular child requires and at what distance it should be placed in order for it to be easily seen. Children should not be expected to work at their near vision threshold, but should be given material that is at least twice their acuity threshold in order that they are not struggling to maintain clarity. When used in conjunction with distance vision testing, near vision testing can also highlight accommodative deficits which are known to exist amongst people with neurological impairments and those with low vision (Lindstedt, 1983, 1986; Duckman, 1984; Woodhouse et al., 1993; Leat, 1996). However, it is important that a comparable test is used for both distance and near acuity measurement. For example, a difference between single letter distance acuity and crowded acuity at near does not necessarily indicate reduced accommodation but may reflect the increased complexity of the near vision task. Near acuity tests also allow assessment of the amount of magnification required by children with low vision and their performance with low vision aids (Chapter 14). In cases of low vision, where crowded print often causes more difficulties than single letter presentation, it is important to be able to measure both types of acuity in order that a suitable print size for crowded tasks can be recommended for school work. The criteria for a good near chart are similar to those for a distance chart, i.e. a logarithmic scale and similar numbers of letters or symbols per line. However, it is preferable to use the N or M notation for measuring near acuity, as these are independent of the distance used. Reduced distance acuity charts are normally calibrated for a particular distance, which is often not the distance at which children read, particularly children with low vision. Near acuity should be recorded as N12 at 20 cm, for example, or 0.2/N12 (i.e. distance over print size).

There are several test charts available to assess near visual acuity in children, many of which are adaptations of distance acuity tests, such as the Lighthouse test, the Ffooks symbols, the LH symbols, reduced Snellen and reduced logMAR charts. The LH symbols are marked in M sizes and both crowded and single symbols are available. Another useful test is the McClure test which provides print in levels of difficulty according to the school grade levels and in simple type faces which are commonly used by children in the early years of school.

CONCLUSION

This chapter has outlined the different types of visual acuity and discussed the advantages and disadvantages of a number of acuity tests available for use with infants and children. Several methods of obtaining resolution acuity estimates in infants have been described, using the Teller or Keeler preferential looking cards. Beyond infancy, tests using picture symbols or letters become more appropriate and a number of these (recognition acuity tests) have been described; where possible, letter matching tests are the preferred method. The Cardiff Acuity Test, based on a resolution task but using pictures rather than plain stripes, provides another possible test for toddlers. Important issues to consider are test repeatability, interocular differences and near vision testing. It is also very important to use age norms specific to a particular test; in this chapter, age norms are provided for several significant acuity tests.

REFERENCES

Adoh, T.O. and Woodhouse, J.M. (1994). The Cardiff Acuity Test used for measuring visual acuity development in toddlers. *Vision Research*, **34**, 555–560.

Atkinson, J., Braddick, O., Pimm-Smith, E. et al. (1981). Does the Catford Drum give an accurate assessment of acuity? *British Journal of Ophthalmology*, **66**, 264–268.

Bailey, I.L. and Lovie, J.E. (1976). New design principles for visual acuity test charts. *American Journal of Optometry and Physiological Optics*, **53**, 745–753.

Banks, M.S. and Bennett, F.J. (1988). Optical and photoreceptor immaturities limit the spatial and chromatic vision of human neonates. *Journal Optical Society of America*, **5**, 2059–2079.

Birch, E.E. and Hale, L.A. (1988). Criteria for monocular acuity deficit in infancy and early childhood. *Investigative Ophthalmology and Visual Science*, **29**, 636–643.

Deves, S., Williams, C., Parker, J. et al. (1996). Visual acuity testing in children up to age 3: normal ranges and comparisons between tests from the 'ALSPAC' study. *Investigative Ophthalmology & Visual Science* (Suppl), **37** (2), S730.

Duckman, R. (1984). Accommodation in cerebral palsy: function and remediation. *Journal American Optometric Association*, **55**, 281–183.

Enoch, J.M. and Rabinowicz, I.M. (1976). Early surgery and visual correction of an infant born with unilateral eye lens opacity. *Documenta Ophthalmologica*, **41**, 371.

Fantz, R., Ordy, J. and Udelf, M. (1962). Maturation of pattern vision in infants during the first six months of life. *Journal of Comparative and Physiological Psychology*, **55**, 907–917.

Fern, K.D. and Manny, R.E. (1986). Visual acuity of the preschool child: a review. *American Journal of Optometry and Physiological Optics*, **63**, 319–345.

Hecht, S. and Mintz, E.U. (1939). The visibility of single lines of various illuminations and the retinal basis of visual resolution. *Journal of General Physiology*, **22**, 593–612.

Heersema, D.J. and van Hof-van Duin, J. (1990). Age norms for visual acuity in toddlers using the acuity card procedure. *Clinical Vision Science*, **5**, 167–174.

van Hof-van Duin, J. and Mohn, G. (1983). Optokinetic and spontaneous nystagmus in children with neurological disorders. *Behavioural Brain Research*, **10**, 163–175.

Hopkisson, B., Arnold, P., Billingham, B. et al. (1991). Visual assessment of infants: vernier targets for the Catford drum. *British Journal of Ophthalmology*, **75**, 280–283.

Kay, H. (1983). New method of assessing visual acuity with pictures. *British Journal of Ophthalmology*, **67**, 131–133.

Klein, S.A. and Levi, D.M. (1985). Hyperacuity thresholds of 1 second: Quantitative predictions and empirical validation. *Journal of the Optical Society of America (A)*, 2, 1170–1190.

Leat, S.J. (1996). Reduced accommodation in children with cerebral palsy. *Ophthalmology and Physiological Optics*, **16**(5), 385–390.

Lewis, T.L., Reed, M.J., Maurer, D. et al. (1993). An evaluation of acuity card procedures. *Clinical Vision Science*, **8**, 591–602.

Lindstedt, E. (1983). Failing accommodation in cases of Down's syndrome. *Ophthalmic Paediatrics and Genetics*, **3**, 191.

Lindstedt, E. (1986). Accommodation in the visually-impaired child. In G.C. Woo (ed.), *Low Vision: Principles and Applications*. Springer-Verlag, New York.

Loshin, D.S. and White, J. (1984). Contrast sensitivity: The visual rehabilitation of the patient with macular degeneration. *Archives of Ophthalmology*, **102**, 1303–1306.

Lovie-Kitchin, J.E. (1988). Validity and reliability of visual acuity measurements. *Ophthalmic and Physiological Optics*, **8**, 363–370.

Mayer, D.L., Beiser, A.S., Warner, A.F. et al. (1995). Monocular acuity norms for the Teller Acuity Cards between ages one month and four years. *Investigative Ophthalmology and Visual Science*, **36**, 671–685.

Mayer, D.L. and Dobson, V. (1982). Assessment of vision in young children: a new operant approach yields estimates of acuity. *Investigative Ophthalmology and Visual Science*, **19**, 566–570.

Mayer, D.L., Fulton, A.B. and Rodier, D. (1984). Grating and recognition acuities of paediatric patients. *Ophthalmology*, **91**, 947–953.

McDonald, M.A., Dobson, V., Lawson Sebris, S. et al. (1985). The acuity card procedure: A rapid test of infant acuity. *Investigative Ophthalmology and Visual Science*, **26**, 1155–1162.

McDonald, M.A., Sebris, S.L., Mohn, G. et al. (1986). Monocular acuity in normal infants: the acuity card procedure. *American Journal Optometry and Physiological Optics*, **63**, 181–186.

McGraw, P.V. and Winn, B. (1993). Glasgow Acuity cards: A new test for the measurement of letter acuity in children. *Ophthalmic and Physiological Optics*, **13**, 400–404.

Norcia, A.M. and Tyler, C.W. (1985). Spatial frequency sweep VEP: Visual acuity during the first year of life. *Vision Research*, **25**, 1399–1408.

Osterberg, G. (1936). A sight-test chart for children. *Acta Ophthalmologica (Kbh)*, **14**, 397–405.

Robinson, J., Moseley, M.J. and Fielder, A.R. (1988). Grating acuity cards: spurious resolution and the "edge artefact". *Clinical Vision Science*, **3**, 285–288.

Salt, A.T., Sonksen, P.M., Wade, A. and Jayatunga, R. (1995). The maturation of linear acuity and compliance with the Sonksen-Silver Acuity System in young children. *Developmental Medicine and Child Neurology*, **37**, 505–514.

Saunders, K.J., Westall, C.A. and Woodhouse, J.M. (1996). Longitudinal assessment of monocular grating acuity: predictive value of estimates in infancy. *Neuro-ophthalmology*, **16**, 15–25.

Shimojo, S. and Held, R. (1987). Vernier acuity is less than grating acuity in 2- and 3-month-olds. *Vision Research*, **27**, 77–86.

Shute, R., Candy, R., Westall, C. and Woodhouse, J.M. (1990). Success rates in testing monocular acuity and stereopsis in infants and young children. *Ophthalmic and Physiological Optics*, **10**, 133–136.

Teller Acuity Cards (TAC) Manual. Dayton, Ohio, USA, Vistech Consultants Inc.

Thompson, C.M. (1987). *Objective and Psychophysical Studies of Infant Visual Development*. Unpublished PhD thesis, University of Aston, Birmingham, UK.

Westall, C. (1991). Eye movements in cortically blind children. *Ophthalmic and Physiological Optics*, **11**, 400.

Wilson, H.R. (1988). Development of spatiotemporal mechanisms in infant vision. *Vision Research*, **286**, 611–628.

Woodhouse, J.M., Meades, J.S., Leat, S.J. and Saunders, K.J. (1993). Reduced accommodation in children with Down syndrome. *Investigative Ophthalmology and Visual Science*, **34**, 2382–2387.

8

Contrast sensitivity

INTRODUCTION

Whereas visual acuity represents the smallest detail that a person can perceive (and is usually measured with high contrast, black on white targets, such as those described in the previous chapter), contrast sensitivity represents the lowest contrast that the visual system can resolve or detect. In the present chapter, following a brief introductory section, we explain the functional and clinical significance of contrast sensitivity, describe what is known about its development and evaluate a number of contrast sensitivity charts in terms of their usefulness with children.

WHAT IS CONTRAST SENSITIVITY?

Contrast sensitivity describes the ability to detect objects (of a variety of sizes) of low contrast, and is therefore measured with low contrast targets (e.g. grey on lighter grey). *Contrast* is defined as the difference between the two grey levels, while *contrast threshold* is defined as the lowest contrast detectable for a given size of stimulus.

Contrast (C) is defined by the equation:

$$C = \left(\frac{I_{MAX} - I_{MIN}}{I_{MAX} + I_{MIN}} \right) \times 100$$

Where I_{MAX} is the intensity of the brightest part of the target and I_{MIN} is the intensity at the darkest part of the target.

The contrast sensitivity (C_s) is the reciprocal of the contrast threshold (C_t).

$$C_s = \frac{1}{C_t}$$

Contrast threshold is traditionally measured with a sine wave grating. This is a series of stripes, the cross-sectional luminance profile of which varies in mathematical fashion (Figure 8.1). Typically, we use either sine wave (sinusoidal) gratings in which the luminance profile is a sine wave, or square wave gratings, in which the profile follows a square shape. As explained in Chapter 1, the spatial frequency of the stripes is defined by the number of cycles in a given distance. It may be measured in terms of absolute distance (e.g. 1 cycle per mm) or, more commonly, in terms of degrees of angular

Fig. 8.1
(a) Three-dimensional representation of the luminance profile of a square-wave grating. Spatial frequency can be defined in cycles per degree subtended at the eye or in cycles per linear distance. If angle $\alpha = 1$ degree, then this grating has a spatial frequency of 2 cycles per degree; if distance $x = 1$ cm, it has a spatial frequency of 1 cycle per cm. (b) Three-dimensional representation of the luminance profile of a sine-wave grating. As for Figure 8.1(a). If angle $\alpha = 1$ degree, then this grating has a spatial frequency of 2 cycles per degree; if distance $x = 1$ cm, it has a spatial frequency of 1 cycle per cm.

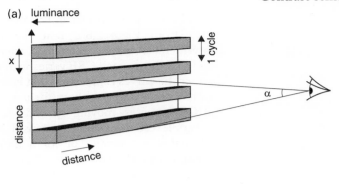

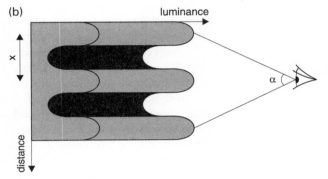

subtense at the eye (e.g. 1 cycle per degree). In some studies on letter detection or reading (see below), spatial frequency is defined in terms of cycles per character width, that is, using the letter width as the reference unit. Contrast threshold is measured by determining the lowest contrast required to detect a grating (or letter) of a certain spatial frequency (or size). The contrast sensitivity of the normal visual system varies with the spatial frequency or the size of the target. The plot (as in Figure 8.2) of contrast sensitivity with respect to spatial frequency for an individual is called the contrast sensitivity function (CSF). It is normally plotted on logarithmic axes, or else the

Fig. 8.2
Typical contrast sensitivity function for different age groups. (Data are taken from Owsley et al., 1983. With kind permission of Elsvier Science Ltd)

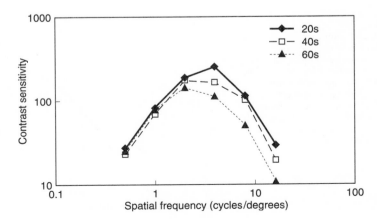

logarithm of the contrast and contrast sensitivity are plotted. It can be seen from Figure 8.2 that the maximum sensitivity is at an intermediate spatial frequency, approximately 4 cycles per degree, and that the average CSF varies with age. In these CSF plots, the area under the curves represents what is visible to the person, while objects with contrast and size above the curve are invisible (contrast decreases as CS increases, moving upwards on the Y axis).

People can lose contrast sensitivity (due to ocular disorders) at all spatial frequencies or for a limited range of frequencies. Two examples are shown Figure 8.3. In one case CS for only high spatial frequencies (fine detail) is reduced. In the other case CS is reduced at all spatial frequencies. The practical significance and the amount of visual disability will be very different in these two cases. The person with loss at high frequencies only will not see fine detail (and therefore will have reduced acuity), but will be able to see the coarse shapes (overall outlines of objects) normally. Magnification will be effective for this person, having the effect of 'shifting' the object along the X axis in the direction of the arrow. The spatial frequency components of the object are made larger and therefore moved from higher to lower spatial frequencies. The spatial frequency components of an object are moved from outside (above) this person's CSF (where they are invisible) to inside their CSF (thus becoming visible). The person with reduced CS at all frequencies will have degraded vision for all objects of all sizes. Low contrast objects, however big, will not be seen. Simply making things bigger (using magnification) will not be effective. An object of medium contrast, represented by the base of the arrow, is still above the CSF function, and is therefore invisible. However much magnification is applied (i.e. however much it is moved to the left in the direction of the arrow) it remains above the CSF and invisible. This person requires an increase of contrast, i.e. the arrow must be moved downwards into the CSF, for the object to become visible. Increasing the contrast of objects is not always possible, however.

Fig. 8.3
Normal CS function, CSF showing significant loss at high spatial frequencies only and CSF showing loss at all spatial frequencies. The base of the arrow represents a target of given contrast which moves in the direction of the arrow when magnification is applied. On the Y axis, as CS increases, the contrast decreases.

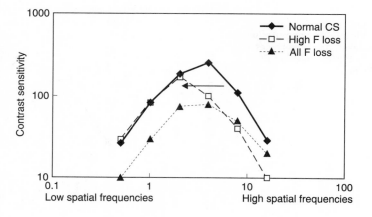

RESEARCH STUDIES

Originally, CS was investigated in research studies, and not used as a clinical measure. It was first measured in the 1960s in some classical studies by Campbell and Green (1965) resulting in the channel theory of vision. This theory suggests the existence of many 'channels' in the visual system, each one being maximally sensitive to a specific spatial frequency. The envelope of the sensitivity of all the channels makes up the CSF. At the same time Hubel and Wiesel were doing their Nobel-prize-winning work on orientation-selective neurons in the visual system (see De Valois and De Valois, 1988). The technique used in these original investigations, and still used in many contemporary laboratory studies, is that of presenting a sinusoidal grating on an oscilloscope screen. The contrast of the grating can be manipulated while the average luminance remains unchanged. The subject is instructed to respond as soon as the grating becomes visible, the contrast being increased from very low contrast which is below threshold. Alternatively, the subject is instructed to say whether the grating is visible in a first or second time period, or at the top or bottom part of the screen. Several repeated measurements are taken for each spatial frequency.

Contrast sensitivity functions have been measured in human observers with normal vision and in those with known eye diseases. For example, glaucoma, cataracts, retinitis pigmentosa, optic nerve abnormality and amblyopia are all known to reduce contrast sensitivity (Leguire, 1991). Some eye diseases (e.g. some cataracts, amblyopia) cause selective loss in the medium and high spatial frequencies, others cause loss at all spatial spatial frequencies (e.g. glaucoma, optic neuritis, cataract), and yet others cause loss mainly at intermediate and low spatial frequencies, as in optic nerve head swelling (Buncic and Tytla, 1989). Some conditions, such as glaucoma, can cause different patterns of CS loss between individuals and at different stages of the disease. Contrast sensitivity has also been used extensively as a tool for furthering our knowledge of the neural basis of some eye disorders. For example, Hess, Campbell and Zimmern (1980) showed that the pattern of CS loss at different luminances is very different in strabismic as opposed to anisometropic amblyopia. In strabismic amblyopia, the CS deficit disappears with decreasing luminance, whereas it remains in anisometropic amblyopia. The deficit was shown to involve mainly the central retina in strabismic amblyopia, but to involve both the centre and periphery in anisometropic amblyopia. Studies such as this gave insight into the neurological functioning in certain eye disorders.

THE FUNCTIONAL SIGNIFICANCE OF CONTRAST SENSITIVITY

Contrast sensitivity has been shown to be related to the performance of many everyday tasks. In fact, good contrast sensitivity is probably more important for many tasks than good visual acuity. Although all the relevant studies have been performed with adult subjects, the results may be applicable to children, and help us to understand and predict the expected visual performance once the CSF is known. It has been shown in a number of studies that aspects of the CSF are able to predict the reading speed obtained with magnification devices in people with low vision (Leat and Woodhouse, 1993; Whittaker and Lovie-Kitchin, 1993). When CS at low and intermediate spatial frequencies is preserved (despite the loss of visual acuity due to an eye disorder), the person is able to obtain good reading speed once the appropriate magnification has been prescribed (Figure 8.3). In contrast, a person with poor CS is unlikely to obtain good reading speed whatever magnification is provided (assuming that the visual fields are not extremely constricted). For fluent reading, not only does the CS have to be adequate to *detect* the print, it has to be good enough to ensure that the print is well *above* threshold. Whittaker and Lovie-Kitchin describe what they call a contrast reserve, which is the ratio of the contrast of the print to the contrast threshold of the person who wishes to read it. Thus a contrast reserve of 2:1 would mean that the contrast of the print is only twice the contrast threshold of the reader. They demonstrated, by means of integrating the results of a number of earlier studies, that a contrast reserve of 3:1 is required for spot reading (40 words per minute), 4:1 for fluent reading (80 words per minute, approximately 2nd year school reading level) and 10:1 for high fluent reading ≥ 160 words per minute, 6th year school reading level). Normal reading is at rates of 200 words per minute or more. In order to read a book or a whole newspaper article, high fluent reading rates are required to sustain interest and enjoyment. There is some controversy about whether fluent reading is required for good comprehension (Legge et al. 1989; Dickenson and Rabbit, 1991). However, we can assume that, for practical purposes, reasonable fluency is required to read longer pieces of written material and that adequate reading speed is necessary for children to succeed in their education and keep up with their peers. By knowing the CS of a child, we can predict the maximum likely reading rate that the child will achieve once she or he has learnt to read. Low vision is not necessarily a barrier to learning to read (Faye et al., 1984), so a child with significantly reduced CS may be able to learn to recognize letters and words; however, the rate of information acquisition by means of visual reading (as opposed to Braille or other sight-substitution techniques) may be limited. Once a child's reading speed drops behind that of his or her peers, albeit because of visual limitations, the child's education in all subjects is likely to suffer (Rosner and Rosner, 1990). Such a child may require supplementary sight-substitution techniques for some of their school work, in order to keep up with the volume of reading required in higher grades. Being able to predict this for the future is helpful so that support, assessments and devices can be put in place without delay when the time comes.

CS has been shown to predict other aspects of daily functioning. Marron and Bailey (1982) showed that CS was helpful, along with central visual field plots, in predicting the mobility of people with visual deficits. CS is also linked with perception of faces (Owsley and Sloane, 1987; Lennerstrand and Ahlstrom, 1989) and with sensitivity to glare (Elliott and Bullimore, 1993). It has also been found to be related to the degree of reported difficulty in performing daily tasks, such as seeing irregularities in the pavement (sidewalk) and watching television scenes (Lennerstrand and Ahlstrom, 1989). Rubin et al. (1994) found that CS was correlated with a wide range of visual tasks such as mobility, bumping into objects, seeing kerbs and edges, and judging distances. Elliott, Hurst and Weatherill (1990) also showed that CS, rather than visual acuity, is correlated with a person's perceived disability. Among people with low vision, CS, rather than visual acuity, determines which is the preferred eye in situations in which only one eye can be used (Loshin and White, 1984). These studies combine to demonstrate that CS is as important as, if not more important than, visual acuity in determining the degree of day-to-day difficulty with visual tasks that a person will experience. Two people with equal visual acuity could have very different CS and the person with the poorer CS will experience far more visual disability.

THE CLINICAL IMPORTANCE OF CONTRAST SENSITIVITY

It has been suggested that measuring CS may help in the diagnosis of certain eye conditions such as strabismus, optic nerve neuritis or glaucoma. Since we are not suggesting that CS measurement should replace other clinical tests such as visual acuity or objective ocular health examination, the real question is, does the addition of CS measurement increase our accuracy or sensitivity of diagnosis or detection of eye disease? Most eye disorders would be detected or suspected by other measurements in an eye examination (such as visual fields, visual acuity or ophthalmoscopy) or by symptomatology. There are very few cases in which an eye disease would be detected by routine measurement of static CS and not by other measures (Elliott and Whitaker, 1992). Arden states that CS is not useful in detecting glaucoma or diabetic retinopathy, nor is it useful in the management of diabetic retinopathy (Arden, 1988). The only pathology which may be detected by reduced CS, in the absence of other signs, is previous optic neuritis (Regan, 1988; Elliott and Whitaker, 1992). In such cases VA might be within normal limits and ophthalmoscopic appearance would often be normal. Older children or adults might complain of a subjective difference of vision between the two eyes, the vision of one eye appearing to be 'washed out'.

There are other cases where CSF changes have been found in the absence of reduced VA. For example, in cases of papilloedema (oedema of the optic disc), which may be caused by increased intracranial pressure, or glioma (tumours) of the optic nerves, measurement of CSF helps confirm the reality of an abnormal ophthalmoscopic picture (Tytla and Buncic, 1988; Buncic and Tytla, 1989).

We do not feel that CS testing is necessary in every child. However, CS assessment has particular value in the functional assessment of children as it relates to subjective visual impairment and to the ability to perform daily tasks. In addition, we recommend that CS should be measured in children suspected of having optic nerve disorders.

Reasons for measuring CS, therefore, are as follows:

1. To aid in diagnosis, e.g. to assess optic nerve function when there is a suspicion of optic nerve disorder.
2. As part of a full functional visual assessment, in order to:

   • give advice regarding contrast of objects and environmental adaptations
   • predict whether a child may require sight-substitution techniques in the future
   • explain a child's difficulties even though acuity may be relatively preserved
   • predict the need for orientation and mobility instruction
   • determine which eye to use for a monocular telescope
   • assess sensitivity to glare
   • assess the value of a spectacle prescription; Haegerstrom-Portnoy (1993) suggests that some children with visual impairments may obtain an improvement in CS without any improvement in VA.

Generally, it is low and intermediate spatial frequencies which have been found to correlate with function. For this reason we are interested in measuring CS at lower spatial frequencies. In addition, we assume that VA has already been measured, so that measuring CS at higher frequencies gives little more information.

DEVELOPMENT OF CONTRAST SENSITIVITY

Contrast sensitivity has been measured in infants using preferential looking techniques (Chapter 6) and visual evoked potentials or VEPs (Chapter 13). The methods underlying both these techniques were designed to determine the lowest contrast that an infant reliably detects stimuli of a range of spatial frequencies. At 2 months of age the CS curve shows reduced sensitivity across all spatial frequencies. Also, the peak of the response is shifted to the left, towards lower spatial frequencies, as is the high spatial frequency cut-off representing the acuity limit (Banks and Salapatek, 1976). The area under the CSF is significantly less than that found in adults. This means that the visual world of infants will be void of many of the rich textures available to adults; low contrast and high spatial frequency information will be invisible to the infant. Atkinson, Braddick and Moar (1977) demonstrated significant developmental changes in the CSF between the ages of 5 weeks and 8–12 weeks. During development the peak sensitivity shifts to the right towards higher spatial frequencies, as does the high frequency cut-off and therefore the acuity limit. This means that in early infancy, as development progresses, infants are able to detect stripes with less contrast as well as to detect smaller stripes. Even so, in the Atkinson et al. (1977) study, even the infants who demonstrated the higher sensitivities were not performing at an adult level: they gave reliable responses to contrast levels of 7% and above in comparison with adults, who might detect contrast levels of less than 0.5%. These studies used preferential looking techniques to assess contrast sensitivity, but results obtained using VEPs show some similarities. Norcia, Tyler and Hamer (1990) measured CSFs to gratings reversing in contrast using the sweep VEP (Chapter 13). They studied CSFs of 48 infants from 2 to 40 weeks old. The age range associated with the most rapid period of development of the VEP CSF is similar to that found with preferential looking techniques (see above). Norcia et al. (1990) found that CS increased by a factor of 4–5 at all spatial frequencies tested between 4 and 9 weeks of age. They also demonstrated that beyond 9 weeks the CS to low spatial frequencies remained constant while that to high spatial frequencies continued to increase. Movshon and Kiorpes (1988) explained the development of the infant CSF in terms of simultaneous horizontal and vertical scaling of the CSF without a change in shape of the function. Norcia et al. (1990) found that the CSF continues to develop until at least 30 weeks of age. Westall et al. (1992), using a preferential looking technique, also found the most rapid development of CS to be in the first 6 months. In summary, in infancy there is an early rapid development of overall sensitivity, with a further slow increase in sensitivity to high spatial frequencies until early childhood. Figure 8.4 shows the CSF measured in three different age groups using a preferential looking staircase technique.

Fig. 8.4
Mean contrast sensitivity (plus and minus 1 standard deviation) for different age groups of children: 3–6 months (+), 6–18 months (○), over 30 months (▲). Contrast sensitivity assessed by FPL.

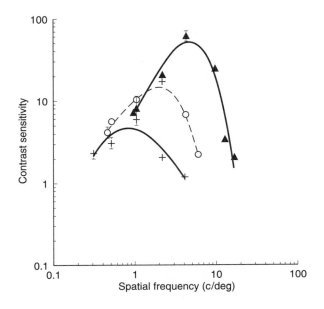

There have been several different investigations into the CSF of young children. The results are variable between studies (Bradley and Freeman, 1982), and it is probable that not all techniques used were appropriate for young children. We will mention three studies, all of which took into account the suitability of the test for children. Atkinson, French and Braddick (1981) designed a novel technique for the measurement of CS in children aged 3–5 years. Black and white gratings were mounted on two cubes, horizontally on one and vertically on the other. The cubes were separated by a screen. The task of the child was to run down the alley to the cube with the 'standing up' stripes, under which a present was concealed. The success of testing visual functions in toddlers is very dependent on the use of imaginative games such as this, and this is borne out by the results of that study. Children were each assigned to one of four groups: 3–3.5 years, 3.5–4 years, 4.0–4.5 years and 4.5–5 years. There was a steady increase in CS with age, with adults having slightly higher CS across all spatial frequencies tested (the mothers of some of the children served as control subjects). There was also little difference in the highest spatial frequency detected across age groups, with most of the children being able to detect a high contrast, 30 cycles per degree grating. Using a more conventional psychophysical procedure Bradley and Freeman (1982) measured CS in children from 22 months to 16 years. Reliable results were found for children over 3.5 years, but the technique failed for toddlers under the age of 2.5 years. Abramov et al. (1984), taking advantage of the children's imagination, used the novel 'rocket ship psychophysics' technique described in Chapter 6 and were very successful in testing children aged 5–8 years. The Abramov et al. and the Bradley and Freeman studies both found the CS of children to be slightly lower compared with adults. Bradley and Freeman found that the CS of the youngest group (2.5–4.5 years) was within 3.5 log units of the adult, and for the middle spatial frequencies the CS of even the youngest children was found to be close to that recorded in adults. However, CS, particularly at the high and low spatial frequencies, continued to increase up until the age of 8 years.

Later in this chapter we review clinical contrast sensitivity tests either designed for, or which can be adapted for use with, children. As for the testing of any visual function it is always desirable to collect 'normal control' data before using the test clinically. Once the normal limits of CS for a specific test are known, then clinical data can be interpreted correctly.

Development of CSF as related to development of the visual pathways

In Chapter 1 we described the development of the photoreceptors, the fovea and the higher visual pathways and the reader is encouraged to refer to that chapter for clarification of the following discussion. We discussed the growth of the cone outer segments which, in infancy are much fatter and shorter than in the adult and therefore capture less light. Banks and Bennett (1988) and Wilson (1988) discuss how increased quantal catch might explain some of the increase in overall sensitivity of the infant CSF during development. The early increase in the length of the cone outer segments, as well as the increase in foveal cone density probably provide the bulk of the reason for the early rapid phase of development of the CSF. The high frequency cut-off (representing visual acuity), which shifts to higher spatial frequencies during development, may be a result of the developing fovea. Development of the myelination of the optic nerve and optic tract, as well as cortical development, may also contribute to CSF development, although Movshon and Kiorpes (1988) explain the early development of the CSF by reference to peripheral mechanisms (perhaps originating in the photoreceptors). There has been recent discussion in the literature about whether, during early development, there is a shift towards higher spatial frequency preference of spatially tuned channels. For example, does a channel tuned to 2 cycles per degree at birth become tuned to 9 cycles per degree in adulthood? Data providing evidence for and against this hypothesis can be found in Peterzell, Werner and Kaplan (1993) and Shannon, Skoczenski and Banks (1996). These two papers, plus a paper describing the development of the CSF in monkeys (Kiorpes and Kiper, 1996) contain the most recent information and theories of CS development for the reader wanting more detailed analyses. The continued development of the CSF into childhood may be due to visual or neurological factors, as well as to non-visual factors such as attention (Bradley and Freeman, 1982).

CLINICAL MEASUREMENT OF CS

As we have seen, CS does not reach adult levels until the age of 8 years. If the CS results of a younger child are found to be lower than that of an adult it should not be inferred that there is a CS deficit. Abramov et al. (1984) very eloquently explain why age-matched norms are required for the same test to be able to reliably detect real differences in sensitivity. Since there are not age-related normal data for every test described below, we strongly advise practitioners to collect their own age-matched control data on children under 8 years.

The earliest measurements of CS in infants were undertaken using oscilloscope-presented stimuli and a preferential looking format. Typically, two screens were employed, on one of which was presented a sine-wave grating of pre-determined spatial frequency and contrast. An observer, naive to the position of the grating, guessed its position from the child's looking responses. In adults, also, the original measures of CS were taken with oscilloscope-presented gratings. It is, perhaps, unrealistic to expect clinical practices to purchase such equipment or, indeed, to have time for such testing. Therefore, for both adults and, more recently, for children, various chart tests of CS have been developed. The ideal chart test of CS would be relatively inexpensive, easy and quick to use, repeatable, valid and not excessively space-occupying. Age norms should be available, together with some idea of the significance of certain levels of reduced CS for visual function. As will be seen below, for many of the chart tests of CS we do not have age norms for the paediatric population, nor do we have data regarding the functional relevance of certain levels of CS in children, so that we are currently forced to extrapolate from adult data.

Earlier versions of such charts used a photographic process to create gratings of various contrasts. This leads to great expense and difficulty controlling the exact contrast achieved. More recently still, dot matrix printing has been used, whereby the contrast depends on the density of dots and is thus less expensive to produce. Another development has been the change from the use of gratings to either letters or, for children, faces or shapes. The most common of these charts are reviewed below.

The Vistech grating chart (VCTS – Vision Contrast Test System)

These are photographically produced sine wave gratings of varying spatial frequency and contrast, printed on one large chart. Various versions of the chart exist. The gratings also vary in orientation and the observer's task is to indicate whether the gratings are vertical or tilted to the right or the left. The test is intuitively appealing in that a score for each spatial frequency is obtained which can be plotted to form a CSF. However, the repeatability of the chart has been called into question (Rubin, 1988; Reeves, Wood and Hill, 1991; Elliott and Bullimore, 1993). The reasons for the poor repeatability may be as follows:

1. A criterion-free method is not used, i.e. the person is allowed to say that he or she cannot see the stripes, so if one observer tries harder than another to guess, the result is a better CS result.
2. Only one response is required for each spatial frequency/contrast value so one lucky guess can unduly influence the result and this leads to greater variability. As all scientists know, more than one measure is required to obtain an accurate result (see Chapter 6) and on the better types of VA charts, there is more than one letter at each acuity level.
3. There is a choice between three orientations of the grating, therefore the chance performance rate (the chance of getting the answer correct by guessing) is 33%, which is high.
4. The chart does not use a log scale and therefore there are larger changes in contrast between some gratings than others.
5. The small area of the grating may lead to variability in the results in people with central scotomas (field defects).

In addition, the highest contrasts are not high enough for use with some people with low vision. In fairness, it must be added that the validity of the Vistech chart is acceptable, that is, it does seem to measure what it proposes to measure (Woo and Leat, 1995). A recent version of the chart has tried to correct these problems. It is called the

FACT (Functional Acuity Contrast Test). It uses sine waves that decrease in 0.15 log contrast steps with a smoothed edge to the grating patches and with larger grating areas. There are three charts in order to improve reliability (Ginsburg, 1996). However, going through the procedure three times means that it is no longer a fast test. In addition, these changes do not deal with one of the main objections which is that it is not criterion free.

Finally, although the VCTS has been used successfully with some preliterate children by asking them to hold a pencil to match the orientation of the gratings (Woodhouse, personal communication), it is to be expected that young children would often confuse the orientation, as with the Illiterate E. The repeatability of the test with children is therefore likely to be even poorer than with adults and so we do not recommend its use.

The Pelli–Robson chart

The Pelli–Robson (PR) chart uses dot-matrix printed letters, of decreasing contrast with three letters at each contrast level. The size of the letters remains constant (6/34 Snellen letter size). The person is asked to read the letters, starting from high contrast and proceeding to progressively lower contrast until the limit of visibility is reached. The idea of using letters to measure contrast sensitivity was suggested because people are used to reading letters in an eye examination, it is fast and the use of letters provides an almost criterion-free method. Since there are 26 letters in the English alphabet, the chance performance rate becomes a little less than 4%. In fact only 10 letters of reputedly equal visibility are used on the PR chart, but the testee is not made aware of this fact. Letters are also much easier to print than sine wave gratings.

The design of the PR chart (Pelli, Robson and Wilkins, 1988) was based on the work of Ginsberg (1978) and Legge et al. (1985). The latter showed that most of the higher and intermediate spatial frequency information of letters can be eliminated before reading performance is affected. In other words, people can still read words which are substantially blurred. This is another indication that we do not need good acuity to be able to read, if the letters are large enough (see above). Their results showed that reading speed only started to be compromised once spatial frequencies of 2 cycles per character width and lower were eliminated. Pelli et al. used this information and assumed that detection of letters at contrast threshold is determined by CS at 2 cycles per character. They assumed that the most useful part of the CSF to measure lies at the intermediate spatial frequencies, at the peak of the function, which is typically at 4 cycles per degree for a normal observer. They therefore composed the PR chart of letters which subtend 0.5 degrees at 3 m (2 cycles per letter = 2 cycles per degree if the letters subtend 1 degree, 2 cycles per letter = 4 cycles per degree if the letters subtend 0.5 degree). Nowadays, the PR chart is more commonly used at a testing distance of 1 m, particularly for low vision observers. In this situation, in theory, the chart is a measure of low spatial frequencies, around 1.3 cycles per degree. This has been confirmed by Woo and Leat (1995).

The method of scoring this chart has been modified since it was first introduced. Originally, the observer's CS was taken as the last line of letters on which the observer could correctly identify two out of three letters. It has since been shown that repeatability is improved if each letter is given a score. We can do this because the chart has a true logarithmic scale, the change in log contrast sensitivity being 0.15 for each contrast step (half octave steps), and there are three letters at each contrast. Thus each letter becomes 'worth' 0.05 log contrast sensitivity. Thus, if the observer misses one letter at a given contrast sensitivity level, 0.05 is deducted from the score. If the observer correctly identifies one additional letter of the next group, 0.05 is added. An 'O' mistaken for a 'C' (or vice versa) is not regarded as an error.

There have now been many studies of, and using, the PR chart and it is becoming the standard for measuring CS clinically. It has been shown to have good repeatability (Rubin, 1988; Elliott, Sanderson and Conkey, 1990; Elliott and Bullimore, 1993) and has been shown to predict reading performance (Woo and Leat, 1995; Leat and Woo, 1997). It has also been found to be useful in the assessment of glare disability in people with cataracts (Williamson et al., 1992; Elliott and Bullimore, 1993) and to be predictive of a person's perceived disability, particularly with regard to mobility out of doors, reading and recognizing faces (Elliott, Sanderson and Conkey, 1990). Leat and Woo (1997) measured CS with the PR chart and reading speed in adults with low vision. They found that reading speed (with appropriate optical magnification) was correlated with the PR score. They estimate that a score of 0.75 is required for spot reading and 1.4 for fluent reading (Leat and Woo, 1997). Normal results are a monocular CS of 1.8 or better between the ages of 20 and 50 years (Elliott, Sanderson and Conkey, 1990), but there are no known norms for children at present.

Obviously, the PR chart can be used for older children who can name letters in which case it would be the chart of choice for measuring CS. Another reason we have spent a while discussing the origins of the PR chart, the significance of the findings and its repeatability is that a number of charts have been more recently developed for children, based on the principles of the PR chart. Since there are, as yet, few data using these charts for children, each lab has to collect its own aged-matched control data, in order to decide the criterion for normal and abnormal. For functional purposes, however, for example to determine what reduction in CS will cause a significant lowering of reading speed, we are forced to refer to the adult data above. This is far from ideal and adult data applied to the case of a child must be interpreted with caution. However, by interpolation, we may infer that a child with a logCS of 0.75 or less will have limited potential for fluent reading. Alternatively, a child with a full, almost normal adult, level of CS would be expected to have good reading potential with appropriate magnification.

To conclude, the advantages of the PR chart are as follows:

1. A true logarithmic scale.
2. Starts at high contrast, therefore suitable for people with very poor CS.
3. Good repeatability.
4. Many studies performed so that the significance of findings is known.
5. Relates to daily visual tasks.
6. Quick to use with observers who are used to reading letter charts.

The Regan low contrast letter charts

We will mention these charts, not so much because we envisage them being used for children, but because readers may have come across mention of them in the literature. These were the first contrast sensitivity charts to use letters rather than gratings. However, the letters on one chart are all of the same contrast and vary in size, in a similar way to a visual acuity chart. In fact, this test is really a test of low contrast acuity rather than contrast sensitivity, although CS can be inferred from the results. The chart originally used five contrast levels (10, 22, 31, 64 and 93%), but now three levels are available (4, 7 and 96%). For clinical use the intermediate (7%) chart is recommended (Regan, 1988). There are data to support the assumption that the chart is mainly a measure of high and intermediate spatial frequencies (Owsley et al., 1990; Woo and Leat, 1995).

The Waterloo low contrast chart

This is similar to the Regan charts with the exception that only one contrast level, 10%, is available. The positioning of the letters is different, but the principle is basically that of the Regan chart, i.e. it is a test of low contrast acuity. Similarly to the Regan charts, it is mainly a measure of high and intermediate spatial frequencies (Woo and Leat, 1995).

LH symbols

These charts use the LH shapes (circle, square, house and apple) instead of letters and are based on the PR chart concept. However, there are five shapes per contrast level and the symbols are a 6/9.5 acuity size, which is significantly smaller than the PR letters when held at 1 m. In addition, the contrast steps do not form a true logarithmic scale, ranging from 0.22 to 0.4 log units between contrast levels. These differences make the results very difficult to compare with the PR chart and also mean that the single letter scoring does not hold. There is a matching response card for use with non-verbal children or those who do not know the shapes.

Cambridge low contrast gratings

The Cambridge low contrast gratings consist of 11 plates (plus one demonstration plate) of dot-matrix printed square-wave gratings (Wilkins, Della Sala and Nimmo-Smith, 1988). The plates are arranged in a book: there is one grating per page with the opposite page being equi-luminant but with no grating. The contrast of the gratings varies between 11% and 0.1% and the spatial frequency is 4 cycles per degree at a testing distance of 6 m. The position of the gratings is randomized, on the left or right page, and the task of the observer is to respond to the position of the gratings. The test can also be performed with the pages held vertically, in which case the gratings will either be on the bottom or top page. This latter method may be easier for children who confuse left and right. Thus, this test is suitable for preliterate children who can respond by pointing or by verbalizing (up/down), or even by eye movements (preferential looking).

A testing distance of 6 m was originally suggested. However, for low vision observers a closer working distance will be necessary, for example, 1.5 m, at which the gratings become 1 cycle per degree. As stated above, we are generally interested in measuring intermediate and lower spatial frequencies, and this is an additional reason for using the Cambridge gratings at a working distance closer than 6 m. The method of use is to start with the highest contrast grating (demonstration plate) and the observer responds regarding the position of the grating, being asked to guess if unsure (i.e. it is a two-alternative forced-choice procedure). Progressively lower-contrast gratings are displayed until the observer makes an error. The plate on which the first error is made is recorded. The examiner goes back four plates and starts the descending trials again. This procedure is done four times resulting in four plate numbers. The final four plate numbers are summed and the CS is read off a table supplied. It is important to ensure that the descending series does not always commence with the same plate, as the observer may start to learn the sequence. The original suggested procedure, to go back four plates, was made on the assumption that an error will not always be made on the same plate. However, the examiner can also introduce more variability if necessary by going back more than four plates or by turning the book through 180 degrees in order to change the sequence. We do not have substantial data for children with this test. However, it has been found that, for 10–19 year olds, at a test distance of 6 m, the lower limit of normal at the 95% confidence limit is a total score (sum of plates) of 22, which corresponds with a CS of 130 (Wilkins, Della Sala and Nimmo-Smith, 1988). Any lower score would be suspected as abnormal.

The Cambridge gratings have been compared against CS as measured on an oscilloscope. Woo and Leat (1995) found that the Cambridge gratings were a good estimate of contrast sensitivity for low spatial frequencies, when used at a distance of 1 m, as would be expected from theory. It was also found that CS, as measured with the

Cambridge gratings in a group of low vision observers, did correlate with reading speed (with the appropriate optical magnifier). Their results predict that a CS of at least 120 is required for fluent reading.

Mr Happy

Mr Happy is a test of CS developed for children by Bailey at the University of Berkeley, California, and is based on preferential looking responses. It is a dot matrix printed smiley face on one card and this is held alongside a blank card. Thus it can be used in a preferential looking manner. The face is made up of contours 12 mm wide, which is slightly wider than the 10 mm letter widths of the Pelli–Robson chart. The contrast levels are roughly in logarithmic steps, although the step sizes are larger than for the PR chart, being in octave steps, and there are an additional few contrast levels included (Table 8.1). This test promises to be very useful for children, although few data are currently available. A preliminary study showed that 96% of normally-sighted children aged 2–3 years were able to respond to the lowest contrast level (1.6%) while 100% of those aged 3–5 could do so (Fisher, Orel-Bixler and Bailey, 1995).

Table 8.1 Contrast levels of the Mr Happy test. Contrast levels in bold are those which are additional to the logarithmic scale

Contrast %	CS	LogCS
80	1.3	0.1
44	2.2	0.35
25	4	0.6
10	10	1.0
8	**12.5**	**1.1**
6.3	**16**	**1.2**
5	20	1.3
3.2	32	1.5
1.6	64	1.8

The method of use is similar to the Hiding Heidi test (see below). It is important that a large enough testing distance is used so that the child cannot resolve the individual dots which make up the face pattern. For most children with normal vision, this means a test distance of 3 m, but 1 m is a common testing distance used for children with low vision.

Hiding Heidi

This test, developed by Hyvarinen, is similar to the Mr Happy test, but with fewer contrast levels (Table 8.2). It is not dot-matrix printed, but uses actual printed grey levels. As with Mr Happy, two cards are held and the child is asked to choose the one with the face. The response can be pointing, verbalizing or preferential looking. One slight disadvantage is the fact that the face is made up of lines of more

Table 8.2 Contrast levels, CS and logCS for the Hiding Heidi CS Test

Contrast %	CS	LogCS
100	1	0
25	4	0.6
10	10	1
5	20	1.3
2.5	40	1.6
1.25	80	1.9

than one width and this makes it difficult to know which line widths are being used for detecting the face. However, the main outline of the face subtends the same angle as the letter stroke widths of the PR letters, therefore at 1 m we can assume that the spatial frequencies being detected are similar to those of the PR chart. It is certainly a test of low frequency contrast sensitivity when held at this distance. By this argument, the data gained from the PR chart can be applied to Hiding Heidi. Thus a logCS of less than 0.75, = contrast threshold of less than 10%, would predict a maximum reading speed of 40 words per minute.

There are few instructions regarding the mode of use of these tests. We therefore suggest the following for the Hiding Heidi cards. Use a working distance of 1 m. Start with the highest contrast and present the face card and the control (absent face) card (Figure 8.5). If the child responds clearly and correctly, go to the next lowest contrast. Randomize whether the control card is right or left. (This can be done by turning away from the child and then turning back holding the card.) Continue until a wrong or unclear response is obtained. Repeat the card with the previous contrast. Take the CS as the lowest contrast at which clear and correct responses are obtained. Usually with this procedure, the examiner will be aware of where the face is. To use this test in a forced choice preferential looking format, the examiner can either shuffle the cards without looking until unaware of where the face is, or use another observer who does not know on which side the face is presented.

It will be noticed that this procedure is very similar to that used with acuity preferential looking cards except that, in the case of the Teller cards, it is usual to decrease the acuity by one octave (a factor of 2), which means using every other card, since the Teller card acuity decreases in 0.5 octave steps (Chapter 7). In the case of the Hiding Heidi cards it will be noted that the contrast decreases by a factor of two (approximately) between each card (i.e. the half-octave steps are missing). Thus, by using every card, we are using the same size steps as when we use every other Teller card.

Cardiff Contrast Test

A new test, yet to be released onto the market, is the Cardiff Contrast Test. The principle, and method of using the test, is the same as that described in Chapter 7 for the Cardiff Acuity Test. The test uses the

Fig. 8.5
Child performing Hiding Heidi
contrast sensitivity test.

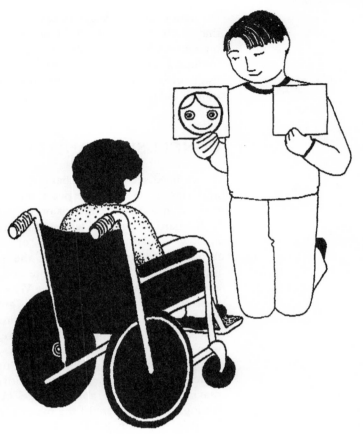

principle of preferential looking, where a child looks towards, or
points to a picture positioned near the top or bottom of a card. The
test has been designed for use with children too young for the Pelli–
Robson test. It has 14 contrast levels from 67.4% to 0.75%, with the
contrast doubling every two steps. This represents a CS of 1.56 to
133.33, in logarithmic steps, which is equivalent to the Pelli–Robson
chart. There is only one size of target, equivalent to 2 cycles per
degree at a viewing distance of 50 cm. Readers are encouraged to look
out for this new test.

A new adaptation of the Vistech chart

Adams et al. (1992) suggest an interesting use of the Vistech chart.
They used the grating patches of the Vistech to form a preferential
looking test. They cut out the Vistech grating patches and stuck them
on a grey card, similar in size to a Teller acuity card. On one side was
the grating patch and on the other side a luminance-matched patch (a
very low contrast grating which is below the adult's threshold). These
are used with a similar procedure to acuity card testing (Chapter 7).
This use of the Vistech allows repeated presentations at each spatial

frequency, should that be necessary, as the card can be rotated. Using this method, Adams and Courage (1993) showed an increase in binocular CS at each spatial frequency and a shift of the peak to higher frequencies over the age range 3–36 months. The testing (at 5 spatial frequencies) took an average total time of 12 minutes for the 36 month olds.

CONCLUSIONS AND RECOMMENDATIONS

As we have seen in this chapter, contrast sensitivity is of functional importance, in some respects more so than visual acuity. Nevertheless, in terms of child vision care, there are limitations at present with regard to available tests and norms. We feel that a measure of CS at low spatial frequencies is of more interest than at higher frequencies. This is based on the results of many studies which indicate that CS at intermediate and low frequencies is relevant to everyday life. Additionally, since VA will have already been measured, measuring CS at higher frequencies gives little additional information. Therefore we recommend that for literate children the Pelli–Robson would be the chart of choice. For preliterate children and for others who are not able to respond to letters, we recommend either the Mr Happy or the Hiding Heidi test. Purchase of these tests (PR plus either Mr Happy or Hiding Heidi) would allow testing in the maximum age and ability range currently possible with clinical testing. The suppliers of the major tests discussed in this chapter are listed in Appendix 8.1.

REFERENCES

Abramov, I., Hainline, L., Turkel, J. et al. (1984). Rocket-ship psychophysics, assessing visual function in young children. *Investigative Ophthalmology and Vision Science*, 2, 1307–1315.

Adams, R.J. and Courage, M.L. (1993). Contrast sensitivity in 24- and 36-month-olds as assessed with the contrast sensitivity card procedure. *Optometry and Vision Science*, 70, 97–101.

Adams, R., Mercer M.E., Courage, M.L. and van Hof-van Duin, J. (1992). A new technique to measure contrast sensitivity in human infants. *Optometry and Vision Science*, 69, 440–446.

Arden, G.B. (1988). Testing contrast sensitivity in clinical practice. *Clinical Vision Science*, 2, 213–224.

Atkinson, J., Braddick, O. and Moar, K. (1977). Development of contrast sensitivity over the first 3 months of life in the human infant. *Vision Research*, 17, 1037–1044.

Atkinson, J., French, J. and Braddick, O. (1981). Contrast sensitivity of preschool children. *British Journal of Ophthalmology*, 65, 525–529.

Banks, M.S. and Bennett, P.J. (1988). Optical and photoreceptor immaturities limit the spatial and chromatic vision of human neonates. *Journal of the Optical Society of America*, 5, 2059–2079.

Banks, M.S. and Salapatek, P. (1976). Contrast sensitivity function of the infant visual system. *Vision Research*, 16, 867–869.

Bradley, A. and Freeman, R.D. (1982). Contrast sensitivity in children. *Vision Research*, 22, 953–959.

Buncic, J.R. and Tytla, M. (1989). Spatial contrast sensitivity impairment in optic nerve head swelling. *Neuro-ophthalmology*, 9, 293–298.

Campbell, F.W. and Green, D.G. (1965). Optical and retinal factors affecting visual resolution. *Journal of Physiology*, **181**, 576–593.

De Valois, R.L. and De Valois, K.K. (1988). Spatial Vision. In *Oxford Psychology* series No.14. Oxford/New York, Oxford University Press.

Dickenson, C.M. and Rabbit, P.M.A. (1991). Simulated visual impairment: effects on text comprehension and reading speed. *Clinical Vision Science*, **6**, 301–308.

Elliott D.B., Hurst, M.A. and Weatherill, J. (1990). Comparing clinical tests of visual function in cataract with the patient's perceived visual disability. *Eye*, **4**, 712–717.

Elliott D.B., Sanderson, K. and Conkey, A. (1990). The reliability of the Pelli–Robson contrast sensitivity chart. *Ophthalmic and Physiological Optics*, **10**, 21–24.

Elliott D.B. and Whitaker, D. (1992). How useful are contrast sensitivity charts in optometric practice? Case reports. *Optometry and Vision Science*, **69**, 378–385.

Elliott, D.B. and Bullimore, M.A. (1993). Assessing the reliability, discriminibility, and validity of disability glare tests. *Investigative Ophthalmology and Vision Science*, **34**, 108–119.

Faye, E.E., Padula, W.V., Padula J.B. et al. (1984). The low vision child. In E.E. Faye (ed.), *Clinical Low Vision*. Boston/Toronto, Little, Brown, pp. 437–475.

Fisher, S., Orel-Bixler, D. and Bailey, I. (1995). Mr Happy contrast sensitivity test: a behavioral test for infants and children. *Optometry and Vision Science*, **72** (Suppl), 204.

Ginsberg, A.P. (1978). Visual information processing based upon spatial filters constrained by biological data. PhD dissertation. Cambridge University. Reprinted as AFAMRL Tech Rep 78-129 Library of Congress 79-600156.

Ginsberg, A.P. (1996). Next generation contrast sensitivity testing. In B.P. Rosenthal and R.G. Cole (eds.) *Functional Assessment of Low Vision*. St Louis, Mosby.

Haegerstrom-Portnoy, G. (1993). New procedures for evaluating vision functions of special populations. *Optometry and Vision Science*, **70**, 306–314.

Hess, R.F., Campbell, F.W. & Zimmern, R. (1980). Differences in the neural basis of human amblyopias: the effect of mean luminance. *Vision Research*, **20**, 295–305.

Kiorpes, L. and Kiper, D.C. (1996). Development of contrast sensitivity across the visual field in macaque monkeys. *Vision Research*, **36**, 239–247.

Leat, S.J. and Woo, G.C. (1997). The validity of current tests of contrast sensitivity and their ability to predict reading speed in low vision. *Eye*, **11**, 893–899.

Leat, S.J. and Woodhouse, J.M. (1993). Reading performance with low vision aids: relationship with contrast sensitivity. *Ophthalmic and Physiological Optics*, **13**, 9–16.

Legge, G.E., Pelli, D.G., Rubin, G.S. and Schleske, M.M. (1985). Psychophysics of reading–I. Normal vision. *Vision Research*, **25**, 239–252.

Legge, G.E., Ross, J.A., Maxwell, T. and Luebker, A. (1989). Psychophysics of reading – VII. Comprehension in normal and low vision. *Clinical Vision Science*, **4**, 51–60.

Leguire, L.E. (1991). Do letter charts measure contrast sensitivity? *Clinical Vision Science* **6**, 391–400.

Lennerstrand, G. and Ahlstrom, C. (1989). Contrast sensitivity in macular degeneration and the relation to subjective impairment. *Acta Ophthalmologica*, **67**, 225–233.

Loshin, D.S. and White, J. (1984). Contrast sensitivity. The visual rehabilitation of the patient with macular degeneration. *Archives of Ophthalmology*, **102**, 1303–1306.

Marron, J.A. and Bailey, I.L. (1982). Visual factors and orientation-mobility performance. *American Journal of Optometry and Physiological Optics*, **59**, 413–426.

Movshon, J.A. and Kiorpes, L. (1988). Analysis of the development of spatial contrast sensitivity in monkey and human infants. *Journal of the Optical Society of America*, **5**, 2166–2172.

Norcia, A.M., Tyler, C.W. and Hamer, R. (1990). Development of contrast sensitivity in the human infant. *Vision Research*, **30**, 1475–1486.

Owsley, C., Sekuler, R. and Siemsen, D. (1983). Contrast sensitivity throughout adulthood. *Vision Research*, **23**, 689–699.

Owsley, C. and Sloane, M. (1987). Contrast sensitivity, visual acuity and perception of 'real world' targets. *British Journal of Ophthalmology* **71**, 791–796.

Owsley, C., Sloane, M.E., Shalka, H.W. and Jackson, C.A. (1990). A comparison of the Regan low-contrast letter charts and contrast sensitivity testing in older patients. *Clinical Vision Science* **5**, 325–334.

Pelli, D.G., Robson, J.G. and Wilkins, A.J. (1988). The design of a new letter chart for measuring contrast sensitivity. *Clinical Vision Science*, **2**, 187–199.

Peterzell, D.H., Werner, J.S. and Kaplan, P.S. (1993). Individual differences in contrast sensitivity functions: the first four months of life in humans. *Vision Research*, **33**, 381–396.

Reeves, B.C., Wood, J.M. and Hill, A.R. (1991). Vistech VCTS 6500 charts – within- and between-session reliability. *Optom Vis Sci.*, **68**, 728–737.

Regan, D. (1988). Low-contrast letter charts and sinewave grating tests in ophthalmological and neurological disorders. *Clinical Vision Science* **2**, 235–250.

Rosner, J. and Rosner, J. (1990). In *Pediatric Optometry*, 2nd edn. Boston, Butterworths.

Rubin, G.S. (1988). Reliability and sensitivity of clinical contrast sensitivity tests. *Clinical Vision Science* **2**, 169–177.

Rubin, G.S., Roche, K.B., Prasda-Rao, P. and Fried, L.P. (1994). Visual impairment and disability in the elderly. *Optom Vis Sci.*, **71**, 750–760.

Shannon, E., Skoczenski, A.M. and Banks, M.S. (1996). Retinal illuminance and contrast sensitivity in human infants. *Vision Research* **36**, 67–76.

Tytla, M.E. and Buncic, J.R. (1988). Optic nerve compression impairs low spatial frequency in man. *Clinical Vision Science*, **2**, 179–186.

Westall, C.A., Woodhouse, J.M., Saunders, K. et al. (1992). Problems measuring contrast sensitivity in children. *Ophthalmic and Physiological Optics*, **12**, 244–248.

Whittaker, G.S. and Lovie-Kitchin, J. (1993). Visual requirements for reading. *Optometry and Vision Science*, **70**, 54–65.

Wilkins, A.J., Della Sala, L. and Nimmo-Smith, I. (1988). Age-related norms for the Cambridge Low Contrast Gratings, including details concerning their design and use. *Clinical Vision Science*, **2**, 201–212.

Williamson, T.H., Strong, N.P., Sparrow, J. et al. (1992). Contrast sensitivity and glare in cataract using the Pelli–Robson chart. *British Journal of Ophthalmology*, **76**, 719–722.

Wilson, H.R. (1988). Development of spatio-temporal mechanisms in infant vision. *Vision Research*, **28**, 611–628.

Woo, G.C. and Leat, S.J. (1995). Contrast sensitivity assessment in low vision and the validity of current tests of contrast sensitivity. Proceedings of 10th Asian Pacific Optometric Congress, Singapore.

Appendix 8.1

Contrast sensitivity test suppliers

Cambridge Low Contrast Gratings; Clement Clarke International Ltd., Airmed House, Edinburgh Way, Harlow, Essex CM20 2ED. Tel. (UK) 01-279-635232; or 3128 East 17th Ave., Suite D, Columbus, Ohio. Tel. (US) 1-614-478-2777 or 1-800-848-8923.

Hiding Heidi Contrast Sensitivity Test; Vision Associates, 7512 Dr Phillips Boulevard, Orlando, FL 32819, USA. Tel. 407-352-1200. Fax 407-352-5632.

LH Low Contrast Symbols; Vision Associates, 7512 Dr Phillips Boulevard, Orlando, FL 32819, USA. Tel. 407-352-1200. Fax 407-352-5632 or from the Lighthouse Inc. 36-02 Northern Boulevard, Long Island City, NY 11101. Tel. 718-937-6959 or 1-800-453-4923. Fax 718-786-0437.

Mr Happy Contrast Sensitivity Test; Precision Vision, 721, N Addison Rd., Villa Park, IL 60181, USA. Tel. 708-833-1454. Fax 708-833-1520.

Pelli–Robson Chart; Clement Clarke International Ltd., Airmed House, Edinburgh Way, Harlow, Essex CM20 2ED. Tel. (UK) 01-279-635232; or 3128 East 17th Ave., Suite D, Columbus, OH. Tel. (US) 1-614-478-2777 or 1-800-848-8923.

Vistech Gratings; VTCS from Vistech Consultants, 4162, Little York Rd., Dayton, OH 45414-5829, USA. Tel. 513-454-1399. Fax 513-454-1355.
The newer FACT version of this chart is available from Stereo Optical Co., 3539, N Kenton, Chicago, IL 40583. Tel. 1-8001354-7848. Fax 606-259-4926.

Waterloo Low Contrast Letter Chart; Now available from the Waterloo Optometry Student Society, School of Optometry, University of Waterloo, Waterloo, Ontario N2L 3G1.

Regan Low Contrast Letter Charts; Paragon Services, 148, Davis Drive, Beaverbank B4G 1E2, Nova Scotia, Canada. Tel. 902-865-4216. Fax 902-865-8587.

9

Binocular vision

INTRODUCTION

In this chapter we describe the binocular processes of human vision, the visual system that emerges from normal and abnormal binocular development, the development of binocular mechanisms and the clinical testing of binocular vision. The chapter begins with a basic overview to give the non-specialist a baseline knowledge of terminology and definitions. Eye-care practitioners may want to skip over the section on binocularity and the visual pathway, but will hopefully learn new information relating to the development of binocular vision and stereopsis. The section on clinical testing of stereopsis should give some ideas about which tests to use in the oculovisual assessment of infants and toddlers.

We will cover basic information about the cover test and popular tests of sensory fusion and stereopsis. We will not describe the details of measuring and interpreting the sensory adaptations to binocular vision that has not developed normally; these details can be found in other texts concentrating on binocular testing (Griffin, 1976; von Noorden, 1996).

BINOCULARITY AND THE VISUAL PATHWAY

Binocular vision is normally single vision; we do not usually perceive double images. Yet we have two eyes, and our visual perception arises from two retinal images. This phenomenon is so natural to us that the naive observer is not surprised by it (von Noorden, 1990). Perhaps this should be much more surprising: how can two retinal images combine to create the perception of one? The singleness of vision is maintained even when we move our eyes. We can look right, left, up, or down and our visual world is still one of unity. We can easily lose this unity, however: by looking at a small object with both eyes open and placing a finger gently on the lateral side of one eye to push the globe of the eye slightly, we can experience double vision.

Before continuing, it may be important to refresh our knowledge of the visual pathways (Chapter 1, Figure 1.8). The optics of the eye create an image on the retina. The retina then transmits signals via the optic nerve to the optic chiasm, where there is partial decussation – a crossing of some, but not all, of the nerve fibres. The nasal fibres (those from the side of each eye closest to the nose), but not the temporal fibres (those closest to the temples), cross before continuing to the brain. This partial decussation effectively means that the left visual field – the part of the image carried by the nasal fibres (that is, the nasal projections) of the left eye and the temporal projections of the right eye – 'travel' or project to the right visual cortex, and the right visual field projects to the left visual cortex.

Remember that each eye's projection remains separate up to the level of the visual cortex. The primary visual cortex (the first visual area of the brain, V1) is where the projections from the right and left eye combine upon the binocular cells of the visual cortex.

Corresponding and non-corresponding retinal points

The horizontal separation of the eyes causes each eye to view the world from a slightly different vantage point. The resulting difference in monocular perceptions means that objects at different depths stimulate different retinal areas. Points on the right and left retinae that respond to the same visual direction are *corresponding points;* images that fall on corresponding points are perceived as coming from the same location in our field of view. Retinal points of the left and right retinae that do not correspond are disparate points; they respond to differing visual directions. Objects closer to the observer than the point of fixation are seen in crossed disparity and objects farther than the point of fixation are in uncrossed disparity.

When the child looks at the toucan (Figure 9.1a) he will see a toucan with a large beak. He will also notice a tree in the background. When he looks at the toucan's left eye, he would see that the tip of toucan's beak is a little in front of the toucan's eyes, and the tree is behind the toucan's eyes.

What is happening on the retina to give this picture? If the child were to gaze into the toucan's left eye (point E; Figure 9.1a, top), then retinal images of the toucan's eye (E) would fall on the child's fovea (labelled as e; Figure 9.1b). These retinal points correspond. Objects to the right and left of any point of fixation (point E in this specific case) which lie along a specific concave surface – the horopter (Figure 9.1b) provide images to the right and left eyes which correspond. Binocular cells of the visual cortex that respond to a disparity of zero would be activated and single binocular vision with sensory fusion results. Objects nearer or further than the point of fixation, e.g. point B (the toucan's beak) and point T (the tree), would stimulate disparate retinal areas. The beak B (imaged at retinal point b) is seen in crossed disparity. The tree T (imaged at retinal point t) is seen in uncrossed disparity. If the disparity is small, the object would still be seen with binocular single vision, but at a different depth plane to the point of fixation. For example, object B which lies within 'Panum's Fusional area' has a small disparity. This area encompasses those disparate retinal points, stimulation of which results in singleness of vision with the ability to judge relative depth. Once the disparity exceeds the range of disparities that excite binocular cells of the visual

Fig. 9.1

(a) The toucan has a big beak (B), and there is a tree (T) behind the toucan. The child is sitting, looking at the toucan. Specifically, the child is gazing into the left eye (E) of the toucan. **(b)** This figure shows how the toucan and the tree are imaged on the retinae of the child. The retinal image of the toucan's left eye is labelled (e), beak (b) and tree (t). Rays from E fall on the right and left eye fovea; these points are corresponding. Rays from B fall on points in the right and left eyes which are disparate. The disparity is small enough to allow B to be seen in binocular single vision, but in a different depth plane to E. Rays from T also fall on disparate retinal points in each eye. The disparity is larger than Panum's fusional area, resulting in a loss of singleness of vision. While gazing at the toucan's left eye, the child will see two trees.

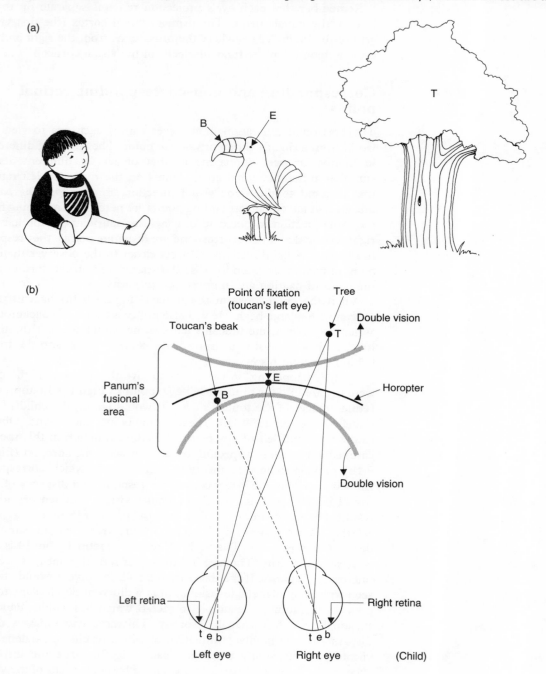

cortex (e.g. point T), and therefore lies outside of Panum's fusional area, then double vision (diplopia) of tree T results.

As we saw in Chapters 7 and 8, an object must be more than a certain size and contrast level in order to be seen. Likewise, in stereoscopic depth perception, an object must exceed a minimum disparity to be seen in depth – *the stereo-threshold*. This varies according to the type of visual stimulus, and also varies between individuals according to factors such as age and the presence of certain ocular conditions. Under ideal conditions the stereo-threshold can be as small as 7 seconds of arc. A stereo-threshold of 15 to 30 seconds found in clinical tests is considered excellent (von Noorden, 1996, p. 27).

Unlike other visual processes, there is also a maximum disparity for the detection of depth. If a disparity exceeds this amount, then double vision (diplopia) results, and the perception of depth diminishes. The upper limits of the range of single binocular vision represent the limits of Panum's fusional area. Panum's fusional area depends on many factors. In the midline, it can be a few minutes to over one degree of arc, but to the right and left of the midline it may be as much as several degrees.

The retinal image of an actual object covers a finite area on the retina; the concept of corresponding retinal points expands to that of corresponding retinal areas. When the retinal image of an object falls on corresponding retinal areas, binocular cells of the visual cortex responding to zero disparity are activated; the object will be seen as one fused surface. When the image of an object falls on disparate retinal areas, then either it is seen in depth, or diplopic images are seen, depending on the degree of disparity.

BINOCULAR SINGLE VISION

Normal functioning of sensory fusion, motor fusion and accommodative vergence will usually mean that binocular depth perception (stereopsis) will be possible.

Sensory fusion

When the retinal images of an object fall on corresponding retinal areas, binocular cells of the visual cortex that respond to zero disparity are activated. A single, fused, percept with no depth will then be seen.

When right- and left-eye foveal images are similar in size and shape, the visual cortex fuses the two images into a single percept. Binocular single vision depends on the capability of brain mechanisms to combine the two retinal images from an object into a single visual image. Such a mechanism is called *sensory fusion*.

Motor fusion

As demonstrated by our experiment on causing diplopia (see p. 216, pressing on globe), binocular single vision also depends on accurate registration of the movements of the two eyes. This precise motor coordination is called *motor fusion*. The disparity vergence system (see Chapter 12) is responsible for precise motor fusion, which acts to maintain sensory fusion. When an object of interest does not coincide with the point of intersection of the two visual axes, binocular cells responding to the resulting disparity trigger disparity vergence eye movements. The eyes then either converge or diverge to fixate on the object (see Chapter 12 for a more detailed description).

Accommodative vergence

Accommodation is the increase in the dioptric power of the eye required to see a near target clearly. Linked to the change in accommodation is a change in vergence acting to bring the lines of sight of the two eyes in line with the near target (Chapter 12). This type of vergence is called accommodative convergence, as opposed to the disparity vergence eye movements mentioned under Motor fusion. Ideally, accommodation and convergence would be in precise register – the amount of accommodation required for precise focus at a specific distance having an equivalent convergence requirement for precise alignment of the visual axes. This is rarely the case. The convergence that each of us makes to a specific change in accommodation may be larger or smaller than that actually required. The accommodative convergence/accommodation (AC/A) ratio is the amount of convergence measured in prism dioptres per unit (dioptre) change in accommodation.

Stereopsis

Retinal disparity, which results in the perception of depth, is the basis of stereopsis (stereoscopic vision). Stereopsis allows us to perceive depth independently of monocular cues such as relative size, overlap and perspective.

VISUAL ALIGNMENT AND OCULAR DEVIATIONS

Normally the axes of the two eyes intercept at the object of regard. Sometimes, however, the eyes are misaligned. A misalignment of the visual axes is called strabismus or heterotropia (tropia for short): one eye fixates the object accurately, while the other turns in another direction (Figure 9.2).

When the visual axis points inwards, or over-converges, this is called an esodeviation or esotropia. Alternatively, the visual axis may point out or under-converge: this exodeviation is called an exotropia.

Fig. 9.2
Child with strabismus. Notice how
the right eye is turned inwards.

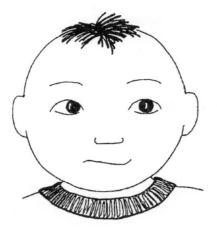

Other types of strabismus are hypertropia (one eye pointing upwards) or hypotropia (one eye pointing downwards).

Strabismus may be comitant (sometimes described as concomitant), which means having the same angle of deviation in all directions of gaze, or incomitant (may be described as inconcomitant), having different angles of deviation according to the direction of gaze. Comitant strabismus may result from developmental abnormalities of the sensory binocular vision system and its links to the oculomotor system. Incomitant strabismus results from abnormalities of the extraocular muscles or their innervation. As this chapter is concerned with the development of the sensory binocular system, comitant deviations are discussed here.

The strabismus might be present all the time (constant), or just occasionally (intermittent). A child might have a strabismus for all targets (near or distant), near targets only or distant targets only. The strabismus may affect one eye only, or either eye may turn at different times (alternating strabismus). For example, a child with esotropia might have a right esotropia, a left esotropia, or an alternating esotropia. In the latter case there is alternation between which eye turns in.

Some forms of ocular deviation are detectable in people with normal binocular vision. A heterophoria (phoria for short) is a latent deviation of the visual axes. If visual fusion is disrupted, for example by a cover being placed over one eye, the eyes may take up a position of slight convergence (esophoria) or divergence (exophoria). Small amounts of phoria are common in a visually normal population; it is very unusual to find a person with orthophoria (no deviation).

An esodeviation is the latent (esophoria) or manifest (esotropia) convergent misalignment of the visual axes. Esodeviations are the most common form of misalignment in childhood. Similarly, an exophoria is the latent divergence of the visual axes, and exotropia is the manifest deviation. Hyperphorias refer to latent vertical deviations which are uncommon in a visually normal population.

Misalignment of the visual axes are described in units of prism dioptres or in degrees. A prism dioptre is the power of a prism that displaces the visual axis by 1 cm at a distance of 1 m, and is equivalent to 0.57 degrees of arc. Both units, prism dioptres and degrees, are used in this chapter.

STRABISMUS

Infantile or early-onset strabismus

Strabismus that occurs before 6 months of age is called infantile or early-onset strabismus (von Noorden, 1996, p. 308). Typically, the strabismus is convergent (esotropia) and the angle of strabismus is large, over 30 prism dioptres. Infantile strabismus is more commonly alternating and is usually not associated with a refractive error larger than normal. In contrast, exotropia present in the first 6 months of age is rare and may be associated with neurological impairment (American Academy of Ophthalmology, 1994, p. 301).

Early-onset strabismus is frequent in children with neurological disorders. For example, up to 30% of children with cerebral palsy or hydrocephalus have strabismus (American Academy of Ophthalmology, 1994, p. 289).

Acquired strabismus

Esotropia occurring after 6 months of age is defined as acquired strabismus (von Noorden, 1996, p. 321). The most common type of acquired esotropia is accommodative esotropia, of which there are two types, refractive and non-refractive. The first type is associated with high hyperopia (Chapter 5) and a normal accommodative convergence/accommodation ratio (AC/A ratio—see below). The second type is associated with a high AC/A ratio. In the first category of esotropia, a spectacle prescription incorporating the appropriate lenses of positive power (Chapter 5) reduces the accommodation exerted. This is then associated with a reduction in accommodative vergence, and therefore a reduction in the angle of esotropia (Chapter 14). The second type manifests mainly at near and requires modification of the AC/A ratio. This could be accomplished by refractive correction of the near esotropia with bifocals or drugs which modify the AC/A ratio.

Other children may have become esotropic because of a prior esophoria at near distances which the fusion mechanisms cannot continue to control; the phoria decompensates resulting in an esotropia.

Von Noorden (1996, p. 344) quotes studies that have found that the prevalence of exodeviations is about one-third that of esodeviations. Exotropia is defined as the basic type when exodeviation is the same at both far and near distances. Divergence excess exotropia occurs when the exodeviation is greater for distance sight than near. Conversely, convergence insufficiency exotropia exists when the near exodeviation is greater than the distance exodeviation. The exodeviation may be a constant exotropia, an intermittent exotropia or an exophoria.

Jampolsky (cited in von Noorden, 1996, p. 344) has found that exotropia usually begins as an exophoria. A suppression scotoma forms (a 'blind spot' resulting from the fact that the brain suppresses part of the image arising from one eye); this inhibits sensory fusion, which causes the exophoria to decompensate into an intermittent or constant exotropia. Another relatively common form of exotropia is sensory exotropia due to monocular or binocular deprivation. Also, constant exotropia may result from a third-nerve palsy.

Children with exodeviations may present to the eye-care practitioner with obviously divergent visual axes. In cases of intermittent exotropia or exophoria, they may present with symptoms of eyestrain, double vision, headaches, or difficulty with prolonged reading.

Small angle strabismus/microtropia/monofixation syndrome

Readers may have come across different terminologies relating to strabismus with a small angle. There is much overlap between the different definitions, and different investigators may strongly advocate one of these labels.

Small angle strabismus and microtropia

A microtropia is strabismus with an ultra small angle (see von Noorden, 1996, pp. 326–330). The misalignment may not be detectable by the cover test (explained later in this chapter). Poor vision in one eye (amblyopia) is usually present and some degree of binocularity may be present, and stereopsis may be absent or reduced. A microtropia is a common finding after surgical alignment for early onset esotropia. In fact, a microtropia is considered a desirable outcome of strabismus surgery. The borderline between small angle strabismus and microtropia is poorly defined and confusing: von Noorden quotes some investigators who consider an angle of strabismus under 5 degrees to be a microtropia, while others would consider this to be a small angle strabismus.

Monofixation syndrome

There is a very large overlap between monofixation syndrome and microtropia, with von Noorden classifying monofixation syndrome as a type of microtropia. However, monofixation syndrome may occur in the absence of strabismus. It is associated with an inherent inability to fuse images focused on each macula. A small central scotoma of one eye is evident under binocular viewing, whereas peripheral fusion is normal (Parks, 1969). The clinical picture associated with monofixation syndrome varies. The child may have had strabismus or anisometropia. Sometimes, there is no strabismus, but a unilateral macular lesion may be apparent ophthalmoscopically. Sometimes, neither strabismus nor a macular lesion is evident. There is usually amblyopia (monocular visual loss), which may vary from less than two lines difference between the eyes (on a standard acuity chart) to more moderate levels of amblyopia. Stereopsis is present, but reduced. The amblyopic eye may, or may not, fixate with a non-foveal retinal area (eccentric fixation). Whatever the aetiology, a child with monofixation syndrome will not demonstrate fusion between the maculae of the two eyes.

When strabismus is associated with monofixation syndrome, the angle measured by the simultaneous cover test is small (less than 8 prism dioptres), and is usually increased when binocular fusion is disrupted with the alternate cover test (see later section). The type of strabismus present is usually esotropia. Peripheral fusion and some degree of stereopsis are present in monofixation syndrome; disparity vergence is normal; and the eyes continue to maintain their alignment for years. Monofixation syndrome should therefore be considered a minor binocular problem and a successful outcome of surgery for infantile strabismus. Indeed, in a study of infants with early-onset strabismus who had their eyes surgically aligned before 24 months of age, 12 out of 28 developed monofixation syndrome (Botet, Calhoun and Harley, 1981). This is a much higher proportion than in those whose eyes were aligned after this age.

DEVELOPMENT OF BINOCULAR SINGLE VISION AND STEREOPSIS

Binocular single vision and stereopsis cannot be demonstrated in newborn human infants, but they develop fairly quickly within the first few months. The development of binocular single vision and stereopsis have been studied by both behavioural (Chapter 6) and electrophysiological (Chapter 13) techniques.

Sensory fusion and stereopsis have been recorded using dynamic random-dot correlograms and dynamic random-dot stereograms, respectively (Braddick et al., 1980; Julesz, Kropfl and Petrig, 1980; Skarf et al., 1993). For details, see High-Tech for Assessing Binocular Single Vision and Stereopsis at the end of this chapter. Briefly, with the child wearing some form of glasses to separate the images to the two eyes, the correlogram alternates between two states, fused and unfused. Likewise, the stereogram alternates between disparate and fused states.

These two types of stimuli have been used for both electrophysiological (visual evoked potentials, VEP) and behavioural (forced-choice preferential looking, FPL-see Chapter 6) studies (Braddick, 1996). The stimulus for a correlogram test of FPL would consist of a display, one half of which contains an anti-correlated pattern, whilst the other half contains checks alternating between correlated and anti-correlated (Braddick, 1996). Likewise, for an FPL stereogram test, one half of the display would contain elements with a binocular disparity, while the other half would contain a fused pattern.

Sensory fusion

Infants do not respond to VEP dynamic random-dot correlograms before about 8 weeks of age and the mean age for the onset of significant correlogram response is 10 weeks (Braddick 1996).

Studies using behavioural responses agree well with those using electrophysiological responses from infants. In a longitudinal study, Smith et al. (1988) tested the same infants with both FPL and VEP techniques. They found a strong correlation between the age of onset of a correlogram response by FPL and by VEP.

Stereopsis

Visual evoked potentials have also been used to study the development of stereopsis (Petrig et al., 1981; Braddick and Atkinson, 1983; Eizenman et al., 1989; Skarf et al., 1993). Onset of stereopsis using VEP has been found to be between 10 and 19 weeks (Petrig et al., 1981). Longitudinal studies have found that the youngest age that infants respond positively to a dynamic random-dot stereogram is about 8 weeks (Braddick, 1996). The mean age of onset has been found to be 10.7 weeks (Braddick, 1996).

Preferential looking techniques have also been widely used to investigate the development of stereopsis. FPL has been used to test for stereopsis using dynamic random-dot stereograms (Smith et al., 1988; Birch and Hale, 1989; Broadbent and Westall, 1990).

Held, Birch and Gwiazda (1980) and Birch, Gwiazda and Held (1982) have successfully measured the development of stereopsis using FPL with a line stereogram rather than the dynamic random-dot stereogram. The child wears polarized glasses, and is seated in front of two displays. One of the displays consists of three vertical bars with no disparity. The second display also contains three bars, but the middle bar has a binocular disparity. If stereopsis is present the child will preferentially look towards the display with the disparate stimulus.

Longitudinal studies using a variety of these techniques agree that stereopsis emerges between 3 and 5 months of age. Usually, no consistent response is found under 10 weeks of age, but after 11 weeks, some infants are able to discriminate stereoscopic depth (Birch, 1993).

Once stereopsis has been established, stereoacuity improves rapidly. Birch and coworkers (1982) used FPL, in response to the three-bar line stereogram, to assess the development of stereopsis. They found that once stereopsis was established, stereoacuity increased rapidly, going from 58 minutes of arc to 1 minute in 4–5 weeks. Stereoacuity of 1 minute of arc was reached by 8–12 months of age. Birch and Hale (1989), using an operant staircase procedure (Chapter 6), found the median stereoacuity to have reached 40 seconds of arc (the smallest disparity tested) by 31–36 months.

Correlations between onset of sensory fusion and onset of stereopsis

Petrig et al. (1981) were the first to suggest that the onset of cortical binocular fusion precedes stereopsis. Eizenman et al. (1989) found the onset of positive VEP to correlograms to precede that for stereograms. Smith and co-workers (1988) found little difference between the onset of correlogram and stereogram response. Braddick and Atkinson (1983) argue that it is difficult to interpret differences between stereopsis and fusion unless comparisons are made using closely similar stimuli and the same infants are tested by both procedures.

Mechanisms responsible for the development of binocular vision and stereopsis

The development of binocular processes depends on a number of factors. First, the sensory visual pathways must be functioning. The onset of binocular interactions is associated with increased resolution and sensitivity of the retina (Banks and Bennett, 1988; Wilson, 1988).

Held (1993) proposes a model for the development of stereopsis. In the mature visual system, the visual cortex (layers II to VI) is organized into vertical columns where cells above and below each other have similar properties. There are columns specific to different visual stimulus parameters, for example, columns are organized according to ocular dominance, i.e. right eye vs. left eye dominance. Signals entering the visual cortex, at layer IV (the input layer) come predominantly from either the right or left eye. Layers II, III, V, and VI contain binocular cells and receive input from layer IV (Daw, 1995). However, in early development, axons from both the right and left eyes synapse onto the same cells in layer IV, according to a theory proposed by Held (1993). These cells would therefore not carry information as to the origin (right eye or left) of any signal. Subsequently, the ocular dominance columns segregate and cells in layer IV retain eye-of-origin information. At this stage some cells outside of layer IV, at subsequent levels of visual processing, would respond to identical (corresponding) right and left retinal images while many other cells would respond to the stimulation of disparate retinal images.

This model is based on the finding that, before they demonstrate stereopsis, infants prefer interocularly rivalrous gratings over fused gratings (Shimojo et al., 1986). This may be because the rivalrous grating would present the binocular cells with a grid possessing more contours than a fused grating. This is the stage when disparity sensitivity begins. Later in development, binocularly fused gratings are preferred to rivalrous gratings, and disparity tuning begins. Hickey and Peduzzi (1987) have demonstrated well-formed ocular dominance columns in a 6-month-old infant, but poorly defined columns in the visual cortex of a 4 month old. From the studies of Birch and

Hale (1989), we have learnt that stereoacuity is improving during this time.

Also, the development of binocular single vision must be accompanied by the development of the disparity vergence control system. During development, sensory-oculomotor interaction undergoes considerable refinement. Eye movements appear to be conjugate most of the time in very young infants and active adjustments to convergence have been shown to occur by 1 month of age (Chapter 12). A feedback loop linking the binocular sensory system and the oculomotor systems evolves during the first few months of life, and it is possible that mechanisms for the development of this interaction are in place at birth. If the feedback loop between sensory and oculomotor systems were defective or absent, it would be impossible to achieve and maintain proper alignment of the eyes and strabismus would result.

Sensitive period of development

There is a sensitive period for the development of binocularity, during which connections to binocular neurons are in a plastic phase and can be broken down and re-formed. According to Banks, Aslin and Letson (1975), the sensitive period for the development of binocular vision starts a few months after birth and peaks between 1 and 3 years of age. If binocular anomalies have not been detected by this time, then treatment at a later stage will be less effective, whereas if treatment is started in the sensitive period, there is more chance of improvement.

Results from strabismic surgery in human infants suggest that binocular function is more likely to develop if the visual axes are aligned at an early age (Ing, 1983). Ing (1983) showed that 100% of the infants with early-onset esotropia who had surgery before 6 months showed peripheral fusion responses as determined by the Worth four-dot test at a near range and/or gross stereoacuity (200 to 3000 seconds of arc). In this study, infants who had surgery before age 2 were more likely to exhibit evidence of binocularity than those who had surgery later than this. A more recent study by Wright et al. (1994) showed that out of seven infants with early-onset esotropia who had had strabismus surgery between the 13th and 19th week of life, two achieved a stereoacuity of 40 seconds of arc as determined by the Titmus fly test (described later) and central fusion according to the Worth four-dot test at a distance (6 m).

The pros and cons of early surgery can be found in Chapter 14, but there does seem to be a greater consensus nowadays that if a child is to achieve some degree of binocularity, strabismus needs to be detected and treated before 2 years of age.

Binocular vision in the presence of strabismus

In human infants there have been reports of binocular vision in the presence of strabismus. Using preferential looking techniques and prismatically correcting the angle of deviation, Stager and Birch (1986) found that 60% of 4-month-old infants with early-onset esotropia demonstrated stereopsis, although this figure declined to 20% at 14 months. At the same time, the percentage of infants with normal binocular visual experience who demonstrate stereopsis increases from 60% to 100%. Interestingly, sensory fusion appears to be less disrupted than stereopsis by abnormal binocular experience. Responses to correlograms have been recorded from infants and children with esotropia (Eizenman et al., 1996; Westall et al., 1998a; 1998b). In all cases the angle of esotropia was corrected with Fresnel prisms. All children had periods of limited (or no) normal binocular visual experience. These data suggest that the sensory substrate of fusion is fairly robust against abnormal visual experience and is less affected by these experiences than the sensory substrate that supports stereopsis.

INTERACTIONS BETWEEN BINOCULAR SENSORY AND OCULAR ALIGNMENT SYSTEMS

Failure of the binocular sensory or the eye-movement system to develop normally can be associated with a number of visual or motor anomalies, such as strabismus, amblyopia, latent nystagmus, asymmetric optokinetic nystagmus (OKN, see Chapter 12), dissociated vertical divergence and ocular albinism.

In the first few months of life, the sensory visual system and oculomotor system are developing. Normal interactions between these developing systems result in the development of normal binocular vision and ocular alignment. Undetected abnormal interactions will often result in strabismus and amblyopia.

One of the most dramatic sensory anomalies found in strabismus is amblyopia, which is reduced visual acuity of one eye (von Noorden, 1996, p. 216). In a visual-impairment study (Flynn, 1991) sponsored by the National Eye Institute, amblyopia was found to be a leading cause of monocular visual loss in the 20–70+ age group, surpassing diabetic retinopathy, glaucoma, macular degeneration, and cataract.

CLINICAL ASSESSMENT OF OCULAR ALIGNMENT

In an infant or child, strabismus may be very apparent, or the angle of strabismus might be small enough not to be noticeable. Occasionally, there may appear to be strabismus where none actually exists; this is called a pseudostrabismus. Pseudostrabismus may be due to a facial asymmetry or epicanthal folds (von Noorden, 1996, p. 163). An epicanthal fold is a fold of skin, more pronounced in some infants than others, running downward from above the eye at the side of the nose. It makes the pupils of the eyes appear close to the nose, thereby simulating strabismus. Although we gain much through simple inspection of the eyes, it is often not sensitive enough to detect and quantify the presence of strabismus. Therefore specific tests must be used.

Cover test

There are three types of cover test: the cover/uncover test, the simultaneous prism-cover test, and the alternate cover test (American Academy of Ophthalmology, 1994, p. 271). The cover test requires the subject's attention and co-operation – not always available from small children. The target for the near cover test is one that requires the child to accommodate. A spot of light is not adequate. Small, brightly coloured toys or pictures may get a child's attention, especially if the examiner is able to create imaginative stories around the chosen target. The cover test should be done with and without the child wearing his or her glasses because a spectacle prescription can make a large difference to the presence or absence of strabismus, and to its size.

Cover/uncover test

This test is used to detect the presence of strabismus or phoria and with experience can be used to estimate the angle of deviation. The child is encouraged to look at the fixation target. It is usually easier to use a near fixation target for young children. However, the cover test should be done for both near (33 cm) and distance (6 m or 20 ft) fixation whenever possible. A cover (an occluder or a cover paddle) is placed in front of one eye of the examinee (Figure 9.3) while the examiner watches for movement of the uncovered eye: if the uncovered eye moves, the child probably has strabismus. The cover is removed as the examiner carefully watches for movement of the

Fig. 9.3 Cover test.

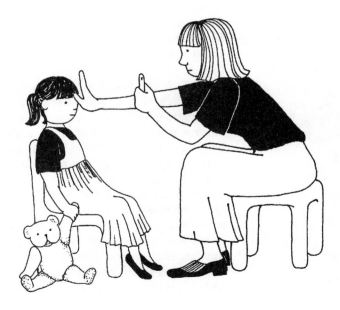

previously covered eye: if movement is seen only when the cover is removed, then a phoria is present. A phoria (the latent misalignment of visual axes) is detected only when binocular vision, and therefore fusion, has been interrupted. It is important to do the cover test, covering each eye in turn in order to detect a strabismus of either eye.

Monocular (right or left) strabismus. The eyes are misaligned before the cover is introduced. If the dominant (undeviated) eye of a child with one deviated eye is covered, then the strabismic eye will move to take up fixation. The eye will move in the direction opposite to the strabismus. A child with a right esotropia shows an outward movement of that eye when the left eye is covered; at the same time, the eye under cover will have moved inwards. When the cover is removed, the strabismic eye again takes up its deviated position and the eye previously under the cover moves out and fixates. When the strabismic eye is covered, no movement will be observed; the strabismic eye will stay in the deviated position. Thus to check for a right strabismus, the left eye is covered while the right eye is observed, and vice versa to check for left eye strabismus. If, when the cover is placed in front of the fixing eye of an infant or young child with strabismus, the child tries to push the cover out of the way, and the eye not being covered shows nystagmoid or searching eye movements, it is probable that the child has a deep amblyopia (von Noorden, 1996, p. 170).

Alternating strabismus. The cover test might be used to compare fixation preference in cases of alternating strabismus. If, during the cover test of each eye in turn, fixation quickly and freely alternates between the two eyes, then it can be assumed that the child has no fixation preference. This is the preferred state before surgical correction of strabismus (Chapter 14). If one eye is preferred – that is, one eye is the non-deviating eye for a larger proportion of the time, and especially if the other eye is slower to take up fixation – then it can be assumed that one eye is dominant and there may be some amblyopia present.

Phoria. If the child has a phoria, the eyes will be straight before the cover/uncover test. After the cover test there will be a momentary misalignment which then recovers back to orthophoria. Once the cover is placed in front of one eye, there will be deviation of that eye because of the interruption of fusion mechanisms. The eye not able to see the target takes up the position of phoria under the cover. If the eye is turned inwards, this is an esophoria; if turned outwards, an exophoria. When the eye is uncovered, it can be seen to move in the direction opposite to the phoria. A child with an esophoria will show an outwards movement of the eye that had been previously covered. Sometimes a child starts out with a phoria, but after prolonged testing the latent deviation dissociates into a manifest strabismus. This demonstrates that the child's fusional mechanisms are not coping well with intermittent disruptions.

The simultaneous prism-cover test

This test is used to quantify the amount of manifest deviation (strabismus) found with the cover/uncover test. It is an associated type of cover test, meaning that binocular vision, and therefore some degree of fusion, is allowed intermittently. The presence of a phoria therefore has little effect on the deviation. The result from the simultaneous prism-cover test will bear a closer resemblance to the amount of heterotropia the child exerts in his or her everyday environment. The child, wearing her or his correcting spectacles, is encouraged to look at a small coloured target held 33 cm from the child's eyes. As the fixing eye is covered, a correcting prism is immediately brought in front of the deviating eye. The test is repeated using increasingly higher prism power until no movement of the eye under the prism is observed. Again, if possible, the test is repeated for distance fixation.

The alternate cover test (prism and cover test)

This is a type of dissociated cover test, allowing no binocular fusion. The test measures the total deviation, both latent and manifest. The child is encouraged to look at a small, brightly coloured target. The cover is alternately placed in front of each eye, and passed back and forward several times. The eye care practitioner determines whether an eso- or exodeviation is present. An esodeviation results in a movement of the eyes 'against', i.e. in the opposite direction to, the cover, while an exodeviation results in a same direction or 'with' movement. A prism is held in front of one eye, with its base in for exodeviations and base out for esodeviations. The prism power is increased while the cover is alternated between the right and left eyes, until no movement is seen during the alternations. The amount of prism power required to neutralize the deviation is the measure of the total deviation: phoria plus tropia. The test is repeated for distance fixation, and the result with and without glasses is recorded.

The alternate cover test is very useful in helping with the diagnosis of monofixation syndrome. If a small angle of strabismus (less than 8 prism dioptres) has been found via the simultaneous prism-cover test, then it is important to do the alternate cover test. In the monofixation syndrome, the angle will often be larger when the eyes are dissociated and peripheral fusion mechanisms cannot function.

If the child is co-operative, the alternate cover test should be done in the secondary and tertiary directions of gaze: up, down, right, left, and the four oblique positions (see Griffin, 1976, p. 7). This test should be done with the child fixing with one eye, and then the other (von Noorden, 1990, p. 367). If the angle of strabismus is different in different directions of gaze, then the child has an incomitant strabismus. If the incomitancy is caused by a recent muscle paresis, a motor deficiency will be seen in the field of action of the paretic muscle (see Alpern, 1969, for a detailed text on actions of the extraocular muscles). Diagnosis of a long-standing paresis is complicated but important, because a recent paresis may indicate a serious health problem (von Noorden, 1990, p. 366).

Corneal light reflex test

This type of testing is not as accurate as the cover test, but it is useful in assessing ocular alignment in young infants or children who do not co-operate sufficiently for the cover test, or who have poor fixation.

Hirschberg test

In the Hirschberg test a penlight is held in front of the child's eyes. The corneal reflection of the light is observed. If the reflection is more towards the nasal side of the deviated eye exotropia is present, while if the light is more towards the temporal side the child has esotropia. Hirschberg calculated that each 1 mm of offset of the corneal reflex is equivalent to 7 degrees (15 prism dioptres) of misalignment (see von Noorden, 1996, p. 180). Since this time, others have argued over the precise mm/degree conversion factor. A value of 12 degrees per mm is more often used, although values ranging from 10.7 to 15.6 degrees per mm displacement have been reported (see von Noorden, 1996, p. 181). Difference would be accounted for by different reference landmarks, test distance (40 or 50 cm) or different calibration methods. This information presents the reader with the idea that this is rather a crude test.

Modified Krimsky's test

The modified Krimsky's test is another of the corneal light reflex tests. A penlight is held 33 cm from the child's dominant eye (if the dominance is known). The corneal reflex from the deviating eye will be shifted in the opposite direction to the deviation. Prisms are placed in front of the dominant eye. The power of prism that centres the reflex in the deviating eye is a measure of the approximated angle of deviation.

For more details on cover tests and corneal reflection tests, see American Academy of Ophthalmology, 1994, pp. 271–274.

Calculation of the AC/A ratio

The AC/A ratio can be calculated from a knowledge of the distance and near ocular deviations. The deviation is measured for distance fixation (greater than 6 m or 20 ft) with the child wearing her or his full spectacle correction. This is assumed to be the angle of deviation with zero accommodation. The deviation is then measured for near (33 cm) fixation. It is assumed that the convergence required will be linked to the amount of accommodation exerted. The AC/A ratio is derived from the equation:

$$AC/A = \frac{PD + dev_n - dev_d}{D}$$

PD is the interpupillary distance measured in cm, dev_n and dev_d are the near and distance deviations; and D is the near fixation distance in dioptres. In these calculations esodeviations are considered to be positive, and exodeviations negative. The normal range of AC/A ratio should be close to the PD in cm. Values above this indicate excessive accommodative convergence; values below this indicate insufficient accommodative vergence (von Noorden, 1996, p. 90).

CLINICAL ASSESSMENT OF SENSORY ADAPTATIONS

Suppression and amblyopia are two of the sensory adaptations that occur with strabismus; a third is anomalous retinal correspondence.

Tests of sensory fusion

Children with comitant early-onset strabismus may not see double, even though the visual axes are misaligned and objects are imaged on disparate retinal points. This is because one eye's retinal image has been suppressed by the brain. If the child has had a constant strabismus for a long period of time, then the suppression of one eye's image will be deep. If one eye's image is deeply suppressed and that eye is not used, then the visual function of that eye may decrease, leading to amblyopia. Children with untreated strabismus and suppression are likely to have amblyopia in the deviated eye. This chapter will only discuss a clinical test of sensory fusion that is suitable for infants and young children.

4-dioptre base-out prism test

If an object's retinal image is shifted in one eye with respect to the other and normal binocular fusion mechanisms are present, the eye receiving the shifted rays will change its vergence in order to regain bifoveal fixation. At least, this is the scenario if suppression is not present. This is the basis of the prism cover test. Prisms bend rays of light.

The child fixates a pen-light. A small prism (4 prism dioptres, base out) is held in front of, for example, the left eye. In the left eye, the retinal image of the fixation spot has shifted, and the fixation light appears shifted to the right. Both eyes move to the right. A movement of the left eye to the right indicates an absence of suppression. If suppression is present, the eye does not move. This movement is immediately followed by an adduction (movement inward) of the right eye. This is because the previous rightwards movement of both eyes resulted in a shift in the retinal image of the right eye. If suppression is not present in the right eye, this retinal shift is noticed, and the motor vergence system attempts to correct this (von Noorden, 1996, p. 212). If normal binocular vision is not present, and the child is able to ignore (suppress) the image to one eye, then these refixation eye movements are not made. Unfortunately, there may be many false negatives with this test, i.e. cases of supression may go undetected, so usefulness with infants is limited.

Other tests of suppression that are used with children over 3 years of age include the Worth four-dot test, the Red Filter ladder, synoptophore tests and polarizing tests. A description of these tests can be found in von Noorden's text (1996, pp. 211–216). Von Noorden warns that the testing environment in most of these tests is very different from our day-to-day visual environment. Bagolini lenses provide a more natural testing environment, but are not suitable for young children.

Tests for anomalous retinal correspondence

If the angle of strabismus has been fairly stable, the child may avoid double vision by a re-coupling of retinal visual direction information. If the visual axes are misaligned, then the fovea from one eye may receive the same retinal image as a peripheral point from the other eye. In time the coupling between the previously corresponding foveas may shift, and the fovea of the fixing eye may become coupled to the peripheral point instead of the fovea of the misaligned eye. This is called anomalous retinal correspondence (ARC). A microtropia is an example of strabismus that is commonly associated with ARC. The tests for anomalous retinal correspondence are many, and can be found in von Noorden (1990, Chapter 13, pp. 255–273). Most of these tests are not suitable for infants and young children.

TESTING FOR STEREOPSIS

In our usual visual environment, small differences in monocular retinal images, caused by the horizontal separation of the two eyes, result in the ability to see in three-dimensional depth. Stereoscopic tests often make use of this: if slightly different images are presented to each eye, artificially creating a retinal disparity, three-dimensional depth can be perceived.

Separating right and left eye images

Separation of the image to each eye is therefore a fundamental part of testing for stereopsis. It can be accomplished by a number of different techniques, described below.

Separation using spectacles

Anaglyphic separation, using coloured filters.   Glasses incorporating a red filter over one eye and a green filter over the other allow the separation of red/green elements in a red/green display (Figure 9.4). Red/green images are displayed on a video monitor or on plates in book form. In the display red dots are accompanied by green dots; each eye's image of these dots will be identical even though one eye receives red dots only and the other receives the green dots only. In a stereo test selected areas of the green dots are separated relative to the red dots. Each eye's image will be slightly different, falling on disparate retinal areas. Stereopsis will therefore result.

Fig 9.4
Child wearing red/green glasses to separate the images to the two eyes in order to test stereopsis. The mechanism involved is explained in the text in the section 'Separating right and left eye image'.

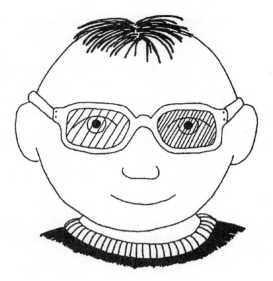

Vectographic separation using polarized filters. The vectographic stimulus is imprinted on Polaroid material, with each eye's target being polarized 90 degrees with respect to the other. Glasses incorporating Polaroid lenses, with one lens receiving horizontally polarized light and the other lens receiving vertically polarized light are used with the polarized displays. As with anaglyphic separation parts of the display received by each eye will be identical, and in other parts horizontally polarized images will be shifted relative to the vertically polarized images. The shifted images will create a disparate pattern when viewed through the polarized glasses.

Liquid-crystal glasses (LCG). Liquid-crystal glasses (LCG) are a very successful means of separating the images to each eye (Eizenman et al., 1989; Skarf et al., 1993; Westall et al., 1998). Each eye's image is separated in time by a technique called alternating field stereoscopy. The LCG are synchronized with the changing (30 Hz) frames on a television monitor, such that the left shutter is open only when the left eye's image is displayed on the screen and the right shutter only when the right eye's image is displayed. The advantage of LCG over red/green glasses is that the transmission of the LCG is higher; this means that the infant's eyes are more visible. Also, the stimulus intensity at the eyes is higher, resulting in higher-amplitude VEP signals than can be recorded with red/green glasses.

Types of glasses. When glasses are required for the separation of each eye's retinal image, the more imagination that goes into the design of the spectacles, the more likely the toddler is to wear them. For example, we have used fun frames, pipe-cleaner glasses or swimming goggles with coloured lenses. Of course, caution must be taken to ensure the sharp ends of the pipe cleaner glasses have been covered to protect the infant.

Separation of the images to each eye without spectacle lenses

Real-depth stereopsis.   Some tests of stereopsis have targets that are actually separated in depth so that no glasses need to be worn. This is a great asset in testing toddlers. The Frisby stereotest (see description below) is a real-depth test. The disadvantage of real-depth tests is that monocular depth cues may confound the result. These depth cues include motion parallax, accommodation, and perspective cues. The monocular cues are minimized by holding the test plates still, by encouraging the child to hold his or her head still, and by controlling the illumination and glare. Some investigators have found that monocular cues result in an under-detection of binocular anomalies (Simons, 1981), whereas others have found that monocular cues are not apparent and that all children with binocular anomalies will fail the Frisby stereotest (Manny, Martinez and Fern, 1991).

Prism separation.   The Lang stereotest displaces the images to each eye by small cylindrical lenses on the surface of the test card. Again, glasses are not needed. This makes the Lang stereotest far easier to perform on the difficult-to-test toddler age-group.

Clinical tests for stereopsis

The TNO stereotest
In the TNO sterotest (Figure 9.5), the images to each eye are separated by means of red/green glasses. This is an example of using anaglyphic separation to produce the appearance of depth. The test is produced as a booklet and is made up of screening plates, three quantitative plates, and a suppression test. The screening plates consist of a butterfly and geometric shapes. These plates, which test

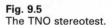

Fig. 9.5
The TNO stereotest.

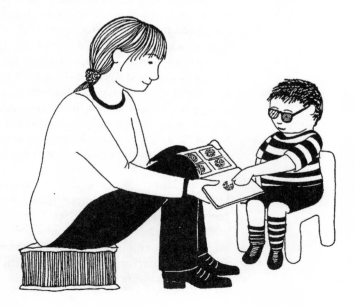

for the presence or absence of stereopsis, are called the qualitative plates. When viewed monocularly, the pictures just appear to be random red and green dots; binocularly, the images appears to stand out. There is also a monocular picture on this page; this helps when instructing the child and is less demoralizing for those children without, or with reduced, stereopsis. The booklet pages are held by the tester directly in front of the child, 40 cm away. At that distance, the disparity of the qualitative targets subtends 33 minutes of arc.

The series of plates called the quantitative plates measures stereoscopic acuity; they show a circle with a pie-shaped sector, or wedge, in a different depth plane. The child is encouraged to point to the missing sector. The stereograms vary in the orientation of the wedge and the degree of disparity, from 15 to 480 seconds of arc when the test is held at 40 cm.

The Frisby stereotest

The Frisby stereotest is made up of three clear Perspex plates of varying thickness: 6, 3 and 1 mm. This test is an example of a real-depth stereotest. On one surface are four 6 cm squares of random dot patterns. One of the squares has a 3 cm diameter circle missing, which is printed on the reverse of the plate. When it is viewed on a uniform white background, the four squares of random dots can be seen; but only those able to detect the disparity created by the thickness of the plate are able to perceive the circle. The plates can be turned over to change the disparity from crossed to uncrossed. At 40 cm, the disparities tested are 340, 170 and 55 seconds of arc.

Each plate of the test is held by the examiner in front of the child. It is particularly important that the plates are kept still: any movement results in monocular artefacts caused by the different relative motions of the surround and the circle. The child is encouraged to point to the circle, or to 'find the ball'. The plate is then rotated, putting the circle into a different quadrant. The test is repeated several times to ensure a consistent response.

A modification of the Frisby stereotest method has given us better results with young toddlers and infants. On a clear piece of Perspex the same size as the Frisby plates, a circle containing the same blue random-dot elements was drawn in one quadrant. This practice plate was shown to the child before using the disparity plates. If the child pointed to the 'ball', she or he was rewarded by a squeak from a hidden toy. The squeak reward was used throughout testing with disparity plates (Saunders, Woodhouse and Westall, 1996).

The Lang stereotest

The Lang stereotest is a card covered with fine parallel cylindrical strips. Beneath each cylinder are two fine picture strips. When viewed binocularly by a person with stereopsis, a star, cat, and car can be perceived in depth. At 40 cm, the disparities are 600 (star), 1200 (cat), and 550 (car) seconds of arc. The Lang stereotest II, a modification of the original test, consists of three figures seen in depth: a moon (200 seconds of arc), a car (400 seconds), and an elephant (600 seconds), along with a star that is monocularly visible.

The Lang test card is held by the examiner directly in front of the child. The child passes the test if he or she is able to point to, or try to grab, one of the shapes. The responses can be checked by turning the card 90 degrees, which eliminates the disparity cues.

Stereo Smile test

This is a new stereo test (Stereo Optical Co. Inc., Chicago), which depends on vectographic separation, and is suitable for infants and young children (Ciner, Schanel-Klitsch and Herzberg, 1996). A 25 by 55 cm card is covered by a random-dot pattern with a random-dot 'Happy Face' to the right or left of the centre of the card. There are two cards with disparities of 480 and 120 seconds of arc when tested at 55 cm, which become 120 and 60 seconds of arc when tested at 1.1 m. Preferential looking type methods are used to determine if stereopsis is present (Chapter 6). In addition the set contains a non-stereo training card, with a smiley face on a random-dot pattern, which is used to prepare the child for testing. Ciner et al. found stereoacuity improved from 5 minutes of arc (6–17 months) to 4 minutes of arc (18–23 months) and to one minute of arc after 30 months. With their three bar target Birch, Gwiazda and Held (1982) found stereo-acuity to have reached 1 minute of arc by 8–12 months of age. The discrepancy between techniques may reflect the difference in stereo-acuity measured with a line stereogram vs stereo-acuity measured with a random dot stereogram.

The Stereo Smile test could prove to be a very useful test for screening and testing infants and young children. Readers are encouraged to look out for studies which evaluate this new test.

Titmus stereotest

The Titmus stereotest is a commonly-used test for stereopsis using vectographic separation of the images to each eye. The child wears polarized glasses. The first test to be administered is usually the fly, a gross stereotest (3000 seconds of arc at 40 cm). The child is asked to touch the wings of the fly. If the child has stereoscopic vision, she or he will grab above the plane of the plate. The Titmus test also contains three rows of animals; one animal in each row has a binocular disparity, and will be seen in depth by a child with stereoscopic depth perception. The child is asked which animal stands out. (Care must be taken with the questions: one of the authors once asked a child which animal jumps out of the picture and she pointed to the rabbits on each row, saying, 'Rabbits jump'.) The disparities of the animals in the three rows are 400, 200, and 100 seconds of arc. Finally, there is the circle test in the Titmus stereotest, with nine sets of four circles. In each of the sets one of the four circles has a disparity and can be seen in depth. The child is asked to 'push down' the circle that stands out (von Noorden, 1996, p. 275). The disparities of the nine sets range from 800 to 40 seconds of arc at 40 cm.

Although widely used, the Titmus stereotest has been criticized because there are monocular cues making it possible for a stereo-blind observer to detect the disparate objects (Simons and Reinecke, 1974).

Randot test

The Randot test is another vectographic test. The test consists of ten rows, each containing three circles (the Randot circles). One of the circles contains a disparity, causing it to be seen in depth by children with stereoscopic depth perception. At 40 cm, the disparities present in each row vary from 400 to 20 seconds of arc. In addition, there are three rows of animals, one in each row having stereoscopic contours. Finally, there are four plates, each containing a random-dot stereogram.

The Randot test has been found to reliably grade stereopsis when stereoscopic acuity is too poor for a child to perform a random-dot stereotest (Simons, 1981).

The Randot preschool stereoacuity test

This recently developed test (1996) is claimed to be appropriate for children as young as 2 years of age. It depends on the ability of the child to recognize a number of simple shapes. The test consists of three booklets, each containing simple pictures on the left hand page and dynamic random-dot stereograms on the right hand page. The task of the child is to point to, or name, the shapes on the left page which contain no depth information. If they are successful with this, they try and find the same shapes (ordered differently) on the right-hand page. These are the test plates, and the shapes are hidden in a random-dot stereogram. There are no monocular cues in the test plates. The first booklet has disparities of 100 and 200 seconds of arc. If the child is able to detect the hidden pictures, then they are shown book 2, with disparities of 60 and 40 seconds of arc. If the child was unable to find the pictures in the first book, they are shown book 3 with disparities of 800 and 400 seconds of arc.

Random-Dot E test

Vectographic separation of each eye's image makes it possible to see the hidden E in the Random-Dot E test if stereopsis is present. One card is a bas-relief of the E on the stereocard. The child is shown this E so he or she knows what to look for. There are another two cards, one of which contains a hidden E in the random-dot background; the other contains only random dots. When the child wears polarized glasses, he or she can distinguish the card containing the E from the other card, if the child has stereoscopic vision. The two cards are held 50 cm in front of the child; the child is asked to identify which cards contains the E. The disparity varies according to test distance; at 2 m, the disparity is 126 seconds of arc.

Table 9.1 Proportion of children passing the Lang, Frisby and Dynamic Random Dot Stereogram (DRDS), showing ranges derived from various studies

Age (months)	Percentages found to pass test		
	Lang	Frisby	DRD
6–12	42–68	20–40	42
12–24	72–75	48–90	30
24–30	~90	88–90	45

Data taken from Broadbent and Westall (1990), K. Saunders (PhD thesis, 1993, University of Wales, College of Cardiff), and Lang and Lang (1988)

Success rates of stereotests in different age groups

Table 9.1 shows the percentage of children, in three age groups, who passed three different stereotests. The Lang and Frisby stereotests did not require glasses. From the table it can be seen that the tests were moderately successful for infants between 12 and 24 months. The dynamic random dot stereogram (a preferential looking type test depending on anaglyphic separation of each eye's image) was not successful for the 12–24 month age group. This is because infants of this age do not tolerate the glasses well. Tests that did not require any glasses were more successful in the 6-month to 2-year age range. By 3 years of age infants wore glasses well, and 90% were able to pass TNO and dynamic random dot stereogram (Broadbent and Westall, 1990).

Reliability of stereotests

Ideally, a test of stereopsis would be failed if a child has strabismus, amblyopia, or suppression. Simons and Reinecke (1974) found the Titmus stereotest to be unreliable in distinguishing patients with binocular problems from those with normal vision. They also found that people with no stereopsis could detect some of the disparate targets; some of the circles appeared different. The best way of avoiding the problem of monocular cues is to use random-dot stereograms. Both Random-Dot E and TNO tests were found to be completely reliable in detecting which children had binocular dysfunction (Simons, 1981). The RDE test was successful if 250 minutes of arc was used as the cut-off between normal and abnormal, but the TNO worked only if the 120-minute arc target was used as the cut-off (Simons, 1981). Simons found that the Frisby stereotest failed to pick up a true binocular dysfunction in some children. The Frisby stereotest benefits from not requiring glasses, but the results are easily contaminated by monocular cues. These may be motion artifacts giving cues to the location of the disparate target, displacement of the figure by tilting the plate, or reflections from the Perspex surface containing the missing part of the pattern (Simons, 1981).

High-tech techniques for assessing binocular single vision and stereopsis

Computer technology has enabled vision researchers to generate novel tests of binocular interaction that can be displayed on TV monitors. The dynamic random-dot correlogram is a computer-generated stimulus consisting of random dots constantly alternating between correlated (fused) and anti-correlated (not fused) phases. The alternation can be perceived only by those with fusion, and provides unequivocal evidence of binocular single vision (Skarf et al., 1993; Westall et al., 1998). In the dynamic random-dot stereogram, a fused background is alternated with a pattern of a known disparity (Petrig et al., 1981; Skarf et al., 1993; Braddick, 1996). The presentation of the correlogram or the stereogram requires the separation of the images perceived by the right and left eyes. Anaglyphic methods or time multi-plexing using liquid-crystal glasses have been used to separate each eye's image in time.

For the correlogram, the dynamic random-dot patterns alternate between two phases: an anti-correlated phase and a correlated phase. In the correlated phase, the random-dot patterns presented to each eye are identical. In the anti-correlated phase, the dot patterns are inverted: a dark dot to one eye corresponds to a bright dot to the other eye. The perception is of a surface alternating between a solid, fused state and a random, snowy state.

The dynamic random-dot stereogram is formed by the alternation between a disparate and a fused stimulus. The perception is of a surface alternating in depth between the surface of the TV screen and a second surface in front of or behind the TV monitor, depending on the amount and direction of the disparity.

These two types of stimuli have been used for both electrophysiological and behavioural studies (Braddick, 1996). For VEP measures, the stimulus (correlogram or stereogram) alternates between two states (presence and absence of the fusion or disparity, respectively) at a known frequency.

The VEP is recorded, and the amplitude of the signal at frequencies corresponding to the stimulus frequency is assessed. If the signal is statistically different from noise, a positive response to the correlogram or stereogram is deemed to have occurred (Skarf et al., 1993; Westall et al., 1998).

FPL testing involves two displays, one containing the correlogram or stereogram, and the other containing identical random dots without fusion (correlogram) or disparity (stereogram). The two patterns may share the same TV monitor (Braddick, 1996), or the separate patterns may be displayed on separate monitors (Broadbent and Westall, 1990). In the latter study, both monitors displayed a dynamic random dot pattern, one of which contained a sector of disparate points in the shape of a square. The square, which would be perceived in depth by a child with stereopsis, could be made to move across the TV monitor. This adaptation added another dimension to get the child's attention.

The concept of a moving stereoscopic form embedded in a dynamic random dot stereogram has been used as a variant of FPL (Fox et al., 1980; Shea et al., 1980; Dobson and Sebris, 1989). The observer is required to judge whether the child is looking to the left or to the right. Recording eye movements using electro-oculogram (see Chapter 12 for details of eye-movement recording) has also been attempted, to help assess if the child has followed the moving disparate form (Leguire, Rogers and Fellows, 1983; Archer et al., 1986; Faubert, 1993).

CONCLUSION

Strabismus, eventually resulting in the disruption of binocular vision, is still a common occurrence in young children. It is becoming increasingly possible, through the use of innovative techniques, to measure stereopsis in infants; failure to demonstrate stereopsis at an age when it would be expected to have developed may be indicative of strabismus. Further testing by the clinician will help to determine what further action is necessary, such as referral or the provision of appropriate refractive corrections at an early age in order to prevent or reduce the strabismus. Research has also shown that early onset strabismus is not necessarily associated with the absence of sensory binocularity; indeed, when surgery is required, early referral resulting in early surgery may mean that a child retains a high degree of binocular function. The eye care practitioner can thus go a long way in preventing the leading cause of monocular vision loss in the 20–70 plus age group – amblyopia. We discuss further the management of binocular anomalies in the final chapter.

REFERENCES

Alpern, M. (1969). Anatomy of eye movements. In H. Davson (ed.), *The eye*, 2nd edn, Volume 3, Chapter 4, New York/San Francisco/London, Academic Press, pp. 27–64.

American Academy of Ophthalmology (1994). *Basic and Clinical Science Course in Pediatric Ophthalmology and Strabismus.* 1994–1995. Section 6. San Francisco, American Academy of Ophthalmology.

Archer, S.M., Helveston, E.M., Miller, K.K. and Ellis, F.D. (1986). Stereopsis in normal infants and infants with congenital esotropia. *American Journal of Ophthalmology*, **101**, 591–596.

Banks M.S., Aslin, R.N. and Letson, R.D. (1975). Sensitive period for the development of human binocular vision. *Science*, **190**, 675–677.

Banks, M. and Bennett, P. (1988). Optical and photoreceptor immaturities limit the spatial and chromatic vision of human neonates. *Journal of the Optical Society of America*, **5**, 2059–2079.

Birch, E. (1993). Stereopsis in infants and its development relation to visual acuity. In K. Simons (ed.), *Early Visual Development, Normal and Abnormal*, Oxford/New York, Oxford University Press, pp. 224–236.

Birch, E.E., Gwiazda, J. and Held, R. (1982). Stereoacuity development for crossed and uncrossed disparities in human infants. *Vision Research*, **22**, 507–513.

Birch, E.E. and Hale, L.A. (1989). Operant assessment of stereoacuity. *Clinical Vision Science* **4**, 295–300.

Botet, R.V., Calhoun, J.H. and Harley, R.D. (1981). Development of monofixation syndrome in congenital esotropia. *Journal of Pediatric Ophthalmology and Strabismus*, **18**, 49–51.

Braddick, O.J., Atkinson, J., Julesz, B. et al. (1980). Cortical binocularity in infants. *Nature* **228**, 363–365.

Braddick, O.J. (1996). Binocularity in infancy. *Eye*, **10**, 182–188.

Braddick, O.J. and Atkinson, J. (1983). Some recent findings on the development of human binocularity: a review. *Behavioural Brain Research*, **10**, 141–150.

Broadbent, H. and Westall, C. (1990). An evaluation of techniques for measuring stereopsis in infants and young children. *Ophthalmic and Physiological Optics*, **10**, 3–7.

Ciner E.B., Schanel-Klitsch, E. and Herzberg, C. (1996) Stereoacuity Development: 6 months to 5 years. A new tool for testing and screening. *Optometry and Vision Science*, **73**, 43–48.

Daw, N.W. (1995). *Visual Development*. New York/London, Plenum Press.

Dobson, V. and Sebris, S.L. (1989). Longitudinal study of acuity and stereopsis in infants with or at risk for esotropia. *Investigative Ophthalmology and Visual Science*, **30**, 1146–1158.

Eizenman, M., McCulloch, D., Hui, R. and Skarf, B. (1989). Development of binocular vision in infants. *Investigative Ophthalmology and Visual Science (Suppl.)* **30**, 313 (abstract).

Eizenman, M., Westall, C.A., Geer, I. and Kraft, S.P. (1996). Binocular fusion in children with strabismus. *Investigative Ophthalmology and Visual Science (Suppl.)* **37**, S2020 (abstract).

Faubert, J. (1993). A new stereopsis test for pediatric vision. *Optometry and Vision Science (Suppl.)* **70**, 89 (abstract).

Flynn, J.T. (1991). Amblyopia revisited. *Journal of Pediatric Ophthalmology and Strabismus*, **28**, 183–201.

Fox, R., Aslin, R.N., Shea, S.L. and Dumais, S.T. (1980). Stereopsis in human infants. *Science*, **207**, 323–324.

Griffin, J. (1976). *Binocular Anomalies, Procedures for Vision Therapy*. Chicago, Illinois, Professional Press Inc.

Held, R. (1993). Two stages in the development of binocular vision and eye alignment. In K. Simons (ed.), *Early Visual Development, Normal and Abnormal*, London, Oxford University Press, pp.250–257.

Held, R., Birch, E.E. and Gwiazda, J. (1980). Stereoacuity of human infants. *Proceedings of the National Academy of Sciences of USA*, **77**, 5572–5574.

Hickey, T.L. and Peduzzi, J.D. (1987). Structure and development of the visual system. In P. Salapatek and L. Cohen (eds). *Handbook of Infant Perception*, Orlando, San Diego, New York, Academic Press, Inc., pp. 1–42.

Ing, M.R. (1983). Early surgical alignment for congenital esotropia. *Journal of Pediatric Ophthalmology and Strabismus*, **20**, 11–18.

Julesz, B., Kropfl, W. and Petrig, B. (1980). Large evoked potentials of dynamic random-dot correlograms and stereograms permit quick determination of stereopsis. *Proceedings of the National Academy of Sciences of USA*, **77**, 2348–2351.

Lang J.I. and Lang, T.J. (1988). Eye screening with the Lang Stereotest. *American Orthoptic Journal*, **38**, 48–51.

Leguire, L.E., Rogers, G.L. and Fellows, R.R. (1983). Toward a clinical test of stereopsis in human infants. *Investigative Ophthalmology & Visual Science*, **24** (Suppl.) 34 (abstract).

Manny R.E., Martinez A. and Fern, K.D. (1991). Testing stereopsis in the preschool child: is it clinically useful? *Journal of Pediatric Ophthalmology and Strabismus*, **28**, 223–231.

von Noorden, G.K. (1996). *Binocular Vision and Ocular Motility: Theory and management of strabismus*, 5th edn. St Louis, Baltimore, Mosby-Year Book.

Parks, M.M. (1969). The monofixation syndrome. *Transactions of the American Ophthalmological Society*, **67**, 609–657.

Petrig, B., Julesz, B., Kropfl, W. et al. (1981). Development of stereopsis and cortical binocularity in human infants: electrophysiological evidence. *Science*, **213**, 1402–1405.

Saunders, K.J., Woodhouse, J.M. and Westall, C.A. (1996). The modified Frisby stereotest. *Journal of Pediatric Ophthalmology and Strabismus*, **33**, 323–327.

Shea, S.L., Fox, R., Aslin, R.N. and Dumain, S.T. (1980). Assessment of stereopsis in human infants. *Investigative Ophthalmology & Visual Science*, **19**, 1400–1404.

Shimojo, S., Bauer, J., Jr, O'Connell, K.M. and Held, R. (1986). Pre-stereoptic binocular vision in infants. *Vision Research*, **26**, 501–510.

Simons, K. (1981). A comparison of the Frisby, Random-Dot E, TNO, and Randot circles stereotests in screening and office use. *Archives of Ophthalmology*, **99**, 446–452.

Simons, K. and Reinecke, R.D. (1974). A reconsideration of amblyopia screening and stereopsis. *American Journal of Ophthalmology*, **78**, 707–713.

Skarf, B., Eizenman, M., Katz, L.M. et al. (1993). A new VEP system for studying binocular single vision in human infants. *Journal of Pediatric Ophthalmology and Strabismus*, **30**, 237–242.

Smith, J., Atkinson, J., Braddick, O.J. and Wattam-Bell, J. (1988). Development of sensitivity to binocular correlation and disparity in infancy. *Perception*, **17**, A57 (abstract).

Stager, D.R. and Birch, E.E. (1986). Preferential-looking acuity and stereopsis in infantile esotropia. *Journal of Pediatric Ophthalmology and Strabismus*, **23**, 160–165.

Westall, C.A., Eizenman, M., Kraft, S.P., Panton, C.M., Chatterjee, S. and Sigesmund, D. (1998a). Cortical sensory responses and monocular optokinetic responses in early-onset esotropia. *Investigative Ophthalmology and Visual Science*, **39**, 1352–1360.

Westall, C.A., Eizenman, M., Chatterjee, S., Smith, K., Panton, C.M. and Kraft, S. (1998b). Using VEPs to assess fusional vergence in children with early onset esotropia. *Investigative Ophthalmology and Visual Science*, **39**, S1101 (abstract).

Wilson, H. (1988). Development of spatiotemporal mechanisms in infants vision. *Vision Research*, **28**, 611–628.

Wright K. W., Edelman P. M., Mcvey J. H. et al. (1994). High-grade stereo acuity after early surgery for congenital esotropia. *Archives of Ophthalmology*, **112**, 913–919.

Appendix 9.1

Suppliers of stereotests

Lang Stereotest; Haag-Streit Service Inc. 6, Industrial Park, Waldwick, NJ 07094, USA

Clement Clarke International Ltd. 15, Wigmore Street, London W1H 9LA, UK

Frisby Stereotest, Clement Clarke; 3128 D East 17th Avenue, Columbus, OH 43219, USA. 1-800-848-8923

Randot Stereotests: Randot Test and Randot Preschool Stereoacuity Test; Stereo Optical Co. Inc. 3539 North Kenton Ave, Chicago, IL 60641, USA

Random-Dot E Stereotest and Stereo Smile Test; Stereo Optical Co. Inc. 3539 North Kenton Ave, Chicago, IL 60641, USA

10

Visual fields

INTRODUCTION

We begin this chapter by explaining the importance of measuring visual fields and describing how fields develop in infancy and childhood. Although measuring fields is an essential aspect of the assessment of functional vision, it is not easy to do in the case of infants and young children. Ways of adapting standard instruments and procedures for use with infants and children are described and the advantages and disadvantages of various methods outlined.

WHAT ARE VISUAL FIELDS?

The visual field is the extent in space in which objects are visible to a stationary eye. As is the case with most visual functions, visual fields can be measured with both eyes together (binocularly) or with one eye at a time (monocularly). The size of the visual field is dependent on the size and brightness of the target used: the larger the target, the larger the visual field up to the maximum limit of the total visual field. The sensitivity to targets tends to increase towards the centre of the visual field, although this is dependent on the overall (ambient) illumination level. Visual fields are usually described in terms of degrees measured from the fixation point. The full extent of the normal adult monocular visual field is 100 degrees temporally, 60 degrees nasally, 65 degrees superiorly and 75 degrees inferiorly.

Visual field defects or scotomas are areas within the visual field where there is a reduction or loss of sensitivity. A central scotoma is when the loss has occurred at and around the fixation point. Hemianopia refers to a loss of one half of the visual field (this could be the right, left, superior or inferior half) and a constriction of the visual field means a reduced total extent of visual field.

There are two basic methods for measuring visual fields – kinetic and static. In kinetic field testing the stimulus is moved from a peripheral position outside the visual field towards the centre until the person first indicates that they can see the target or, in the case of an infant, looks towards the target. In static field testing, the target is presented at a series of predetermined visual field locations and the viewer indicates when and if the target was seen.

WHY MEASURE VISUAL FIELDS?

Some knowledge of the extent of visual fields is a vital part of a functional visual assessment. Constrictions in visual fields may have far more effect on visual performance than visual acuity. In adults, Marron and Bailey (1982) found that visual field loss (as well as contrast sensitivity loss) correlated significantly with mobility while VA was only weakly associated with it. That is, visual fields and contrast sensitivity can give a good prediction of mobility while VA has very little predictive usefulness. Similarly, Pelli (1986) found that contrast sensitivity and visual fields could be reduced to a far lesser extent than could VA before mobility was affected.

Pelli found that mobility was affected when the field was reduced to 7 degrees. However, clinically, we take a slightly more conservative estimate and it is normally accepted that, when the field is reduced to 20 degrees, mobility will be compromised. Traditionally, we think of peripheral field loss as causing mobility difficulties and, indeed, this is the case if extensive field loss is experienced, as in the examples above. However, when equal solid angles of visual field subtended at the eye are considered, loss of the central and inferior and lateral mid-peripheral field are more devastating (Lovie-Kitchin et al., 1990; Flanagan et al., 1993). Lovie-Kitchin et al. (1990) showed that loss of the central region of the visual field (central 37 degrees) has the greatest effect on mobility, followed by the mid-periphery and inferior fields (out to 58 degrees). Loss of the superior peripheral visual field has very little effect.

These studies were all done with adult observers, but there is no reason to assume that young children behave any differently from adults in this respect.

If a constriction of the visual field is found, orientation and mobility training should be considered. It is now felt that this type of training can start earlier in life. The child is taught basic concepts of awareness of the environment, use of light and dark to orientate towards windows and lights and techniques to negotiate stairs and other obstacles. Use of a white cane, if appropriate, would be introduced later.

Reading is greatly affected with a hemianopia, depending on whether there is a right or left visual field loss. Eye movements into a scotomatous area will lack accuracy. Generally, when reading, we make fixations at the first few letters of a word (depending on the length of the word and the location of the previous fixation). The perceptual span (the area from which information can be obtained during each fixation) is asymmetrically placed to the right of fixation for English text and to the left of fixation for Hebrew (which is read from right to left). This perceptual span asymmetry is almost certainly related to the direction that the eyes are moving (Morris and Rayner, 1991). The decision about where to position the eyes after each fixation is related to the up-coming word length, which is in turn based on information gained from parafoveal vision. Thus a right visual field defect close to the parafoveal area will greatly impede this process (for reading in English).

This is confirmed by findings with adults with central scotomas. They place the image of interest on a parafoveal part of the retina, usually adjacent to the edge of the scotoma. This is called eccentric viewing, and this 'new' fovea is called the preferred retinal locus. Most adults with adventitious central visual loss develop a fairly consistent preferred retinal locus and subjects who are artificially given a central scotoma develop the concept of eccentric viewing quite quickly (Whittaker and Cummings, 1986). However, it is generally not easily acquired as an unconscious habit and the person remains aware that they are 'looking off centre'. Although few studies have been done with children, we assume that they also develop a consistent preferred retinal locus. Indeed, the observation that a child views eccentrically can be diagnostic of a central field loss. Those who view eccentrically so as to place their scotoma to the right of each word will read more slowly than those who place the scotoma at some other location (Whittaker and Cummings, 1990). However, a left field defect will impede return saccadic eye movements from the end of one line to the beginning of the next. In general it seems that eccentric fixation in a direction perpendicular to the direction of eye movements gives rise to optimum reading speed (Peli, 1986) and, indeed, most adults choose a preferred retinal locus which is superior to their scotoma which means that they move their scotoma upwards in the visual field (Guez et al., 1993).

Potential reading speed will be affected not only by the position of the preferred retinal locus, but also by its eccentricity, which will be closely related to the size of the central scotoma. Whittaker and Lovie-Kitchin (1993) analysed a number of previous studies and found that there is a maximum possible reading speed depending on the eccentricity of the preferred retinal locus (Table 10.1). Although these data were also gathered from adults with adventitious loss, they give us guidelines as to what may be expected from children with central scotomas, in terms of reading rates.

Older children with such defects may require training while the teachers of younger children require visual field information so that material can be placed on the appropriate side and the child can be placed on the better side of the classroom; for example, a child with a

Table 10.1   Maximum expected reading speed for adult reading in the presence of central scotoma resulting in eccentric viewing

Maximum potential reading speed	Eccentricity of preferred retinal locus	Scotoma diameter
Spot reading (40 words per minute)	>15 degrees	>30 degrees
Fluent reading (80 words per minute)	< 11 degrees	< 22 degrees
High fluent (160 words per minute)	< 2 degrees	< 4 degrees

Table taken from Whittaker and Lovie-Kitchin, 1993

left hemianopia should be placed towards the left-hand side of the class (from the child's point of view).

A central scotoma will affect many aspects of visual performance. While adults with adventitious visual loss will be intensely aware of a central scotoma and require training in eccentric fixation, it is generally assumed that children learn this themselves. Indeed, this seems to be the case and children may have an abnormal sense of 'straight ahead': they may be eccentrically fixating but feel that they are fixating centrally, in contrast with adults with adventitious vision loss who, as mentioned above, are always intensely aware that they are eccentrically fixating. In the case of a child who is already eccentrically fixating, yet unaware of it, it is impossible (and, indeed, unnecessary) to undertake training. Whether children learn to use the optimum eccentric position is not known. A simple explanation to the parents and carers about why the child appears not to make eye contact may be necessary but, in addition, a child may need training about the use of eye contact in conversation. As discussed in Chapter 3, eye contact is an important non-verbal component of social interactions and if it is not maintained by the listener it is often assumed that they are not interested in the conversation, are excessively shy or are talking to someone else (Fichten et al., 1991); the result can be misunderstandings and social isolation. Therefore, although there must be reorientation of carers, those with visual impairment may also need to learn to emit the visual cue of apparent eye contact (Zawilski, 1980; Fichten et al., 1991).

DEVELOPMENT OF THE PERIPHERAL RETINA

As we will see later, the infant's visual field at birth is not equal in extent to the adult field and understanding of this is important. As described in Chapter 1, the general development of the human retina appears to be in a centrifugal direction (spreading peripherally from the fovea). One of the most extensive studies of the developing human retina was by Provis et al. (1985). Cell division (mitosis) occurs over the entire retina in the first 10–12 weeks of gestation, but at 14 weeks it ceases in an area which will eventually become the macula. This ceasing of cell division spreads eccentrically until mitosis is only occurring at the extreme periphery. Mitosis ceases by the thirtieth gestational week. Similarly, the differentiation of the retinal layers proceeds from the centre to the periphery (Horsten and Winkelman, 1962; Provis et al., 1985). There is migration of ganglion cells from the future fovea towards the periphery (Provis et al., 1985) and the enlarging of the ganglion cells into their mature forms occurs first at the developing macula and continues into early neonatal life, especially in the temporal retina which in this respect lags behind the nasal retina. The retinal area increases throughout gestation and into the early postnatal period. However, the rate of this surface increase slows after birth so that there is a smaller increase between

3 weeks and 4 months postnatally; the increase may continue at a slow rate even to the age of 1–2 years (Robb, 1982). This increase in area may be due to migration of the cells, but is more likely to be due to the development of individual cells. There is a greater postnatal expansion of the temporal, compared with the nasal, retina, which results in a denser concentration of cells in the latter.

Since there are limited data available on retinal development in humans, we must turn to animal studies to gain insights into the retinal development of higher mammals. Animal studies result in a greater volume of data which can be gathered in a controlled fashion, i.e. at predetermined developmental ages. In cats and other mammals, the centrifugal pattern of maturation is also present. Although the complement of ganglion cells is present at birth (Johns, Rusoff and Dubin, 1979) there is mitosis in the peripheral retina to produce cells for the inner retinal layers which differentiate as layers after birth. The expansion of the retina in cats has been shown not to be uniform, the periphery continuing to expand later in development than the central region (Lia, Williams and Chalupa, 1987). In the macaque monkey, the extent of the 6-week-old nasal retinal area is 70% that of the adult (Packer, Hendrickson and Curcio, 1990). A 6-week-old macaque is considered developmentally equivalent to a 6-month human.

Although development occurs centrifugally, being initiated at the future fovea, the macular region is not fully developed at birth (Chapter 1) and complete differentiation of the macula does not occur until 2–4 months. The foveal depression is also still immature at birth, the inner nuclear and ganglion cell layers moving aside by 4 months (Abrahamov et al., 1982) to 45 months (Yuodelis and Hendrickson, 1986). The density of cones at the fovea increases during intrauterine development (Diaz-Araya and Provis, 1992) and continues after birth as the cones migrate towards the fovea, becoming longer and thinner. This may continue until as late as 45 months of age (Yuodelis and Hendrickson, 1986), which agrees with visual acuity development measured by psychophysical means (Gwiazda et al., 1980; Fulton, Hansen and Manning, 1981; Mayer and Dobson, 1982). Thus the general pattern of development is in the centrifugal direction with migration of cells in the inner retinal layer in this centrifugal direction. However, the movement of cones is in the opposite direction, centripetally.

The vascularization of the temporal retina is not complete until just after birth, although that of the nasal retina is complete earlier, at 8-months gestation. It is thought that this is the reason that the temporal retina is susceptible to more severe retinopathy of prematurity than is the nasal retina. In addition, there is evidence that the uncrossed contralateral retinal projections (from the temporal retina) may develop later than the crossed projections (nasal retina).

Thus it seems likely that, just as foveal development continues after birth, so does the development of the peripheral retina, and that the increase in visual field measured behaviourally (see below) reflects this development.

NORMAL VISUAL FIELDS IN INFANTS AND YOUNG CHILDREN

Schwartz, Dobson and Sandstrom (1987) used a black double arc perimeter with a black curtain behind it and kinetic techniques to measure fields on infants up to 8 weeks (Figure 10.1). The stimulus (a white styrofoam sphere) was moved by hand from the periphery inwards and the observer, who was behind the curtain, was unaware of its location. The fixation stimulus was a stationary white sphere. The observer indicated when and in what direction an eye movement away from fixation was made. If the eye movement was in the correct direction, this target position was taken as the extent of the infant's visual field. Neonates and 4- and 8-week-old infants showed fields which were significantly smaller than those of adults. While the binocular fields of adults were 60–80 degrees, the infants' fields were 20 degrees for the 4 week olds and 20–40 degrees for the 8 week olds. A number of similar studies have been undertaken (Tronick, 1972; MacFarlane, Harris and Barnes, 1976; Mohn and van Hof-van Duin, 1986) and the general findings are as follows:

1. There is only a slight increase in the extent of the visual field in the first 2 months and it increases more rapidly from 2 to 8 months.
2. The size of infants' fields (up to 8 weeks) is smaller than adults' fields but similar in shape, i.e. at all ages fields are smaller in the vertical meridians than the horizontal.
3. Eight week olds show larger fields than 4 week olds.

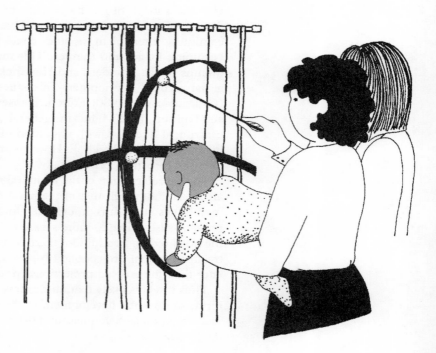

Fig. 10.1
Infant being tested with the double arc perimeter. An observer watches the child's eye movements through a slit or hole in the curtain behind the arc.

4. Surprisingly, neonates have apparently larger fields than 4 week olds. This last finding may be due to infants of 4–8 weeks having attention that is more directed towards one stimulus at a time. When sucking a dummy (pacifier) they show smaller fields than without (MacFarlane, Harris and Barnes, 1976) and when the central stimulus remains while the peripheral stimulus is presented, their attention is less easily transferred to the new stimulus, resulting in smaller apparent field size. This has been described as a 'staring' response, the infant's fixation being apparently locked onto the central fixation target (Mohn and van Hof-van Duin, 1986). For this reason many studies of infant fields have arranged for the central fixation target to be extinguished when the peripheral stimulus is presented. An alternative method of diminishing the effects of the staring response is to allow the infant longer to make their response (Goldberg, Maurer and Lewis, 1993). Maurer and Lewis (1991) suggest that the apparent ineffectiveness of a peripheral stimulus to elicit an eye movement in babies may be because of a preference to make spontaneous eye movements in some directions more frequently than others.

5. There is a monotonic increase in visual fields from 2 to 6 months and a slower increase to 1 year of age, at which point the rate of increase slows again and the visual fields are almost adult-like.

6. There is some evidence that the nasal field (temporal retina) matures more slowly than the temporal field (Lewis and Maurer, 1992), particularly in the first 3 months of life. This difference between nasal and temporal field maturation seems to be evident when static techniques, rather than kinetic ones, are used (Mayer and Fulton, 1993). This difference may be due to the later development of the uncrossed visual pathway, differential maturation of the cones or ganglion cells of the nasal versus the temporal retina, or later development of projections from the cortex to the subcortical centres controlling nasal and temporal eye movements.

7. As with adults, the size of the field measured is dependent on stimulus size and brightness (Lewis and Maurer, 1992).

Mohn and van Hof-van Duin (1986) measured infants' fields using a technique similar to that described by Schwartz, Dobson and Sandstrom (1987) except that the peripheral stimulus was 'jiggled'. The fixation stimulus was also moved until the baby's attention was gained and then it was kept stationary. Using this method, it was found that after 2 months of age the binocular visual field increased rapidly until 8 months and then continued to increase more slowly. However, even by 1 year the fields were still smaller than adult fields in the inferior and horizontal meridians although superior fields were adult-like.

Their data are shown in Figure 10.2. Our results (Dodd and Leat, 1991) using similar apparatus were in good agreement (Figure 10.3). There was an increase with age over the first months of life, but by 10 months the binocular fields were still smaller than adult fields (measured on the same apparatus), being 16% smaller in the superior, 33–40% smaller in the horizontal and 42.5% smaller in the inferior fields.

Several studies have used existing bowl perimeters adapted for use with infants and children. The adaptations have usually involved the use of central flashing LEDs which are extinguished when the static peripheral target appears. The target is considered to be seen when the observer's assessment of the child's eye movement is in the correct direction, the observer usually being unaware of the position of the target. Mayer, Fulton and Cummings (1988) found that the visual fields of infants were 93% of the adult field by the age of 6 months. They used a static technique whereby the fixation stimulus was extinguished when a peripheral pulsing stimulus was presented.

Dodd and Leat (1991) measured fields using a modification of the older Gambs instrument. This has a translucent bowl onto the outside of which stimuli are projected with a hand-held device which slides on the convexity of the bowl. The largest stimulus is equivalent to the largest stimulus on the Goldmann. The perimeter was adapted with flashing fixation LEDs which were extinguished when the peripheral static target was presented, looking responses representing the child's response. Children from 1 year upwards could be tested on this instrument and the results showed that there is a tendency for the measured visual field to increase with age up to 4 years.

Fields measured on a Goldmann perimeter, adapted in a similar manner, appear to increase with age from 2.5 to 4 years and even the 4 year olds have smaller fields than adults along the horizontal meridians (Figure 10.4). Quinn, Fea and Minguini (1991) also found an increase in field size between 4 and 10 years of age using both the Goldmann and double arc perimeters. This increase may be in part because infants and young children maintain a high criterion for making a response compared with adults, that is, they wait until the peripheral stimulus is well within their visual field before responding.

Cummings et al. (1988) used a bowl perimeter with LEDs embedded in its surface to measure fields on children from 2 to 5 years. Flashing LEDs were used as fixation targets and the peripheral stimuli were sequentially illuminated along one meridian of the field, starting with the most peripheral, until the child made a looking response. The observer was naive about the direction of the stimulus. With this apparatus, there was no age effect on the size of the visual field for children of 2 years and upwards and the results for these children were not dissimilar to those of adults. Repeatability was 7% in most cases. The discrepancies between studies regarding whether fields continue to increase after 2 years may be due to numbers of subjects or differences in procedures.

More recently, Mutlukan and Damato (1993) suggest the use of eye tracking devices (which are now becoming quite common in visual field instruments for adults) together with a computer-generated video task in which the child has to track a moving circle, which helps to maintain fixation. When the child is fixating accurately a peripheral target is presented and the child has to signal its presence by pressing

Fig. 10.2
(a) Development of the binocular visual field along the horizontal (left) and vertical (right) meridia (cross-sectional study) measured with the double-arc perimeter. The dashed lines show the results obtained when data from infants who were judged to be staring at the fixation light were excluded from the analysis. Error bars = 2 SEMs. **(b)** Development of the monocular visual field along the horizontal (left) and vertical (right) meridia. Error bars = 2 SEMs. (Reprinted from *Clinical Vision Sciences* Vol 1, Mohn, G. and van Hof-van Duin, J. 'Development of the binocular and monocular visual field of human infants during the first year of life' p. 51–64. © 1986. With kind permission from Elsevier Science Ltd, The Boulevard, Langford Lane, Kidlington OX5 1GB, UK.)

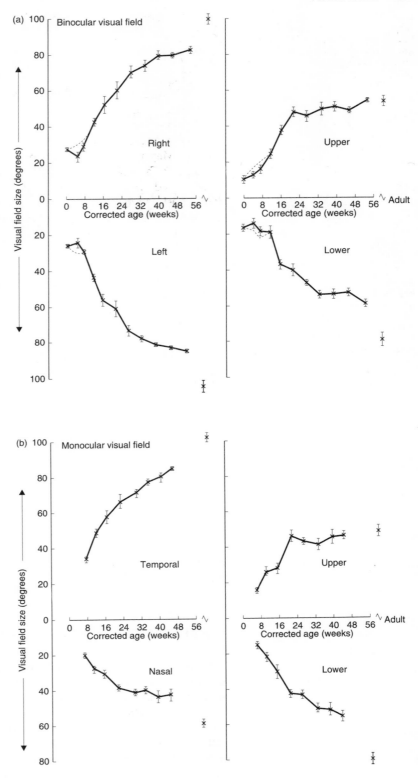

Fig. 10.3
Binocular visual field with respect to age as measured on the double arc perimeter (cross-sectional study). □ = right field, ○ = upper field, △ = left field and ▽ = lower field. Standard deviations are shown.

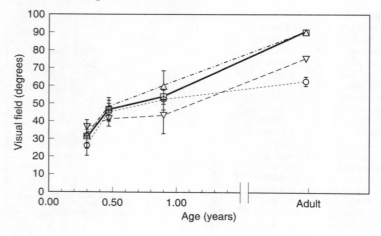

Fig. 10.4
Binocular visual fields measured with respect to age on the modified Goldmann perimeter (cross-sectional study). □ = right field, ○ = upper field, △ = left field and ▽ = lower field. Standard deviations are shown.

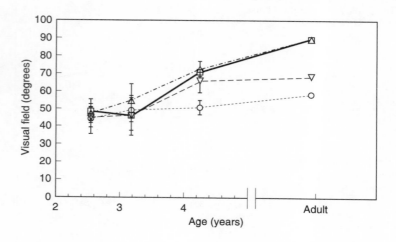

a button on a joystick. The testing thus becomes like a video game and may be effective in children aged 5 years and upwards.

DETECTION OF VISUAL FIELD DEFECTS

The question remains as to whether such techniques are sufficiently sensitive to detect field defects. Luna et al. (1989) (using the arc perimeter technique of Mohn and van Hof-van Duin), found that the test was sensitive enough to show a mean difference between the peripheral fields of infants with grade 3 retinopathy of prematurity (ROP) and infants matched for gestational age and birthweight who did not have ROP; the infants with ROP had significantly smaller fields at 9 months (although at 4 months their fields had been within

Fig. 10.5
Results of flashing LED
perimetry for an infant with
severe hydrocephalus.
(a) Binocular visual field at
14 months. (b) Monocular
fields at 22 months. Dots
represent single correct trials
and thick solid lines
represent the range of
positions at which the
stimuli were not detected.
(From Mayer, D.L., Fulton,
A.B. and Cummings, M.F.
(1988). Visual fields of
infants assessed with a new
perimetric technique.
*Investigative Ophthalmology
& Visual Science,* **29,**
452–459. Reproduced with
permission from Lippincott-
Raven Publishers)

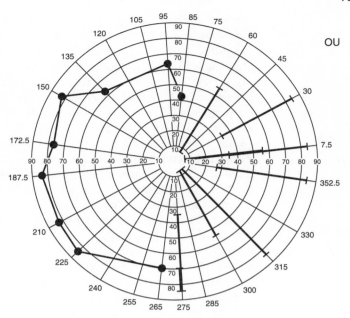

(a)

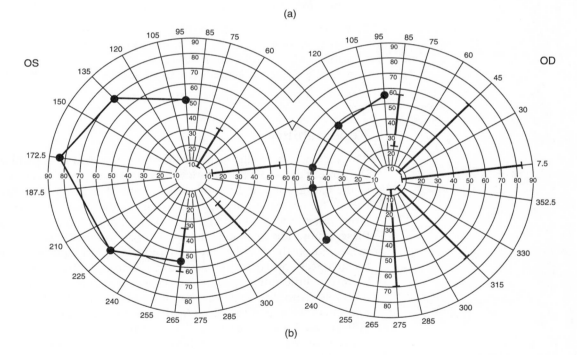

(b)

the normal range for their age and at 18 months they had caught up
with the matched group). Similarly, the mean field size of infants with
perinatal asphyxia is smaller than that for healthy preterm infants
(Luna, Dobson and Getz, 1993). However, clinically, we need to be
able to detect field defects in an individual child, not just determine

average differences between a normal and abnormal population. Cummings et al. (1988) report on a technique using statically presented LEDs and eye movement responses; evidence from one child, aged 12 years, suggested that the technique of eye movement responses is capable of revealing large field defects such as hemianopia. Mayer et al. (1988) report one case of a child at risk for hemianopia which was confirmed by the use of their flashing LED perimeter at 14 months of age (Figure 10.5). Van Hof-van Duin and Mohn (1986) showed that the arc perimeter technique will detect visual field constrictions in infants with visual impairments and in high-risk preterm babies. Infants with white matter disorders or with CNS abnormalities have been shown to have visual fields outside the normal range (Getz, Dobson and Luna, 1993; Mayer et al., 1993). More recently, Luna et al. (1995) showed that the arc perimeter can detect visual field deficits in infants up to 36 months; they found deficits in preterm and full-term infants who had perinatal asphyxia plus CNS abnormalities, but rarely in those with only perinatal asphyxia. More studies are required to answer the question of how sensitive these techniques are to subtle field defects.

Other methods of measuring hemifield defects in children which may become more widely used in the future are listed below:

1. Covert responses such as pupil or heart rate changes. Pupillo-metric responses have been shown to detect optic tract lesions in adults (Mayer and Fulton, 1993).
2. Visually-evoked potentials to targets located in one hemifield.

Repeatability

The absolute size of the visual field can be expected to depend on the instrumentation being used since the size of the targets, the brightness of the background and the brightness ratio of target and background are all factors which are known to affect the visual field in adults. However, the visual field size may be instrument-dependent even if these factors are matched. In our comparison of the same children measured on the Gambs and the Goldmann with equivalent stimuli, the field was consistently larger with the Gambs, although in the adult there was little difference. The Gambs is a simpler instrument than the Goldmann and therefore less intimidating for children and this may effect the size of the visual field measured. However, Quinn et al. (1991) found that there was a good agreement between the total visual field measured on a Goldman bowl and a double arc perimeter, even when different response measures were used.

Other factors which will affect the latency of eye movements towards a peripheral stimulus in infants and therefore influence the measured extent of the visual field are: the presence of a central stimulus; whether the child is sucking a dummy (MacFarlane, Harris and Barnes, 1976); whether the child's chin is held as infants may reponds better with head movements than eye movements alone

(Roucoux et al., 1981); and the frequency of spontaneous non-stimulus related eye movements.

The traditional method of determining the repeatability of visual fields, since only a few thresholds are determined at any one field location or meridian, is the root mean square (Hirsch, 1985). This determines an overall level of expected repeatability by calculating the standard deviation of the differences between first and second observations at each location. Using this technique we were able to determine that there was no significant difference between the repeatability of each of the three techniques we used for measuring visual fields (Goldmann, Gambs and Arc perimeter). The repeatability was of the order of 4 degrees at 7 years old to 10 degrees at 3 years.

Mohn and van Hof-van Duin found a range of repeated measurements of 7 degrees at birth to 14 degrees at 1 month, decreasing gradually to 8 degrees at about 1 year old. This is a fairly large value for repeatability which means that small, subtle field losses will not be detectable in young infants by these methods.

CLINICAL TESTING OF FIELDS IN INFANTS AND YOUNG CHILDREN

General methodology

As with preferential looking, eye movement responses are used to assess infant's visual fields. When a peripheral stimulus is presented within the field, an involuntary fixation response occurs. Therefore the first requisite for testing infants' fields is some means of observing the eyes. Many of the studies have been arranged so that the observer does not know where in the visual field the target is to be presented and makes guesses based on the infant's response. Only if the observer guesses correctly is that stimulus considered within the infant's visual field. This may involve up to four people (not including the baby!): one to hold the child, one to observe the eye movements, one to present the stimulus and one to record the results. Clinically, this is often not feasible. We therefore allow the person who presents the stimulus to also observe the eye movements and only brisk eye movements in the appropriate direction are counted as a response.

Secondly, a more attention-grabbing central fixation stimulus is required as children will not fixate the usual black or white spot. Flashing LED targets can be used and will hold the attention of most infants for 15–25 trials of peripheral stimulus.

A third difference between testing a child and an adult, which follows from their limited attention span, is that less information may be gathered from the child on one occasion.

Fourthly, infants of 4–8 weeks seem to be rivetted in their fixation of the central stimulus and fail to change attention to the peripheral when presented. Therefore, for this age, the central flashing LEDs should be extinguished when the peripheral stimulus is presented which implies static rather than kinetic stimulus presentation. Some studies have also made use of auditory stimuli to encourage central fixation.

Simple apparatus should be used as children are made wary when approaching complicated equipment. They may be distracted by surrounding parts of the equipment such as the bulb house on the Goldmann which can frighten a child, as can the stimulus projection arm which swings behind them; it is better not to move this part of the apparatus until the child is in place.

Binocular visual fields are often measured instead of attempting to occlude one eye. This is particularly appropriate if a functional visual assessment is being undertaken, as we are interested in the field used by the child in normal viewing. For diagnostic purposes a monocular field must be attempted.

Specific clinical methods

A number of existing perimeters can be adapted for use with children. Many bowl perimeters can be used with minor changes.

Goldmann bowl

Cummings et al. (1988) found that the Goldmann bowl perimeter could be used with a repeatability of 10% in most cases with children as young as 2 yr 9 m without any adaptations, simply by using the infant's eye movements as a response. We adapted the Goldmann bowl by removing the detachable telescope. This gives a wider field of view so that one side of the child's head is visible and their eye movements can easily be seen. We replaced the telescope with two LEDs which flash alternately. It is still possible to observe the infant's eyes above the LEDs. A small electrical switch coupled with the Goldman's own switch for presenting the stimulus enables the LEDs to be extinguished when the peripheral target is presented, statically. The youngest child we were able to test with this technique was 2.5 years old (although not as many points were tested as with the slightly older children). Similar adaptations to the simpler Gambs perimeter enabled us to measure visual fields in infants of 1.2 years and upwards.

The clinical routine can be slightly different from research protocols. For practical reasons, the observer also presents the stimulus when the child is centrally fixating. Thus it is possible for one clinician to perform the test. The child either sits on a parent's lap, kneels or sits on a chair or stands, depending on the age. It is fairly easy to determine when the stimulus is presented within the visual field in which case a clear, brisk eye movement in the correct direction is seen. When the stimulus is outside the field and goes undetected, aimless or searching eye movements are made. For older children, constant encouragement to watch the flashing lights is required. Stimuli are first presented for approximately 1 second duration outside the expected field and then every 10 degrees closer

Fig. 10.6
Confrontation test.

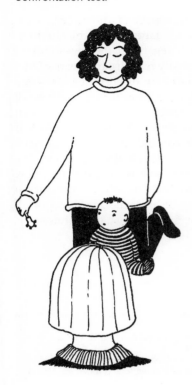

to fixation until a response is made. Then a new meridian is selected. Meridians 30 degrees apart should be tested in pseudo-random order (if too many meridians are attempted, attention and co-operation will be lost before the end of the test). True random order cannot be used due to the necessity to bring the projection arm through the 'gate' in order to complete the second half of the field. The field plot is marked with those positions not seen as well as those seen, e.g. a cross for 'not seen and a tick for 'seen'. The fact that eye movements were used as the response criterion should also be recorded. The advantage of using the Goldmann is that the visual fields plotted are comparable with known adult norms, the stimulus size and intensity being the same as used with adults (we use the V4e stimulus but smaller targets can be used). The disadvantages are that young children are wary of being asked to place their head on the chin rest and are distracted by the projecting arm of the instrument. There is also little contact between the clinician and the child.

Children from the age of 5 or 6 years may be able to respond to the traditional method of visual field plotting with the Goldmann. They enjoy using the buzzer and in fact the test can be introduced as like a computer game. This helps with co-operation!

A number of arc perimeters could be similarly adapted. We adapted an older Gambs perimeter which consists of a translucent bowl with a hand held projection device which slides on the convexity of the bowl. Again it was adapted with flashing LEDs to act as fixation stimuli. Since this instrument was less intimidating to the child, results were obtained with infants down to 1 year.

Confrontation

The confrontation test can be adapted for use with young children and with multiply-challenged older people (Mohn and van Hof-van Duin, 1983; Orel-Bixler, Haegerstrom-Portnoy and Hall, 1989). One examiner sits opposite the child, gains their attention and watches their eye movements. Meanwhile another examiner stands behind the child and brings an internally illuminated target or a white sphere (polystyrene Stycar ball, approximate diameter 3 cm) on a black wand (approximate diameter 3 cm) from behind the child in an arc centred on the child's head (Figure 10.6). If using an illuminated target, the room lights should be dimmed slightly. The eye movements are observed to indicate when the child has detected the target. Since the child will soon become accustomed to one target, it is useful to have at least two targets that can be alternated. This is a very approximate method: auditory cues can 'give the game away', the targets used are usually very large and/or bright, and the contrast against the background is not constant. However, in the multiply-challenged population this will give an approximation of the intactness of the visual field which can be gained in no other way. In children with very minimal visual responses, this is one of a battery of tests designed to determine if there is the ability to make any visual response to a stimulus (van Hof-van Duin and Mohn, 1986) and the test will usually be performed binocularly.

CONCLUSION

Measuring visual fields is an important aspect of functional visual assessment, but it is not easily achieved in infants and young children. Although more research is needed with regard to the development and measurement of visual fields in the early months and years of life, we have provided in this chapter an overview of current knowledge and given some practical suggestions for the clinical measurement of visual fields in infants and young children. Even neonates can generally be tested using an adapted arc perimeter, while a modified Goldmann perimeter can be used with some children from $2\frac{1}{2}$ years upwards. From about the age of 5, some children can use the traditional Goldmann method. Confrontation testing using internally illuminated stimuli or white styrofoam balls as stimuli provides a rough-and-ready alternative which may be of value for those of all ages with multiple impairments and/or minimal visual responses.

REFERENCES

Abrahamov, I., Gordon, J., Hendrickson, A. et al. (1982). The retina of the newborn human infant. *Science*, **217**, 265–267.

Cummings, M.F., van Hof van-Duin, J., Mayer, D.L. et al. (1988). Visual fields of young children. *Behavioural Brain Research*, **29**, 7–16.

Diaz-Araya, C. and Provis, J.M. (1992). Evidence of photoreceptor migration during early foveal development: A quantitative analysis of human fetal retinae. *Vis Neurosci.*, **8**, 505–514.

Dodd, C. and Leat, S.J. (1991). The assessment of visual fields in infants. *Ophthalmic and Physiological Optics*, **10**, 411.

Fichten, C.S., Judd, D., Tagalakis, V. et al. (1991). Communication cues used by people with and without visual impairments in daily conversations and dating. *Journal of Visual Impairment and Blindness*, **85** (9), 371–378.

Flanagan, J.G., Elliott, D.B., Patla, A. et al. (1993). The Waterloo vision and mobility study: Visual correlates of mobility performance in subject's ARM. *Investigative Ophthalmology & Visual Science*, **34**, 790.

Fulton, A.B., Hansen, R.M. and Manning, K.A. (1981). Measuring visual acuity in infants. *Surv. Ophthalmol.* **25**, 325–332.

Getz, L., Dobson, V. and Luna, B. (1993). Grating acuity and visual field development in infants who experienced intrauterine growth retardation. *Investigative Ophthalmology & Visual Science*, **34**, 1420.

Goldberg, M.C., Maurer, D. and Lewis, T.L. (1993). Influence of a central stimulus on infants visual fields. *Investigative Ophthalmology & Visual Science* (Suppl.) **34**, 354.

Guez, J., Le Gargasson, J., Rigaudiere, F. and O'Regan, J.K. (1993). Is there a systematic location for the pseudo-fovea in patients with central scotoma? *Vision Research*, **33**, 1271–1279.

Gwiazda, J., Brill, S., Mohindra, I. and Held, R. (1980). Preferential looking acuity in infants from two to fifty-eight weeks of age. *Am. J. Optom. Physiol. Opt.* **57**, 428–432.

Hirsch, J. (1985). Statistical analysis in computerised perimetry. In Whalen, W.R. and Spaeth, G.L. (eds), *Computerised Visual Fields.* New Jersey, U.S.A, Slack Inc.

van Hof-van Duin, J. and Mohn, G. (1986). Visual field responses, optokinetic nystagmus and the visual threatening response: Normal and abnormal development. In Detection and measurement of visual impairment in pre-verbal children. *Documenta Ophthalmologica Proc. Ser.* **45**, 305–316.

Horsten, G.P.M. and Winkelman, J.E. (1962). Electrical activity of the retina in relation to histological differentiation in infants born prematurely and at full-term. *Vision Research*, **2**, 269–276.

Johns, P.R., Rusoff, A.C. and Dubin, M.W. (1979). Postnatal neurogenesis in the kitten retina. *Journal of Comparative Neurology*, **187**, 545–556.

Lewis, T.L. and Maurer, D. (1992). The development of the temporal and nasal visual fields during infancy. *Vision Research*, **32**, 903–911.

Lia, B., Williams, R.W. and Chalupa, L.M. (1987). Formation of retinal ganglion cell topography during prenatal development. *Science*, **236**, 848–851.

Lovie-Kitchin, J., Mainstone, J., Robinson, J. and Brown, B. (1990). What areas of the visual field are important for mobility in low vision patients? *Clinical Vision Sciences*, **5**, 249–263.

Luna, B., Dobson, V., Carpenter, N.A. and Biglan, A.W. (1989). Visual field development in infants with Stage 3 retinopathy of prematurity. *Investigative Ophthalmology & Visual Science*, **30**, 580–582.

Luna, B., Dobson, V. and Getz, L. (1993). Infants who suffered perinatal asphyxia show decreased visual field size in the first three years of life. *Investigative Ophthalmology & Visual Science*, **34**, 1420.

Luna, B., Dobson, V., Scher, M.S. and Guthrie, R.D. (1995). Grating acuity and visual field development in infants following perinatal asphyxia. *Developmental Medicine and Child Neurology*, **37**, 330–344.

MacFarlane, A., Harris, P. and Barnes, J. (1976). Central and peripheral vision in early infancy. *Journal of Experimental Child Psychology*, **21**, 532–538.

Marron, J.A. and Bailey, I.L. (1982). Visual factors and orientation-mobility performance. *Am. J. Optom. Physiol. Opt.* **59**, 413–426.

Maurer, D. and Lewis, T. (1991). The influence of a central stimulus on newborn's effective visual field. *Investigative Ophthalmology & Visual Science* (Suppl.) **32**, 963.

Mayer, D.L. and Dobson, V. (1982). Visual acuity development in infants and young children as assessed by operant preferential looking. *Vision Research*, **22**, 1141–1151.

Mayer, D.L. and Fulton, A.B. (1993). Development of the human visual field. In K. Simons (ed.), *Early Visual Development Normal and Abnormal*. New York/Oxford, Oxford University Press.

Mayer, D.L., Fulton, A.B. and Cummings, M.F. (1988). Visual fields of infants assessed with a new perimetric technique. *Investigative Ophthalmology & Visual Science*, **29**, 452–459.

Mayer, D., Stewart, J., Raye, K. et al. (1993). Visual fields, acuity and recognition memory in very low birth weight (VLBW) infants. *Investigative Ophthalmology & Visual Science*, **34**, 1420.

Mohn, G. and van Hof-van Duin, J. (1983). Behavioral and electrophysiological measures of visual functions in children with neurological disorders. *Behav. Brain. Res.* **10**, 177–187.

Mohn, G. and van Hof-van Duin, J. (1986). Development of the binocular and monocular visual fields of human infants during the first year of life. *Clinical Vision Sciences*, **1**, 51–64.

Morris, R.K. and Rayner, K. (1991). Eye movements in skilled reading: Implications for developmental dyslexia. In J.F. Stein (ed.), *Vision and Visual Dyslexia*. Boca Raton, CRC Press.

Mutlukan, E. and Damato, E. (1993). Computerised perimetry with moving and steady fixation in children. *Eye*, **7**, 554–561.

Orel-Bixler, D., Haegerstrom-Portnoy, G. and Hall, A. (1989). Visual assessment of the multiply-handicapped patient. *Optometry and Vision Science*, **66**, 530–536.

Packer, O., Hendrickson, A.E. and Curcio, C.A. (1990). The developmental redistribution of photoreceptors across the Macaca Nemestrina (Pigtail Monkey) retina. *Journal of Comparative Neurology*, **298**, 472–493.

Pelli, E. (1986). Control of eye movement with peripheral vision: implications for the training of eccentric viewing. *Am. J. Optom. Physiol. Opt.*, **63**, 113–118.

Provis, J.M., Van Driel, D., Billson, F.A. and Russell, P. (1985). Development of the human retina: Patterns of cell distribution and redistribution in the ganglion cell layer. *Journal of Comparative Neurology*, **233**, 429–451.

Quinn, G.E., Fea, A.M. and Minguini, N. (1991). Visual fields in 4- to 10-year-old children using Goldmann and double-arc perimeters. *Journal of Pediatric Ophthalmology and Strabismus*, **28**, 314–319.

Robb, R.M. (1982). Increase in retinal area during infancy and childhood. *Journal of Pediatric Ophthalmology and Strubismus*, **19**, 16–20.

Roucoux, A., Crommelinck, M., Guerit, J.M. and Meulders, M. (1981). Two modes of eye-head coordination and the role of the vestibulo-ocular reflex in these two strategies. *Developmental Neuroscience*, **12**, 309–315.

Schwartz, T.L., Dobson, V. and Sandstrom, D.J. (1987). Kinetic assessment of binocular visual field shape and size in young infants. *Vision Research*, **27**, 2163–2175.

Tronick, E. (1972). Stimulus control and the growth of the infant's effective visual field. *Perceptual Percept. Psychophys.*, **11**, 373–376.

Whittaker, S.G. and Cummings, R.W. (1986). Redevelopment of fixation and scanning eye movements following the loss of foveal function. In S.R. Hilfer and F.B. Sheffield (eds), *Cell and Developmental Biology of the Eye: Development of Order in the Visual System.* New York, Springer-Verlag, pp. 177–191.

Whittaker, S.G. and Cummings, R.W. (1990). Eccentric eye movements with loss of central vision. In A.W. Johnston and M. Lawrence, *Low Vision Ahead II, Conference Proceedings*, pp. 67–73.

Whittaker, S.G. and Lovie-Kitchin, J. (1993). Visual requirements for reading. *Optometry and Vision Science*, **70**, 54–65.

Yuodelis, C. and Hendrickson, A. (1986). A qualitative and quantitative analysis of the human fovea during development. *Vision Research*, **26**, 847–855.

Zawilski, J. (1980). A guide to better living for the visually-impaired. In *Collection of Resource Materials Related to the Handicapped*. Montreal, Centre for Continuing Education, Dawson College.

11

Colour vision

INTRODUCTION

In considering the assessment of colour vision, the test which first comes to mind is the Ishihara, which is familiar to many members of the public as well as to eye practitioners. However, it was devised for use with adults and has probably been used too uncritically with children in the past. In this chapter we examine the problems in testing children's colour vision and discuss the advantages and disadvantages of a range of tests, including some which are currently under development. First, some general background information is provided, explaining very briefly the nature of colour vision and its development, the difference between inherited and acquired deficiencies and the effects of colour deficiency on children's development. Parents, other carers and teachers will find some particularly useful information in the section entitled 'Educational and everyday problems.' The chapter ends with some broad guidelines for testing children's colour vision.

NORMAL COLOUR VISION AND ITS DEVELOPMENT

Normal colour vision

Human vision, like that of other primates, is based on two types of light-sensitive cells, or photoreceptors. In the periphery of the retina are the rods, subserving low light intensity vision, while the cones, found throughout the retina but concentrated in the fovea centralis, subserve high light intensity colour vision. Vision at low levels of illuminance, when only the rods operate, is without colour (achromatic), whereas in normal daylight maximum colour discrimination is possible.

Most people are trichromats, that is, they have three types of cone containing different types of light-absorbing photopigment. Each photopigment has a unique profile of sensitivity to various wavelengths, although these absorbency spectra do overlap with one another (Figure 11.1). About 10% of the cones are 'blue' cones, responding maximally to the lower wavelengths (around 440 nanometres, nm), while the remainder are about equal numbers of 'green' and 'red' cones, responding maximally to 545 nm and 565 nm

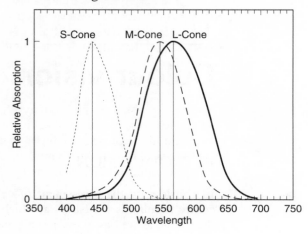

Fig. 11.1
Relative spectral sensitivities of short-, medium- and long-wave receptors. (From Smith, V.C. and Pokorny, J. (1972). Spectral sensitivity of colour-blind observers and the cone photopigments. *Vision Research,* **12,** 2059–2071 and Smith, V.C. and Pokorny, J. (1975). Spectral sensitivity of cone photopigments between 400 and 500 nm. *Vision Research,* **15,** 161–171.)

respectively. It should be noted that the 'red' pigment actually has maximum sensitivity in the yellow, rather than the red, region of the spectrum, but the original colour-name term has tended to stick (Jacobs, 1986; Millodot, 1986). Some workers have advocated replacing the colour-name terms of the cones with S, M and L (short, medium and long wave), and this terminology is being increasingly used.

Any single cone can only signal the number of units of light, or photons, absorbed by its pigment, and cannot of itself distinguish between brightness (or intensity) of stimulation and wavelength. Comparisons of the strength of signal emanating from two or more types of cone is needed to determine colour.

It should be noted that this system alone does not account for the entire range of colours perceived by humans. Non-spectral colours such as pink can be accounted for by opponency theory, whereby there are three independent mechanisms, each composed of a mutually inhibiting pair of colour systems, red-green, yellow-blue and black-white. Historically, the Young–Helmholtz theory of colour vision was based on the principle of trichromacy and the Hering theory on opponency. It is now known that these two theories are not mutually exclusive, but complementary, with opponency coming into play at a higher level of visual processing than the cone receptors, where the pigment-based trichromatic system is located. In considering colour deficiency it is in the trichromatic pigmentary system that deficits appear to be located, although we may note in passing that there is research which suggests that the picture is more complicated than this (e.g. Pokorny and Smith, 1982). (For general reviews of research on colour vision see Jacobs, 1986; Boynton, 1988.)

The development of colour vision

It is only in recent years that techniques have become available which have enabled researchers to determine whether infants respond differentially to different wavelengths of light (e.g. Teller and Lindsey, 1993). Such techniques, all discussed elsewhere in this book, include preferential looking (based on the infant's direction of gaze), operant conditioning (rewarding the infant for performing certain behaviours), inducing optokinetic nystagmus or OKN (automatic stabilizing eye movements in response to a moving visual field) and measuring visual evoked potentials (VEP, electrical activity of the brain in response to visual pattern stimulation). An additional problem in measuring responses to chromatic stimuli is that different colours also differ in luminance (brightness), which must therefore be carefully controlled so that the person cannot discriminate between stimuli on the basis of luminance rather than hue. Various studies have attempted to control for this by matching the luminance of stimuli presented to infants, despite uncertainty as to whether luminance matches are in fact the same in newborns as in adults; however, there is now some evidence that they are similar, at least for stimuli of low spatial frequencies in the region of 0.1–1 cycle per degree (Morrone, Burr and Fiorentini, 1993).

Various studies using behavioural methods have suggested that colour vision is not well-developed at birth (e.g. Adams and Maurer, 1983; Adams, Maurer and Davis, 1986). While some studies suggested that in the early weeks the infant is relatively weak in red sensitivity, others indicated a lack of a short-wave mechanism. These studies led to the suggestion that the newborn's retina effectively functions like peripheral vision in an adult, while by 3 months of age colour vision is well developed, including the ability to divide colours into hue categories, such as blue, red, yellow and green, as adults do, although relatively large stimuli are needed (Bornstein, Kessen and Weiskopf, 1976; Bornstein, 1978; Teller and Bornstein, 1984).

VEP studies support the behavioural evidence that colour vision is absent or weak until several weeks after birth. Prior to about 2 months of age, VEP responses to even high-contrast red-green stimuli (equated for luminance) do not occur (while, on the other hand, responses to luminance stimuli of only 20% contrast produce strong and reliable VEP responses) (Morrone, Burr and Fiorentini, 1993). Allen, Banks and Norcia (1993) have argued that the lack of response to chromatic stimuli can be explained by a general lack of sensitivity of the infant's visual system and is not due to a particular immaturity of the chromatic system. Morrone, Burr and Fiorentini (1993), however, have argued that this general lack of sensitivity is not a sufficient explanation for the limits of infant colour vision and suggest that special neural mechanisms (beyond the receptors) do in fact undergo development during the early weeks of life. Interested readers are referred to these two papers for a fuller exposition of these arguments, which is beyond the scope of this chapter.

It is interesting to note that there is some indication of reduced sensitivity to both shorter and longer wavelengths of light in young adolescents (in comparison with adults). The reason is not clear, but the differences are small, unlikely to show up on standard screening tests and are not thought to be of clinical significance (Hill, 1984).

COLOUR DEFICIENCY

Inherited deficiencies

Deficiencies in colour vision may be either inherited or acquired. Inherited defects are often referred to as 'congenital', although strictly speaking this term covers any condition present at birth, whether inherited or acquired prenatally or perinatally. Inherited colour vision defects are binocular and lifelong, with no presently known treatment. Although a prescribed coloured filter in front of one eye may aid in discriminating between certain colours, it does not restore normal colour vision and interferes with binocularity (Birch, 1985).

Aside from the indications of immature colour vision in young infants and of very slightly reduced sensitivity in older children, the assumption is generally made that the incidence of inherited colour deficiency in children is similar to that in adults – around 8% of males but only about 0.5% of females in a European population. However, a number of studies assessing children directly, including both United States and Australian samples, have found a lower incidence of colour deficiency in boys, of between 6% and 7% (e.g. Thuline, 1964; Walters, 1984). Some adult male populations also have lower incidences of colour deficiency: there is about a 5% incidence in Japanese and Scottish males and 3% amongst Australian aborigines.

Inherited colour deficiency results from the absence or modification of one or more cone pigments, usually red or green. The sex difference in incidence occurs because, genetically, the green and red pigments are encoded on the X-chromosome. A female would need 'colour defective' genes (for the same type of colour defect) on her two X-chromosomes in order to be colour defective, whereas a male with colour defective genetic information encoded on his one X-chromosome would actually be colour defective. A female with only one affected chromosome would have normal colour vision herself but be a carrier of colour deficiency, which could find expression in her children (usually her sons, unless the father also had defective colour vision in which case daughters might also be colour defective).

The blue pigment is not sex-linked, being encoded on chromosome 7 (Tovee, 1992), and very few people have an inherited blue, or tritan, defect, whereby yellows appear grey and orange has a pinkish appearance. However, in the case of acquired deficiency, blue cones are commonly affected, being particularly susceptible to high light intensity and oxygen deprivation. This kind of colour deficiency is therefore of clinical importance. There are variations in blue sensitivity even among people with normal colour vision owing to individual differences in a layer of pigment which overlies the fovea.

Blue sensitivity also decreases with age as a result of changes in the crystalline lens (Birch, 1985).

The most severe form of colour deficiency is monochromacy (achromatopsia), or almost total absence of colour vision, which is very rare, occurring in perhaps 3 people in every 100 000. To these people, the world appears rather as it does on a black and white television.

The next most severe form, in which colour vision is dependent on only two types of cone, is dichromacy. Although it has been reported that dichromats may have an advantage in being able to penetrate camouflage which deceives trichromats (Morgan, Mollon and Adam, 1989), they are generally disadvantaged in a world geared towards trichromacy. Red-green dichromacy, affecting about 25% of those with a colour defect, is commonly referred to as red-green blindness, although the use of such colour-name terms and the word 'blindness' are misleading and often discouraged by writers on colour vision. Dichromacy usually takes one of two forms, protanopia or deuter-anopia (tritanopia being very rare). Protanopes ('red-blind') confuse reds with dark brown, dark greys and black, light greens with light brown, and purplish shades with blue; their sensitivity to the brightness of red is also reduced. Deuteranopes ('green-blind') confuse red, orange and light brown, blues, violets and blue-purples, light greens and magentas.

Less severe deficiencies (anomalies) are protanomaly or red weakness (about 1% males), and deuteranomaly or green weakness (about 5% males). The degree of deficiency of these anomalous trichromats varies from very slight to near-dichromacy. Deuterano-malous and protanomalous individuals can use brightness sensitivity as a compensatory mechanism. Because some children with colour defects may use brightness or other clues (such as the colour-name labels other people attach to particular objects), they may sometimes use appropriately the names of colours which are not in their perceptual repertoire, and this may lead others to believe that such a child does not have a colour defect.

The ability to discriminate between spectral hues is illustrated by the 1931 CIE (Commission Internationale d'Eclairage) chromaticity diagram (Figure 11.2). This locates various standard hues within a triangular 'colour space' with a primary colour (green, blue or red) at each corner (note that these are imaginary, 'pure' colours). The X axis indicates the proportion of red and the Y axis the proportion of green in any hue (the proportion of blue is calculated by subtracting the sum of the proportions of red and green from 1). The areas depicted in this plot show the areas of certain 'groups' of colours. Thus a colour which we would label as pink would have chromaticity co-ordinates which would fall within that area of the graph, but many discriminable hues can be detected within that area by a person with normal colour vision. Congenital protan, deutan and tritan dichromats typically confuse colours along lines which span from one side to the other of the graph, known as 'confusion lines' which lie along colours which are easily discriminated by colour-normal individuals. Those without

Fig. 11.2
The CIE chromaticity space. (Taken from Coren, S. and Ward, L.M. (1989). *Sensation and Perception,* 3rd edn. San Diego, Harcourt, Brace, Jovanovich, reproduced by permission of the publisher.)

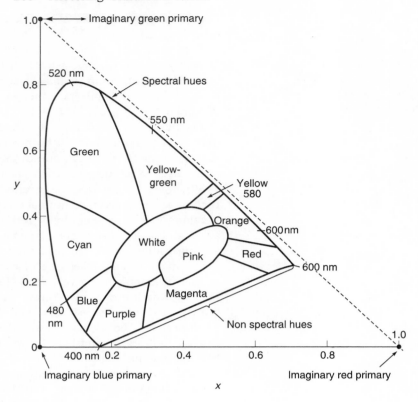

long-wave cones make confusions which lie along lines characteristic of protan deficiency, those without medium wavelength receptors make confusions along deutan lines and those lacking short-wave cones make confusions along tritan lines. Use is made of these confusion lines to select and specify hues used in colour vision tests. For example, the hues used in the Minimalist Test (discussed later in the chapter) are illustrated in Figure 11.3.

It should be noted that the well-accepted view of congenital colour vision defects presented above seems to apply best to small field stimuli, as typically used in colour vision tests. With large fields, most dichromats appear to experience limited trichromacy, based partially on signals from rods (Pokorny and Smith, 1982).

Acquired deficiencies

Acquired, as opposed to inherited, colour vision deficiencies, are clinically important and, unlike inherited deficiencies, may be monocular or asymmetrical in severity between the two eyes (and testing should be done with the two eyes separately if pathology is suspected). They may occur as a result of drugs, toxins, certain disease states or injury. Unlike congenital deficiencies, which remain stable, acquired defects may change as the pathological state

Fig. 11.3
Positions of the probe chips used in the Mollon–Reffin Minimalist test in relation to the CIE chromaticity diagram. Each dot represents a chip lying along a confusion line (protan, deutan and tritan). (By courtesy of Dr John Mollon.)

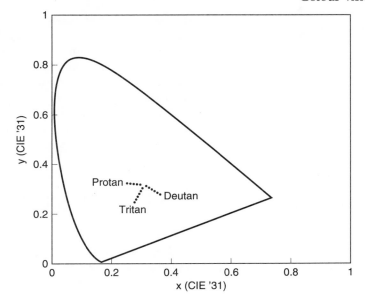

progresses (or remits). If pathology is suspected as the cause of a child's colour vision defect, referral for ophthalmological examination is vital. In addition, acquired colour deficiencies may not fall into the same clear categories as inherited colour defects, although we use the same tests (based on these categories) to test for them (Fischer, 1996). For this reason it is suggested that the names protan, deutan and tritan be used in the case of inherited defects only, with acquired defects being referred to as red-green or blue-yellow.

Acquired red-green defects do occur, and may resemble protan defects (Type I – as in juvenile macular degeneration) or deutan defects (Type II – as in retrobulbar neuritis). However, the 'blue' system is also very commonly affected (Type III, resembling a tritan defect). For example, although Oyama et al. (1991) found both blue-yellow and red-green defects in association with traumatic optic nerve injuries, the blue-yellow system was generally much more vulnerable. In retinitis pigmentosa, blue-yellow defects are also usual, although the red-green system can also be affected if there is sufficient macular involvement. It is often the case in progressive retinal conditions that there is a general loss of ability to discriminate colours which are less saturated (i.e. 'washed out').

The question has been raised as to whether children with diabetes should be screened for colour vision changes which might indicate retinal complications, as these are known to occur in adults with diabetes (again, in the blue system). Mantyjarvi (1991) assessed the colour vision of 9–18-year-old children who had had diabetes for a mean time of nearly 6 years. Significant differences from control children were found, but these only showed up on detailed analysis of their colour vision using an anomaloscope (discussed below) and it still fell within the normal range. Ophthalmoscopic examination and the use of routine clinical vision tests did not reveal any problems. It seems, therefore, that any early changes in colour vision which may be occurring in these children are unlikely to show up through normal clinical methods. The same is true for adults.

It was at one time recommended that children with diabetes should have their colour vision examined to ensure that they could carry out the colour-matching task necessary to check their urine glucose level (Aspinall, Hill and Cameron, 1980). This is of less importance these days, as it is usual for children to monitor their own blood rather than urine for glucose, with the sample being tested electronically.

EFFECTS OF COLOUR DEFICIENCY

Career choice

Pathological conditions aside, there is the question of whether or not it is important to know whether a child has a colour vision defect. A teacher could reasonably expect one or two pupils in a class to be colour deficient. Most would be deuteranomalous ('green deficient'). These figures are based on extrapolation from the adult incidence, but checking whether this is so in practice is not a straightforward matter, as it brings us to the difficult question of what test or tests should be used to assess colour vision in children. We will consider that after first examining the degree to which colour deficiency affects a child's life.

Traditionally, it has not been considered of importance to assess colour vision (apart from in pathological conditions) until an age when career choices become relevant. Occupations such as electronics, vocational driving, graphic design, interior design and the textile and chemical industries may require good colour vision. Some individuals have reported that their colour vision deficiency has prevented them from advancing in their careers, such as a hairdresser who could not go into his own business because he could not select tints, and a printer who was restricted to black and white printing (Steward and Cole, 1989). Some occupations are completely barred to those with moderate to severe colour deficiencies. Such barriers have been in place for railway and maritime occupations for more than a century, arising from concerns about risks of accidents arising from an operator's inability to discriminate between coloured signals. Cole (1991) has drawn attention to the lack of standardization of occupational colour vision standards and procedures, pointing out that in these days of equal opportunities in employment there is a need to be very sure that a colour vision deficiency is truly a barrier to good job performance. Furthermore, technological developments in some industries may make colour a less salient dimension than previously (contrariwise, computerization may make it more so, as discussed later).

Although some industries and authorities will insist on their own testing programme for applicants, the vision care specialist may be able to alert a young person to colour vision difficulties at an early enough stage to guide selection of school subject options leading to particular career paths.

Educational and everyday problems

In the case of younger children, the major question to be considered is whether a colour defect does, in fact, affect their general development or education. A number of studies suggest an association between colour vision and education. Espinda (1971) found that children with colour vision deficiencies tended to have a lower school grade point average than those with normal colour vision. In another study, Espinda (1973) found that more than the expected number of children with colour defects were referred to special programmes for those with learning disabilities. Grosvenor (1977) reported poorer primary school reading performance, while Dannemaier (1972) found that secondary school children with defective colour vision had more difficulty with the biology course and were (not surprisingly) poorer achievers in the subject. More recently Hurley (1994) has described a case study which suggests that colour vision deficiency can impair literacy acquisition.

Others, however, have reported no association between colour deficiency and school achievement. Differences in findings may be partly due to different methods used for assessing colour vision, some of which are not appropriate for children at certain ages (Hill, 1984). Furthermore, some writers have suggested that the reported association between learning problems and colour vision deficiency are due to children with learning disabilities failing the tests for reasons other than colour deficiency, such as difficulty in discriminating a figure from its background (e.g. Justen and Harth, 1976). Dwyer (1991) examined the colour vision of children who were about 12 years old and who had learning difficulties, using a battery of tests to overcome any problems they had in performing particular tests. She found that almost 20% of the boys with learning difficulties were colour defective, half having a moderate to severe defect. This does seem to suggest a real association between colour deficiency and learning problems although, as Dwyer discusses, learning problems are likely to involve numerous factors, and it is not possible to conclude simplistically that colour problems cause learning problems. Nevertheless, as she says, a child who is experiencing learning problems for other reasons may be further handicapped by a colour vision defect.

It does seem reasonable to suppose that young children with colour defects might meet educational problems when materials are colour-coded, for example, in reading materials or mathematics, when different colours of letters or blocks are sometimes used to help explain concepts (Waddington, 1965). As Dwyer (1991) notes, colour is used in classrooms to stimulate interest and attention, to increase motivation and to convey instructional messages. In fact, children who have learning problems are especially likely to be presented with such materials, as colour-cueing is regarded as useful for developing discrimination skills in children who are having difficulty in learning to distinguish letters or numbers. Colour pervades the curriculum in other ways too, such as colour-coding of such things as library book categories or work sheets. Indeed, as Dwyer (1983) has noted, 'Students are required to . . . use color either creatively or systematically in many areas of the curriculum.' Older children themselves have reported particular problems with maps, with coloured chalk on blackboards, with litmus paper and with reading teachers' marks on their books, and feel limited in their career choices (Carpenter, 1983).

There is also evidence that a colour defect can lead to practical problems in everyday life. Children have reported difficulty in seeing traffic lights and brake lights when cycling, difficulty with board games and snooker, in choosing clothes which match and in seeing colour television distinctly. Some reported that certain foods had colours which looked unattractive to them, including cheese (very dark), radishes (orange) and spinach (black) (Carpenter, 1983). The increasing use of microcomputer technology in education and other settings is also likely to create problems for those with colour deficiencies: for example, they may have difficulty with spreadsheet headings or be unable to distinguish the coloured sections on a piechart (Adkins and Pease, 1991). If this problem occurs, it can be overcome by changing the colour scheme of the computer.

It may be that many children overcome their problems to a large extent, particularly in the case of mild defects, by using alternative cues such as brightness or copying what other children do. However, as discussed by Dwyer (1991) young children may not have yet developed such strategies at a time when colour is important in their learning, and it is possible that those with more general learning problems will have greater difficulty in developing such strategies. Art teachers are often aware of children who have colour vision problems, as revealed by paintings such as red ploughed fields and pale green skin, but teachers are in general unaware of children's colour vision problems (Carpenter, 1983). It therefore seems worthwhile testing early so that teachers can be informed and make adaptations (for example, using shape-coding instead of colour-coding, and avoiding the use of hard-to-distinguish colours on blackboards and whiteboards) and be less likely to blame a child for what appear to be silly mistakes or uncooperative behaviour.

Hill (1984) has recommended that colour vision testing should feature in the assessment of any child who is experiencing learning problems. In addition, colour vision testing is an important part of a functional visual assessment for children with low vision and/or multiple impairments. It is known that in adults many low vision conditions give rise to either a red-green or a blue-yellow defect and the same may be expected for children with low vision. Indeed, one study showed that 75% of children with low vision failed at least one of four colour tests (Kalloniatis and Johnston, 1990) indicating a high percentage of colour defects in this population, as expected on the basis of adult data. Although we know little of the percentage of children with multiple disabilities who have colour vision difficulties, there is some evidence of a higher than usual prevalence of red-green defects (Perez-Carpinell, de Fez and Climent, 1994).

Children's understanding of colour vision deficiency

It may also be important to help a child with a colour vision deficiency to come to some kind of an understanding of it. Most children questioned by Carpenter (1983) could not explain the cause of their colour defect, and this is quite in accord with research on children's understanding of health-related issues, which indicates limited understanding in young children (Chapter 3). Even by secondary school age children may have little awareness of or understanding about colour deficiency, feeling uncomfortable about it or even regarding it as an illness. This was indicated by a study in Italy by Gallo and Nardella (1991). They found that many students were unaware of their own colour deficiency, especially if it was not very severe, although some with slight defects were aware of them while others with strong defects were not. They also reported that the young people were reluctant to admit to being different, and that those with normal colour vision, when shown plates unreadable by those with normal colour vision (Ishihara test, plates 18–21) often showed embarrassment and even disorientation and asked afterwards for reassurance as to their normality. The reaction to testing of those previously unaware of their colour blindness ranged from slight uneasiness to complete denial, while those who already knew they had a colour deficiency were restless about performing the test. Those with normal colour vision regarded colour blindness as an 'illness', which might further reinforce the feelings of those with colour vision deficiencies regarding being abnormal. Carpenter (1983) also reported that older boys seemed more reluctant than younger ones to admit to having problems as a result of colour vision deficiency. These findings support earlier suggestions that colour vision deficiencies may affect a child's psychological development (Bacon, 1971; Snyder, 1973), although better-designed research in this field is needed (Wilkinson, 1990).

Given the importance of the developmental task of older children in building good peer relationships, it is not surprising to find that those with colour vision difficulties may be uncomfortable with being 'different'. Children with colour deficiencies may therefore benefit from counselling to help them understand their condition and come to terms with any negative feelings it engenders. That counselling would be effective is suggested by the finding that children with older siblings or other relatives with similar problems adjust to their difficulties at an earlier age than eldest or only children (Waddington, 1965).

TESTING CHILDREN'S COLOUR VISION

Problems in designing colour vision tests

Many tests of colour vision, with various advantages and disadvantages, have been developed over the years, and continue to be developed. One important consideration in designing a test, or choosing one clinically, is the purpose of testing, whether to screen for congenital defects, or to make a detailed assessment of vision for occupational purposes or because an acquired defect is known or suspected to exist.

Most tests, such as the well-known Ishihara, have been designed to screen the general population for congenital red-green defects (Birch, 1991), and have been designed to be quick to use and portable. To be totally effective as a screening tool, a test should be passable only by those with normal colour vision and 'failed' only by those with deficiencies. In reality this is not possible, and the aim is for a minimal number of false positives (those with normal colour vision who fail the test) and false negatives (those with a deficiency who nevertheless pass the test). The confidence with which one can make a decision of colour vision normality is always greater than the confidence with which one can decide that a person is colour vision defective (Hill and Aspinall, 1980) and this is especially true for children. False positives are a real problem in designing tests for children, since if the task is a difficult one for children they may fail it despite having normal colour vision. False negatives are an issue with regard to the sensitivity of the test – since there are degrees of colour deficiency the designer has to decide what is an acceptably low level of deficiency which could be allowed to pass. In general, a screening programme should be aimed at identifying those with normal colour vision, with the remainder being 'doubtfuls' – people who would benefit from further assessment, preferably using an alternative test.

There are two other, basic, problems which a colour vision test must overcome. One is the fact that some individuals with colour vision defects can nevertheless make some discriminations using brightness as a cue. The other is that it may be possible to identify a patch of colour by detecting the edges of the patch – an edge artefact. These two problems were overcome in 1876 by Stilling, who introduced pseudoisochromatic (i.e. 'falsely the same colour') plates. These can be likened to mosaics, made up of discrete patches of colour. A person with normal colour vision can detect a figure contrasting with the background while a person with a colour defect either cannot distinguish it or sees an alternative pattern. Edge artefacts are not a problem because the figure to be identified does not have an edge (each patch has its own), and brightness cannot be used as a cue because the brightness of the coloured patches varies.

There are also technical problems to be addressed concerning the nature of the colour source, whether this be pigmented papers (in which case the light is reflected) or a direct light source. For the production of tests which used pigmented papers, standardized (Munsell) colour samples are available.

There are circumstances in which there is a need not just to screen for colour deficiency, but to investigate the colour vision of an individual in detail. It may be important for occupational purposes, for research, or for clinical reasons to be able to specify both the nature and the extent of a colour vision defect (whether it is mild or severe). Blue-yellow defects as well as red-green defects may need investigating because of their importance in pathological conditions, and colour vision testing can aid in differential diagnosis, in monitoring change and in assessing functional vision.

Ideally, sophisticated psychophysical testing of acquired colour vision deficiencies should be done (King-Smith, 1991), but such methods are not yet in common clinical use. Furthermore, when it comes to testing children, the demands of most such tests are beyond their capabilities. Testing of acquired colour vision deficiencies in both adults and children is still therefore heavily reliant upon tests which are, in essence, simplified versions of psychophysical methods but based on pigment colours (Birch, 1991). Unfortunately, since clinical colour vision tests have primarily been designed to screen for congenital red-green colour vision defects, these may be used inappropriately in the case of acquired defects. For example, the commonly-available Ishihara has been used uncritically to assess acquired deficiencies, despite its lack of a tritan plate (Krastel and Moreland, 1991).

Tests of colour vision

Below we give a brief description of some of the types of instruments for assessing colour vision that have been commonly used over the years (Birch, 1985, 1991). We will then discuss the usefulness of various tests with children, and finally describe some of the most recent tests which hold particular promise for use with children.

Anomaloscopes

An anomaloscope is a spectral colour-matching instrument based on the fact that red and green light when mixed appears the same as monochromatic yellow light (the Rayleigh match). The viewer either adjusts controls to achieve a match between the two halves of a split field (Nagel anomaloscopes) or is required to comment on a match presented by the examiner who then makes adjustments as necessary (Pickford–Nicolson or Nagel anomaloscope). An anomalous trichromat will choose red-green ratios outside the normal, narrow range, a deuteranomalous person choosing more green and a protanomalous person more red. Protanopes and deuteranopes can match any red-green ratio with yellow, the two types being distinguished by the relative luminances needed in the comparison field. The Nagel anomaloscope is sensitive and accurate, but expensive. The Pickford–Nicolson anomaloscope is widely used, but is less accurate, being relatively more affected by room lighting, the expertise of the examiner and examiner–examinee communication. Although not routinely in clinical use because of high cost and level of special expertise needed to use it, the anomaloscope is regarded as the definitive test for screening and diagnosing inherited protan and deutan defects. Indeed, it is the only test which can accurately distinguish between dichromats and trichromats. There have been attempts to develop anomaloscopes to screen for tritan defects and these have achieved some success.

Pseudoisochromatic plates

Based on 'mosaic' patterns, as described earlier, the best known pseudoisochromatic test is the Ishihara, which consists of a series of 'plates', or coloured designs, in book form. The first plate has an orange figure which is detectable even by those with colour deficiencies, and is used to explain the test; failure on this plate would indicate lack of understanding, pretence of colour defect or gross visual pathology. Subsequent plates contain numerals which may or may not be detectable depending on the nature of the individual's colour vision. The Ishihara is a good screen for congenital protan and deutan defects; however, the severity of the defect is not measured (although a person just failing the test can be considered to have a mild defect). It does not screen for tritan defects. Neither does it distinguish between protan and deutan defects even though there are plates which are claimed to do this. As well as the numeral plates there are also 'trails' or 'wavy line' plates, which the testee can trace (using a paintbrush to avoid soiling the plates). These so-called 'illiterate' plates are designed to be used if the person cannot produce verbal responses or has difficulty in identifying numerals. These plates have often been used with young children. A simplified Ishihara, the Ishihara test for Unlettered Persons (IUP), includes circles and squares to be identified verbally, and these have proved successful with 4–7 year olds provided repetitions are permitted (Birch and Platts, 1993). A number of other pseudoisochromatic tests have either been designed especially for use with children or have often been used with them, including the AO-HRR (geometric shapes), Farnsworth F2 (to screen for blue-yellow as well as red-green deficiencies), Guys (developed at Guys Hospital London, with templates to match letters against), the Matsubara (Japanese-style pictures) and the Velhagen Pflugertrident (letter E in various orientations with a template to be matched with the target) and the SPP-1 and the SPP-2. As later discussion will show, the fact that a test has been specially designed for use with children does not guarantee its usefulness, and unfortunately some of the best tests are now out of print, including the AO-HRR and the Farnsworth. The AO-HRR is nevertheless discussed below as many practitioners still have access to this test and it is sometimes referred to in research reports. It should be noted that different printings of pseudoisochromatic plates have different validity.

Arrangement tests

These use the concept of arranging a series of colours in a specified order, people with colour deficiencies making errors in the sequence. These tests were designed for occupational purposes, and are not screening tests but are used to diagnose and grade the degree of colour deficiency, and are therefore also of clinical use, especially in investigating acquired colour vision defects. The Farnsworth–Munsell 100 hue test (FM 100-hue) involves placing 85 colour sample discs in order in four boxes; manual scoring of this test is tedious. The D-15 panel test uses only 15 discs, giving typical errors in the case of protan, deutan and tritan defects; there is also a desaturated version (using paler hues) which can be used in conjunction with the standard version. The City University test is derived from the D-15, has both saturated and desaturated versions, but is not itself an arrangement test; in booklet form, each page displays a central circle of colour surrounded by four other coloured circles and the testee has to choose the closest match (one is a near correct match indicating normal colour vision while the other three lie along confusion lines for protan, deutan and tritan-type defects).

Lanterns

These are specifically designed for colour vision testing for those wishing to enter industries such as aviation which necessitate the accurate detection of coloured signals. They are many and varied and to be found on the premises of statutory licensing authorities and some research laboratories. Ordinarily, vision care practitioners do not have access to them and may not understand them (Cole, 1991).

Usefulness of tests with children

Although the desirability of screening children for colour vision defects can be argued, this has not been easy to do in the past, despite attempts to produce tests specifically designed for children. A major problem is that the difficulty of the tasks often means that children with good colour vision will fail a test. To be suitable for screening purposes, a test must be manageable by the majority of children at the age in question to avoid the production of false positive results. To be suitable for assessing an acquired defect, not only must the child be able to manage the task, but it should provide information about yellow-blue as well as red-green defects and should provide quantitative as well as qualitative information.

Hill (1984) analysed the types of tests available into different levels of complexity. The simplest tests would merely involve detection of a stimulus, as was done in the experiments on infants' colour vision described earlier, using techniques based on preferential looking and other behavioural responses, on OKN and VEP. Such tests were limited to laboratory use at the time of Hill's review and this is largely still the case (although later some promising recent developments will be discussed). The next level of complexity identified by Hill consists of discrimination tests, involving 'same-different' judgements, as in the case of the anomaloscope. Resolution tests come next, such as the wavy lines of the Ishihara, followed by identification (matching) such as Guys. Finally come the most demanding tests, requiring manipulation of stimulus properties such as naming of shapes and numbers and problem solving, which would include the Ishihara numbers, the AO-HRR, the City and the arrangement tests. Hill acknowledges that this classification is not 'pure', and that a particular test could fall into another group depending on exactly how it was carried out.

It is only possible to determine whether a test is suitable for screening children of a particular age by comparing the test with another which is accepted as being a good test, and validating it against this baseline. Hill says that the Pickford–Nicolson anomaloscope is suitable as a validating instrument for children from the age of 4, who are able to make the necessary same-different judgements. He claims support for its use from a study with boys with intellectual impairments, which identified a percentage of colour vision deficiency very similar to the 8% of the adult male population (by contrast, about 30% of such boys fail the Ishihara). Although the Nagel anomaloscope is in some respects a better instrument than the Pickford–Nicolson, it has been reported as being more difficult for young children to use because it involves viewing the target with a telescopic system, and Verriest (1981) recommended that it should not be used below the age of 12. However, Dwyer (1991) apparently used the Nagel successfully with her sample who, although their mean age was 12 years, had learning disabilities, and so would be performing cognitively at a younger age level. Her success may have been aided by her technique: she presented the task as a game in which the child had to identify the colour and brightness of the two halves of the moon, with the tester manipulating the settings and using a bracketing method (Chapter 6).

Hill validated a number of colour vision tests against the Pickford–Nicolson anomaloscope for children of various ages. He acknowledged that the minimum ages that he suggests for the various tests to be suitable for screening will be considered conservative by many practitioners. Although the Ishihara wavy line plates are often used with young children, Hill presents evidence that they are not, in fact, suitable for screening children under the age of 8 years. This means that, given the tests available at the time of his review, there was no readily available screening test that could be used with children below this age – a concerning fact given the arguments for identifying colour deficiencies well below this age. Hill recommends that identification tests not be used for screening below 10 years, and interpretation tests, such as the Ishihara figures, not until 12 years. However, in a clinical, rather than a screening situation, a test may be used at a younger age: if a child passes, there is little doubt that colour vision is normal, but a failure may enable only a guarded diagnosis to be made until the child is older.

Hill's work illustrates the difficulty that has existed in assessing young children's colour vision. Tests are either specialized laboratory ones (such as anomaloscope and VEP), have poor screening efficiency (such as Guys), are too difficult for many young children (such as Ishihara numbers) or are not intended as screening instruments as well as being difficult for young children (such as the arrangement tests).

Even tests specially designed or recommended for use with children should be used with caution. The poor screening efficiency of Guys is one example. Another is the the Velhagen Pflugertrident test, recommended for screening kindergarten children in the former German Democratic Republic: this has been found to be unreliable, with a proportion of children with colour vision defects passing the test and young children (4–7 years) having difficulty with the matching task involved (Birch and Platts, 1993). Both this test and the Ishihara for Unlettered Persons (IUP) were designed to classify colour defects as protan or deutan but, using these tests, Birch and Platts were able to classify fewer than half the colour defects in their sample. They concluded that the IUP test can be used for screening red–green defects in young children if the methodology is flexible, but that detailed examination of colour defects, in terms of type and severity, cannot be carried out until the child is older and able to cope with the more difficult arrangement tests.

The AO-HRR, although long out of print, is still used by many practitioners. Although its value as a screening tool for children under 10 is limited (Hill, 1984), with half of 4–5 year olds failing the test (Verriest, Uvijls and Malfroidt, 1981), it retains some clinical value in the case of acquired defects in young children (especially if relaxed administration procedures are used, such as allowing children to trace rather than name the shapes): it includes protan, deutan and tritan plates, and permits the degree of defect to be assessed.

The City test is another which should not be undervalued in its potential use with young children, despite Hill's (1984) suggestion that it requires fairly complex cognitive skills. Sullivan, Shute and Westall (1990) found that 4 year olds made only a small percentage of errors. It seems possible, therefore, that Hill's analysis of the skills required is over-complex, and that the children simply treat it as a perceptual matching task. The City is not very sensitive in that children with mild colour defects can pass it (indeed, as discussed earlier, it is not intended as a screening test), but it should serve the purpose of screening out those children whose defect is most likely to be handicapping.

Testing the colour vision of a child with low vision is particularly problematic, since pseudoisochromatic plates require a reasonable acuity level, and children with severe visual impairment tend to look at them from a very short distance. Hedin (1983) recommends the use of the D-15 with children above the age of 5–6, as the task is possible even with severely impaired acuity, and will disclose yellow-blue defects and scotopic (rod-based) visual behaviour. The only caution here is that children may tend to become bored with the test and take less care with their placements towards the end of the colour sequence and this would appear to indicate a blue-yellow deficit. Another recommendation is to use the Pickford–Nicolson anomaloscope with over-10s. These recommendations seem out of line with Hill's, whereby the anomaloscope can be used at a much younger age than the D-15. Given the difficulty of testing the colour vision of children with normal acuities, it seems that testing those with low vision is an even less exact science at present, although the Mollon–Reffin Minimalist test is promising (see below).

Promising developments for testing young children

Preferential looking: for screening

In his 1984 review, Hill mentioned colour-vision tests based on direction of gaze as being confined to the laboratory. Since then, a preferential-looking based screening test has been developed (Pease and Allen, 1988). It consists of four pseudoisochromatic plates, and the testee has simply to look or point at the target. They demonstrated that with children aged 3–6, the percentage failing the test was in much closer accord with known adult levels of colour deficiency in comparison with the other pseudoisochromatic tests they used, the Farnsworth F-2 (a single-plate test for red-green and blue deficiencies) and the AO-HRR screening plates.

In another study, their test was used with primary-school children (aged 4–7) and compared with the Ishihara numbers and wavy lines and the City test (Sullivan, Shute and Westall, 1990). The value of the preferential-looking based test was again demonstrated in this study as the youngest children made a low percentage of errors on it in comparison with the Ishihara tests, and it was also effective at picking up children with colour vision defects (as indicated by their performance on the entire battery of tests). The preferential-looking test also has the advantage over the Ishihara in being quick and simple.

The test is not without disadvantages, however. The value of the tritan plate remains unknown at present, but it seems that some caution should be exercised in its use in acquired defects as it is based on the specifications of the Farnsworth F-2 plate, which has been shown to be unreliable for detecting tritan-like defects. Furthermore, it does not give information about degree of defect, as does the AO-HRR.

Despite the potential of this test as a quick screening device for red-green defects in young children, it has unfortunately never appeared on the market, although the keen practitioner can make up his/her own cards by reference to Pease and Allen's (1988) paper. Readers should also be alert to the possibility of new preferential-looking based tests becoming available.

A 'Minimalist' test: for acquired defects

Another recent promising development for the detailed assessment of colour vision deficiency is the Mollon–Reffin 'Minimalist' test

(Mollon, Astell and Reffin, 1991a), which is still under development. This is intended as a rational reduction of existing arrangement tests of colour vision. The authors set out to develop a test that would give a quantitative and qualitative assessment of colour discrimination, but would be much more rapid to administer and score than the 100-hue test. They sought a simple task which could be done at a bedside and would place minimal demands on a patient's concentration, cognitive ability and dexterity, thus being potentially useful with young children as well as frail and neurologically impaired adults.

Their minimalist test is an 'odd-one-out' task, measuring directly the confusions among sets of coloured chips of varying saturation and which lie explicity along the confusion lines of the three types of congenital dichromat (Figure 11.3). The examiner adds one coloured chip to a pool of achromatic (grey) chips of varying lightness and mixes it randomly with them. The distractor chips serve the purpose of ensuring that the task cannot be solved on the basis of differences in perceived lightness. The person is asked to identify the coloured chip with a pointer (Figure 11.4). As in the first Ishihara plate, the first chip used is a saturated orange, which does not lie on any confusion line, to demonstrate the task and identify pretence or gross pathology. Then, a simple staircase procedure (Chapter 6) is used to establish the number of the chip on each confusion line which can be reliably distinguished from the distractors. For an adult with normal vision the procedure takes only about 1 minute, and for a person with a colour defect, only a little longer.

Fig. 11.4
Child performing the Mollon–
Reffin Minimalist test.

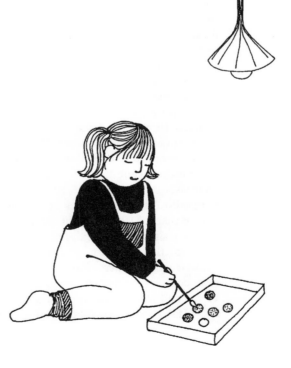

The test is sensitive enough to permit the detection of changes over time (e.g. as a result of drug dosages or recovery from optic neuritis). However, the test does not reliably detect and separate protanomalous and deuteranomalous observers, and cannot in its present form serve as a screening test for congenital deficiencies. Its value lies in monitoring acquired colour deficiencies (an alternative to the 100-hue or desaturated D-15) and in classifying dichromats into protan or deutan types (an alternative to the standard D-15) (the authors note that these limitations apply because of the spectral properties of pigments, and would not apply to a test based on similar principles using raster, light-source, displays). Its low acuity requirements also suggest its usefulness with those with low vision.

The instructions for use of the Mollon–Reffin test that accompany version 0.7 (1994) claim that it can be used with children as young as 3, although evidence for this was not presented in the referenced 1991 paper. Evidence for validation with children is still needed, therefore, and two of the present authors have work under way on this. Our preliminary results with preschool and early school-age children are promising enough to convince us of the value of giving this relatively untried test some depth of coverage here.

High-tech developments

Computerization of colour vision testing (computer-controlled raster displays), for both congenital and acquired deficits, is under development by the same workers as above (Mollon, Astell and Reffin, 1991b). The problems of edge artefacts and luminosity cues are solved as in pseudoisochromatic plates by the use of discrete patches of colour with their own contours and varying randomly in luminosity. The mosaic target forms a Landolt C (Chapter 7). The testee presses one of four response buttons to indicate the location of the gap. The test gives complete separation of protan and deutan observers. Modification might allow testing of infants by using targets that appear to move and monitoring the infant's eye movements.

Computers can also be valuable in another way, in simplifying the analysis of the results of certain colour vision tests. For example, Steinschneider and Polotsky (1991) have described a programme for IBM-compatibles which analyses D-15 results. It gives numerical and graphical presentation of results, and data may be saved for further analysis.

Finally, VEP techniques are showing promise. Ver Hoeve, France and Bousch (1996) evaluated a VEP sweep method for assessing colour vision anomalies. Although much work remains to be done to develop the technique, their study provides some preliminary evidence of validity: they found VEP responsivity to be consistent with colour vision status in individuals with normal colour vision, in verbal children with red-green deficits (as assessed by tests such as the AO-HRR) and in an infant with suspected achromatopsia.

CONCLUSIONS: HINTS ON TESTING CHILDREN'S COLOUR VISION

Cole (1991) has noted that optometrists and ophthalmologists are not always as knowledgeable about defective colour vision nor as skilled in its diagnosis as they should be, and that the difficulty is compounded by the fact that there is no simple standard for colour vision (comparable with Snellen acuity) which a single test can address. As we have seen in this chapter, the situation is even more complicated when it comes to children, and it is difficult with the present state of knowledge and technology to suggest a hard and fast protocol. However, the following guidelines, taken in conjunction with the foregoing information, may be helpful:

1. Determine the *purpose* of testing in choosing a test – whether for screening, for detailing colour vision (for educational/ occupational purposes), or for examining pathology.
2. Decide whether *red-green* assessment will suffice or whether assessment for a *blue-yellow* defect is needed. If so, consider preferential looking, AO-HRR (if you have a copy), the Mollon– Reffin or the City; arrangement tests may be used with teenagers and some younger children).
3. Consider the *age/likely ability level* of the child. Tests of choice for the youngest children, if available, are preferential looking and the anomaloscope (with modified procedures), followed by the Mollon–Reffin, the Ishihara wavy line plates and the City. The Ishihara letters and arrangement tests are inadvisable for screening use before 12 years although the Ishihara for Unlettered Persons can be used with young children if a flexible approach is taken. The AO-HRR may also be possible if standard criteria are relaxed.
    A *battery* of tests may be advisable since a child who cannot grasp one test may be able to understand another. If the child passes any one test it suggests the lack of a colour vision problem.
4. Use a suitable *light source*. Tests based on pigmented paper, such as pseudoisochromatic plates and arrangement tests, are affected by this. A standard light box should be used if possible, or else natural daylight (a North-facing window in the Northern hemisphere, South-facing in the South – not in direct sunlight). Ordinary tungsten lamps should be avoided as they will change the apparent hues of the tests and affect their efficiency (however, a standard 200 watt bulb may be used if the testee wears Wratten 78AA filters). Tests should also be stored away from light, as this will cause fading.
5. If initial screening suggests a colour vision deficiency, then a *follow-up test* should be given, preferably a different one; however, if the Ishihara is used for both tests Hill (1984) recommends a delay of at

least several minutes before retesting and presenting the plates in a different, random order.

6. If initial screening suggests a colour vision deficiency, determine *family history*. This can be particularly valuable when the colour vision of a young girl is in question: if both parents are colour defective she is almost sure to be; if the father is colour defective and the mother a carrier, she has a 50% chance of being colour defective (Hill, 1984).

   Family history is also important if testing suggests tritanopia. To rule out autosomal dominant optic atrophy, the child and all family members must have normal acuity and fields and normal optic nerves as determined ophthalmoscopically (Krill, Smith and Pokorny, 1970).

7. Consider the *implications* of any defect. Discussions with child and parent will be needed, and perhaps communication with teachers or referral to general practitioner or ophthalmologist if pathology is implicated. Carers may appreciate details of colour confusions typically made in case of congenital colour deficiency, and coloured filters may assist discrimination in some cases (Haegerstrom-Portnoy, 1990). Advice can also be given regarding environmental modifications and use of colour.

REFERENCES

Adams, R.J. and Maurer, D. (1983). A demonstration of color perception in the newborn. *Paper presented at Meetings of the Society for Research in Child Development, Detroit.*

Adams, R.J., Maurer, D. and Davis, M. (1986). Newborns' discrimination of chromatic from achromatic stimuli. *Journal of Experimental Child Psychology*, **41**, 267–281.

Adkins, M. and Pease, W. (1991). Using color as information in computer displays: problems with perception and communication. *Paper to Annual meeting of International Communication Association, Chicago, IL, May.*

Allen, D., Banks, M.S. and Norcia, A.M. (1993). Does chromatic sensitivity develop more slowly than luminance sensitivity? *Vision Research* **33** (17), 2533–2562.

Aspinall, P., Hill, A.R. and Cameron, D. (1980). An evaluation of the Ames' Clinitest. In G. Verriest (ed.), *Colour Vision Deficiencies*. Bristol, Adam Hilger.

Bacon, L. (1971). Colour vision defect – an educational handicap. *Medical Officer*, **125**, 199–209.

Birch, J. (1985). A practical guide for colour-vision examination: report of the standardization committee of the international research group on colour-vision deficiencies. *Ophthalmic and Physiological Optics*, **5** (3) 265–285.

Birch, J. (1991). Colour vision tests: General classification. Ch. 11. In D.H. Foster (ed.), *Vision & Visual Dysfunction, Vol. 7: Inherited and acquired colour vision deficiencies.* Boca Raton, CRC.

Birch, J. and Platts, C.E. (1993). Colour vision screening in children: an evaluation of three pseudoisochromatic tests. *Ophthalmic and Physiological Optics.* **13**, 354–359.

Bornstein, M.H. (1978). Chromatic vision in infancy. In H.W. Reese and L.P. Lipsitt (eds), *Advances in Child Development and Behavior, Vol. 12.* New York, Academic Press.

Bornstein, M.H., Kessen, W. and Weiskopf, S. (1976). The categories of hue in infancy. *Science*, **191**, 201–202.

Boynton, R.M. (1988). Color vision. *Annual Review of Psychology*, **39**, 69–100.

Carpenter, D.V. (1983). *An Examination of the Difficulties Encountered by Colour Defective Pupils in a Wiltshire School.* M.Ed. Thesis, Bristol University.

Cole, B. (1991). Does defective colour vision really matter? *Conference paper (Sydney, Australia).*

Dannemaier, W. (1972). The effects of color perception on success in high school biology. *Journal of Experimental Education*, **41**, 15–17.

Dwyer, J. (1983). Colour vision in children. Unpublished Master of Educational Studies thesis, Faculty of Education, Monash University.

Dwyer, J. (1991). Colour vision defects in children with learning difficulties. *Clinical and Experimental Optometry,* **74** (2), March/April, 30–38.

Espinda, S.D. (1971). Color vision deficiency in third and sixth grade boys in association to academic achievement and descriptive behavioral patterns. *Dissertation Abstracts International, 32,* 786.

Espinda, S.D. (1973). Color vision deficiency: a learning disability? *Journal of Learning Diseases,* **6,** 163–166.

Fischer, M.L. (1996). Clinical implications of color vision deficiencies. In B.P. Rosenthal and R.G. Cole (eds), *Functional Assessment of Low Vision.* St. Louis, Mosby.

Gallo, P.G. and Nardella, M.P. (1991) Colour vision deficiencies in secondary school students in Italy. In B. Drum, J.D. Moreland and A. Serra (eds), *Colour Vision Deficiencies X. Documenta Ophthalmologica Proceedings Series, Vol. 54.* Dordrecht, Kluwer Academic. pp. 429–440.

Grosvenor, T. (1977). Are visual anomalies related to reading ability? *Journal of the American Optometric Association,* **48,** 510–517.

Haegerstrom-Portnoy, G. (1990). Color vision. In A.A. Rosenbloom and M.W. Morgan (eds), *Principles and Practice of Pediatric Optometry.* Philadelphia, Lippincott.

Hedin, A. (1983). Colour vision and spectral sensitivity in children with visual handicaps. Early visual development, normal and abnormal, *Acta Ophthalmologica,* Suppl. **157,** 53–57.

Hill, A.R. (1984). Defective colour vision in children. In A. Macfarlane (ed.), *Progress in Child Health,* Vol.1. Edinburgh, Churchill Livingstone.

Hill, A.R. and Aspinall, P.A. (1980). An application of decision analysis to colour vision testing. In G. Verriest (ed.), *Colour Vision Deficiencies V.* Bristol, Adam Hilger.

Hurley, S.R. (1994). Color vision deficits and literacy acquisition. *Reading Psychology,* **15** (3), July–Sept., 155–163.

Jacobs, G.H. (1986). Cones and opponency. *Vision Research,* **26** (9), 1533–1541.

Justen, J.E. and Harth, R. (1976). The relationship between figure-ground discrimination and colour-blindness in learning-disabled children. *Journal of Learning Disabilities,* **9,** 96–99.

Kalloniatis, M. and Johnston, A.W. (1990). Color vision characteristics of visually impaired children. *Optometry and Vision Science,* **67** (3), 166–168.

King-Smith, P.E. (1991). Psychophysical methods for the investigation of acquired colour vision deficiencies. In D.H. Foster (ed.), *Vision & Visual Dysfunction,* Vol 7: *Inherited and Acquired Colour Vision Deficiencies.* Boca Raton, CRC.

Krastel, H. and Moreland, J.D. (1991). Colour vision deficiencies in ophthalmic diseases. In D.H. Foster (ed), *Vision & Visual Dysfunction,* Vol 7: *Inherited and Acquired Colour Vision Deficiencies.* Boca Raton, CRC.

Krill, A.E., Smith, V.C. and Pokorny, J. (1970). Similarities between congenital tritan defects and dominant optic nerve atrophy: coincidence or identity? *Journal of the Optometre Society of America,* **60,** 1132.

Mantyjarvi, M. (1991). Nagel anomaloscope findings in diabetic school children. In B. Drum, J.D. Moreland and A. Serra (eds), *Colour Vision Deficiencies X. Documenta Ophthalmologica Proceedings Series,* Vol. 54. Dordrecht, Kluwer Academic, pp. 523–527.

Millodot, M. (1986). *Dictionary of Optometry.* London, Butterworths.

Mollon, J.D., Astell, S. and Reffin, J.P. (1991a). A minimalist test of colour vision. 59–68. In B. Drum, J.D. Moreland and A. Serra (eds), *Colour Vision Deficiencies X. Documenta Ophthalmologica Proceedings Series,* Vol. 54. Dordrecht, Kluwer Academic, pp. 59–68.

Mollon, J.D., Astell, S. and Reffin, J.P. (1991b). Trials of a computer-controlled colour vision test that preserves the advantages of pseudoisochromatic plates. In B. Drum, J.D. Moreland and A. Serra (eds), *Colour Vision Deficiencies X. Documenta Ophthalmologica Proceedings Series,* Vol. 54. Dordrecht, Kluwer Academic, pp. 69–76.

Mollon, J.D. and Reffin, J.P. (1994). *Manual for the Mollon–Reffin Minimalist Test, Version 0.7.* Cambridge, Dept. of Experimental Psychology.

Morgan, M.J., Mollon, J.D. and Adam, A. (1989). Dichromats break camouflage of textural boundaries. *Investigative Ophthalmology and Visual Science,* **30,** Suppl., 220.

Morrone, M.C., Burr, D.C. and Fiorentini, A. (1993). Development of infant contrast sensitivity to chromatic stimuli. *Vision Research,* **33,** 2535–2552.

Oyama, K., Kitahara, K., Hisato, G. and Tamaki, R. (1991). The characteristics of color vision defects in optic nerve injuries. In B. Drum, J.D. Moreland and A. Serra (eds), *Colour Vision Deficiencies X. Documenta Ophthalmologica Proceedings Series*, Vol. 54. Dordrecht, Kluwer Academic, pp. 561–568.

Pease, P. and Allen, J. (1988). A new test for screening color vision: Concurrent validity and utility. *American Journal of Optometry and Physiological Optics*, **65** (9), 729–738.

Perez-Carpinell, J., de Fez, M.D. and Climent, V. (1994). Vision evaluation in people with Down's syndrome. *Ophthalmic & Physiological Optics*, **14**, 115–121.

Pokorny, J. and Smith, V.C. (1982). New observations concerning red-green color defects. *Color Res. Appl.*, 7, 159–164.

Snyder, C. (1973). The psychological impact of being colour blind. *Journal of Special Education*, 7, 51–54.

Steinschneider, T. and Polotsky, O. (1991). Combined computer program for the Farnsworth D-15 and Roth 28-hue tests. In B. Drum, J.D. Moreland and A. Serra (eds), *Colour Vision Deficiencies X. Documenta Ophthalmologica Proceedings Series*. Vol. 54. Dordrecht, Kluwer Academic, pp. 229–234.

Steward, J.M. and Cole, B.L. (1989). What do color vision defectives say about everyday tasks? *Optometry and Vision Science*, **66**, (5), 288–295.

Sullivan, J., Shute, R. and Westall, C. (1990). Colour vision testing in children. *Ophthalmic & Physiological Optics*, **10**, 412–413.

Teller, D.Y. and Bornstein, M.H. (1984). Infant color vision. In P. Salapatek and L.B. Cohen (eds), *Handbook of Infant Perception*. New York, Academic Press.

Teller, D.Y. and Lindsey, D.T. (1993). Infant color vision: OKN techniques and null plane analysis. In K. Simmons (ed), *Early Visual Development: Normal and Abnormal*. New York, Oxford University Press.

Thuline, H.C. (1964). Color-vision defects in American schoolchildren. *Journal of the American Medical Association*, **188**, 514–518;

Tovee, M.J. (1992), Colour Blindness. *The Psychologist: Bulletin of the British Psychological Society*, Nov. 501–503.

Ver Hoeve, J.N., France, T.D. and Bousch, G.A. (1996). A sweep VEP test for color vision deficits in infants and young children. *Journal of Pediatric Ophthalmology and Strabismus*, **33**, 298–302.

Verriest, G. (1981). Color vision tests in children. *Atti Fond Giorgio Ronchi*, **36**, 83–119.

Verriest, G., Uvijls, A. and Malfroidt, A. (1981). *Color Vision Tests in Children, Part II.* **36**, 91–99.

Waddington, M. (1965). Color blindness in young children. *Education Research*, 7, 234–236.

Walters, J.M. (1984). Portsea modified clinical technique; Results from an expanded optometric screening protocol for children. *Australian Journal of Optometry*, **67**, 176–186.

Wilkinson, W.K. (1990). The cognitive and social-emotional correlates of color deficiency in children. *Paper to Annual meeting of Arizona Education Research Organization/Rocky Mountain Education Research Association, Phoenix, AZ.*

12

Eye movements

INTRODUCTION

In this chapter we will discuss different types of eye movements, the development of eye-movement responses, the measurement of eye movements and some of the types of abnormal eye movements. First, some basic explanations are given for those less familiar with eye movement terminology. Readers with more knowledge of eye movements may want to skip this section. Detailed reviews of the developmental stages of eye movements can be found in Aslin (1987), Hainline (1988, 1993), and Schor (1990). A recurring theme in this chapter is that eye movements are essential for vision. For example, the eyes follow the path of moving objects, allowing them to be seen clearly; eye movements allow a new object of interest to be fixated on the fovea for clear vision; and eye movements help stabilize movements of the visual world on the retina.

VOLUNTARY AND INVOLUNTARY EYE MOVEMENTS

Eye movements may be voluntary or involuntary. Voluntary movements are under conscious control; involuntary are not.

Voluntary eye movements are responsible for localizing targets onto the fovea, the most sensitive part of the retina. Because foveal vision is the clearest, we move our eyes to ensure the image of regard falls there.

Involuntary eye movements occur continuously in response to head movements and to movement of the visual environment. These eye movements act to minimize the difference in velocity between the moving visual environment and movement of the retinal image. Without involuntary eye movements, which serve to stabilize and therefore clarify the retinal image, our vision would be reduced to the level of legal blindness. The stationary retinal image produced by a moving object can be likened to the production of a stable image in photography. When we take a photograph, we get a clear image of a moving object only if the camera is focused on the object, and moves with it. This is called panning. The result is a sharp picture of the moving object, with a blurred background. This can be contrasted to the case where the camera is kept still, although the object is moving; in the resulting photograph the background will be sharp, and the moving object blurred. Like panning in photography, involuntary eye movements act to move the eye to follow movement in the visual environment; thus, a sharp retinal image is produced.

Clarity of vision, in a world where we and much of our environment are in a continual state of motion, relies heavily on an interdependent range of involuntary (reflex) and voluntary (intended) eye movements.

CONJUGATE AND DISJUNCTIVE EYE MOVEMENTS

A second way to classify voluntary eye movements is into conjugate and disjunctive movements. The distinction between these two classes of eye movements becomes clear if we imagine viewing a running dog.

Fig. 12.1
Example of conjugate eye movements. A dog is continuously running between two trees, and a child watches the dog. This results in following eye movements. The eye movement trace shows the conjugate, following eye movements from the right and left eyes.

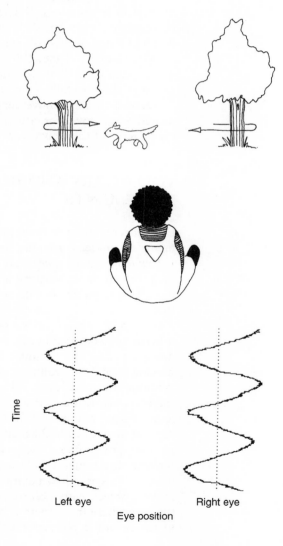

Left eye   Right eye

Eye position

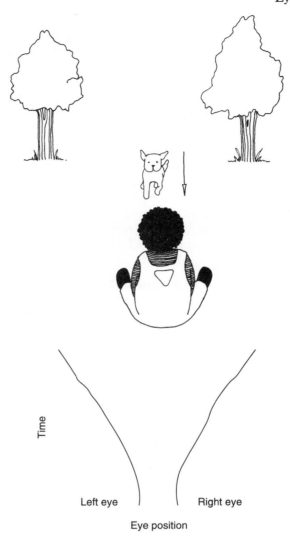

Fig. 12.2
Example of disjunctive eye movements. The dog is running towards the observer. The eye movement traces show the eyes moving in the opposite direction to each other: the right eye moving to the left and the left eye to the right.

If the dog is running across our field of view, in a path that remains the same distance from our eyes, then our following eye movements are approximately *conjugate* and the angle between the visual axes does not change (Figure 12.1). This means that the left and right eyes move together, as if they are yoked together. (The eye movements would be truly conjugate if the dog was follow the arc of a circle, the observer being positioned at the centre of the circle.)

On the other hand, if the dog runs towards us, our eyes move in opposite directions, and the angle between the visual axes changes; the left eye moves to the right and the right eye to the left, and the eyes converge as the dog gets closer (Figure 12.2). If the dog we are watching runs away from us, our eyes diverge. These eye movements are *disjunctive,* or vergence, eye movements.

These are the broad categories of eye movements: voluntary/involuntary, conjugate/disjunctive. We will now describe each subtype of eye movement, and its development in humans, in more detail.

PURSUIT (VOLUNTARY FOLLOWING) EYE MOVEMENTS

Pursuit eye movements are an example of voluntary conjugate movements. Pursuit, or voluntary following, eye movements allow clear perception of moving targets. They allow us to maintain fixation on a moving object. To see a running dog clearly, our eyes move in the same direction and with a similar angular velocity to that of the dog, such that the retinal image stays close to the fovea. Figure 12.1 shows an example of conjugate pursuit eye movement.

Time and velocity characteristics of smooth-pursuit eye movements

If a stationary object at which we are looking moves, a pursuit eye movement is initiated after a fraction of a second (about 1/8 second). This time lag is the latency of the response to an unpredicted target movement. In adults, smooth-pursuit eye movements can occur for velocities as slow as 0.08 degrees/second and as fast as 40 degrees/second (Howard, 1982).

Development of pursuit eye movements

The type and characteristics of the stimulus used to evoke pursuit eye movements have been found to be very important. Infants differ in their responsiveness to pendular motion of a stimulus than to constant-velocity motion. Constant velocity, also known as simple ramp motion, occurs when a target moves in an unpredictable manner from one position to another at a constant speed. Pendular motion occurs when a target moves back and forth across a screen in a predictable manner; the velocity of the pendular stimulus is constantly changing from zero (when the target direction changes) to a maximum value at the screen centre. This is known as sinusoidal motion.

Development of the response to constant-velocity targets
Pursuit eye movements are immature in early infancy, although segments of smooth pursuit movements have been recorded in newborns (Kremenitzer et al., 1979) and in infants 4–6 weeks old (Roucoux, Culee and Roucoux, 1983; Hainline, 1985) by using slow (5–15 degrees/second) constant-velocity targets. By 10–12 weeks of age, infants are able to make following responses to higher-velocity (> 15 degrees/second) constant-velocity targets (Hainline, 1985; Roucoux, Culee and Roucoux, 1983).

Fig. 12.3
Following eye movements to a sinusoidally moving target in a 6-week-old infant, a 10-week-old infant, and an adult. The target is shown by the smooth sinusoidal curve. The 6-week-old infant follows the target with movement steps in the appropriate direction; the 10-week-old infant shows segments of smooth pursuit eye movements and the adult shows accurate pursuit eye movements. (Taken from Aslin, R.N. (1981). Development of smooth pursuit in human infants. In D.F. Fisher, R.A. Monty and J.W. Senders (eds), *Eye Movements: Cognition and Visual Perception*, pp. 31–51. Reproduced with permission from Lawrence Erlbaum Associates Inc.)

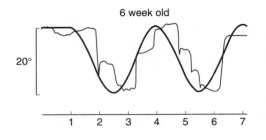

6 week old

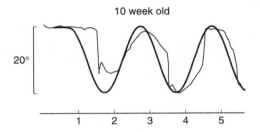

10 week old

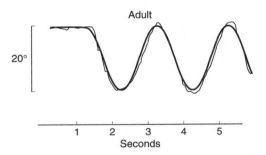

Adult

Seconds

Development in response to sinusoidal motion

Pursuit eye movements to pendular targets in very young infants are brief and intermittent. Under 2 months of age, infants are unable to visually follow targets moving with pendular motion (Aslin, 1981). At birth, infants attempt to track pendular target motion with a number of step-like eye movement responses (saccades – see below), and do not demonstrate true pursuit components to their tracking response until 8–12 weeks (Aslin, 1981). When periods of smooth pursuit eye movements emerge, there are periods of smooth eye movements interrupted by catch-up saccades (Figure 12.3). At 8–12 weeks of age, there is more chance of pursuit eye movements if the angular velocity of the target is less than 10 degrees/second.

These studies have shown that very young infants are able to better follow slowly moving constant-velocity targets than pendular targets. In contrast, although older children and adults are able to follow unpredictable ramp targets accurately, they improve this performance when following predictable pendular targets.

Schor (1990) quotes studies which suggest that by 4–5 years of age, pursuit eye movements have matured, but are still less precise than those of adults. Even by 10 years of age, children's pursuit eye movements are not as precise as those of adults.

292 Assessing Children's Vision

Fig. 12.4
Monocular optokinetic nystagmus in a 2-year-old child measured with electro-oculography. The top trace shows calibration eye movements to a target displacement of 10 degrees. The next two traces are from the right eye, with the target moving to the left and right respectively. The lower two traces are from the left eye. (Taken from Aslin, R.N. (1981). Development of smooth pursuit in human infants. In D.F. Fisher, R.A. Monty and J.W. Senders (eds), *Eye Movements: Cognition and Visual Perception*, pp. 31–51. Reproduced with permission from Lawrence Erlbaum Associates Inc.)

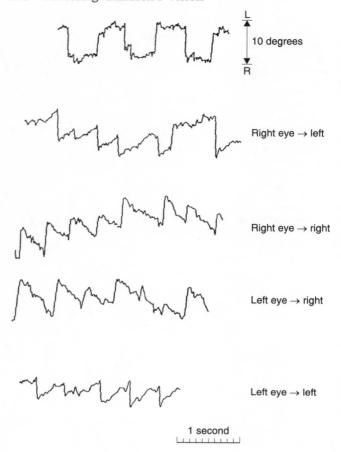

OPTOKINETIC (INVOLUNTARY FOLLOWING) EYE MOVEMENTS

A visual scene moving in one direction across the field of view evokes involuntary, conjugate, rhythmical movements of the eyes called optokinetic nystagmus (OKN). Slow eye movements in the direction of the visual field motion alternate with quick return 'flick' eye movements called saccades (see below) (Figure 12.4). In humans the slow eye phase of OKN may arise partially from activation of pursuit eye-movement pathways. OKN can be observed by watching other passengers looking out of the window of a moving train or car. (For a fuller description of OKN, see Howard, 1982, pages 233–243.)

The stimulus for the slow phase of OKN comes from retinal image movement. Signals from the retina are transmitted via the lateral geniculate nucleus to the visual cortex, where cells that are directionally selective respond to motion, sending signals through other brain centres to the oculomotor nuclei. These signals are then passed to the extra-ocular muscles, causing an involuntary eye movement. The slow-phase eye movement velocity is less than the retinal image velocity; the difference, called the retinal slip velocity, is the stimulus for continued OKN. Any changes in the direction and velocity of the retinal image motion are detected by a change in retinal slip velocity, which signals higher visual centres to modify signals to the extra-ocular nuclei. Thus, OKN is modified by continual feedback from the retina.

The purpose of OKN is to minimize motion of the moving environment upon the retina. Thus, the eye maintains a clear image similarly to the panning technique used by a photographer to obtain a sharp image of a moving object.

Time and velocity characteristics of optokinetic nystagmus

After a latency of about 1/8 second, the mature optokinetic reflex responds to target motion in any direction or orientation with slow following movements interrupted two or three times each second by saccadic refixation in the opposite direction. Slow-phase eye velocities over 40 degrees/second can be reached in adults; and if the area of the moving visual field is large, eye velocities up to 90 degrees/second are possible (Schor, 1990).

Fig. 12.5
Monocular optokinetic nystagmus in a 14-month-old infant with early onset strabismus measured with electro-oculography. The top trace shows calibration eye movements to a target displacement of 10 degrees. The next two traces are from the right eye, with the target moving to the left (temporal-nasal direction) and right (nasal-temporal) respectively (nasal-temporal direction). The lower two traces are from the left eye, temporal-nasal target movement and then nasal-temporal target movement. For either eye, target movement in the temporal to nasal direction results in a typical OKN trace. Target movement in the nasal to temporal direction results in no, or very limited, eye movements. The same kind of asymmetry is seen in infants under 3 months of age.

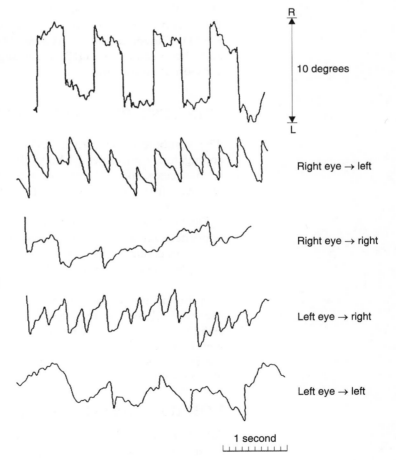

10 degrees

Right eye → left

Right eye → right

Left eye → right

Left eye → left

1 second

Development of optokinetic nystagmus

Reflex optokinetic following responses to large, moving, patterned fields are more easily evoked in infants than are pursuit responses to small isolated targets (Atkinson and Braddick, 1981). However, OKN is immature in young infants: OKN fast phases are less frequent than in adults. Also, in infants under 3 months old, monocular OKN is poorer for stimulus movement in one direction than the other; i.e. OKN is asymmetric. OKN is more likely to respond to visual movement towards the covered eye, i.e. in the temporal-to-nasal direction. Even if OKN is elicited for motion in the nasal-to-temporal direction, the velocity and frequency of the response is less than in the other direction. After about 5 months of age, the OKN of infants becomes symmetric, at much the same time that stereopsis emerges (Naegele and Held, 1982).

Abnormal binocular experience occurring in the first year of life can have a profound effect on OKN. Monocular OKN has been found to be asymmetric in adults with amblyopia (Schor and Levi, 1980; Westall and Schor, 1985). Further research has revealed that asymmetries of both OKN and pursuit systems are associated with early-onset strabismus (Mein, 1983; Tychsen, Hurtig and Scott, 1985; Westall and Shute, 1992; Schor et al., 1997; Westall et al., 1998) and with early-onset monocular (Maurer, Lewis and Brent, 1983) or binocular cataract (Lewis, Maurer and Brent, 1985). Figure 12.5 shows monocular OKN recordings in a 14-month-old child with early-onset strabismus.

THE VESTIBULO-OCULAR REFLEX

The vestibulo-ocular reflex (VOR) is another type of involuntary, conjugate eye movement. The VOR is the eye-movement response to head acceleration. The stimulus for VOR comes, not from visual feedback from the retina, but from the semicircular canals of the middle ear.

During head acceleration, the eyes make slow movements in the opposite direction to head movements. These slow eye movements are interrupted by fast, saccadic corrective eye movements. For example, a leftward movement of the head results in rightward slow-phase eye movement and leftward fast corrective saccades. The purpose of this eye-movement response is to minimize movement of the eyes relative to the visual environment. In other words, the stability of the eyes with respect to the visual environment is closely maintained, helping to stabilize the image on the retina – another of the eye's mechanisms for creating a clear image by panning, as in photography.

VOR time and velocity characteristics

The VOR is initiated earlier than following-type optokinetic and pursuit eye movements, starting less than 1/60 second after a head

Eye movements **295**

movement (Leigh and Zee, 1991, p. 16). The amplitude of the slow-phase eye movements is close to the amplitude of the head movements for sinusoidal head oscillations of frequencies corresponding to natural head rotations (i.e. 0.5–5 cycles/second). The direction of the eye movement is almost precisely opposite to that of the head movement (Leigh and Zee, 1991, p. 18). This means that eye movements and head movements of equal but opposite size occur together, resulting in the stabilization of a stationary image on the retina.

Development of the vestibulo-ocular reflex

The VOR is relatively mature at birth, compared with other eye-movement responses. The anatomical structures are developed and the VOR can be evoked even at birth (Preston and Finocchio, 1993). For more information on determining how VOR time constants change or how the temporal relationship between eye and head position changes during development, see the review by Preston and Finocchio (1993).

In 1 month olds, head acceleration results in VOR slow-phase eye movements of higher amplitude and velocity than are found later in life (see review by Schor, 1990). Preston and Finocchio (1993) referred to a study of their own that showed that the ratio of eye velocity to head velocity is 1.0 in 1–4-month-old infants. This demonstrates a perfect compensatory slow-phase eye-movement response. The ratio of eye velocity to head velocity declines to 0.6 in adulthood, by which time the visually induced compensatory eye movements complement the VOR for the maintenance of visual stability.

Visual feedback has an indirect influence on the VOR during the developing years. This was deduced from a study (Sherman and

Fig. 12.6
Example of conjugate, saccadic eye movements in an adult. The target was a brightly coloured ball which appeared to bounce to the left and right of a computer screen. The ball was visible in one place for almost 1 second, then disappeared and reappeared 20 degrees (horizontally) from the initial target location. After another second the ball jumped back to the original location. The bouncing continued for the duration of the recording.

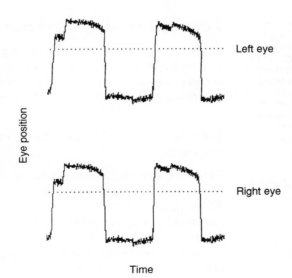

Keller, 1983) of the VOR in adults who were severely visually impaired. The VOR was found to be absent or greatly reduced in adults who were blind from an early age, but not in adults who became blind later in life.

When visual development is normal, there is rapid oculo-visual development, including growth of the eyeball and its contents, during the first few months of life. At this time there is a need for continual accurate calibration of the VOR to maintain a stable retinal image during head movement.

SACCADIC EYE MOVEMENTS

Saccadic eye movements are very fast, conjugate eye movements. The saccadic system is used to centre our gaze on an object of interest rapidly and accurately (Howard, 1982, p. 260). This form of saccade is under voluntary control. When saccadic eye movements are used for refixation, the amplitude of the initial saccade is close to that required to bring the image of the new object of interest onto the fovea. Often a small corrective saccade is required for accurate alignment. Figure 12.6 shows saccadic eye movements recorded from the left and right eyes of an adult to a 20-degree target displacement. The eye movements are conjugate, and small corrective saccades can be seen.

There are also involuntary saccadic eye movements. An example of this is the fast eye-movement component of the optokinetic and vestibular reflex, where saccadic eye movements return the eye to a more central position after each slow eye movement. A second example occurs during inspection of complex scenes, when scanning eye movements allow the observer to maximize her or his visual understanding of the scene. Saccadic eye movements are interspersed between periods of steady fixation (Yarbus, 1967).

Time and velocity characteristics

Saccadic eye movements responding to a sudden shifting of the viewed target are very fast and can reach velocities as high as 1000 degrees/second (Alpern, 1971; Schor, 1990). Saccadic eye movements can be initiated about 1/5 second after the shift in the target.

Development of saccadic (refixation) eye movements

Refixation saccades have been recorded in 1- and 2-month-old infants (Aslin and Salapatek, 1975; Roucoux, Culee and Roucoux, 1983). These investigators found their saccadic eye movements to be immature compared with those recorded from older children or adults.

Saccadic eye movements in very young infants usually start with an initial fast eye movement, in the appropriate direction but with a

FIGURE 12.7
Saccadic eye movements in a 2-month-old infant for a target jumping 20 degrees from one location to another. (Taken from Aslin, R.N. (1981). Development of smooth pursuit in human infants. In D.F. Fisher, R.A. Monty and J.W. Senders (eds), *Eye Movements: Cognition and Visual Perception*, pp. 31–51. Reproduced with permission from Lawrence Erlbaum Associates Inc.)

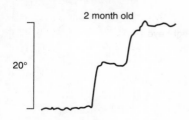

2 month old

20°

much smaller amplitude than would be required to direct the eyes towards the new target location; this saccade is said to be *hypometric* (Figure 12.7). Because of this, more refixation saccades are required to bring the image of the peripheral target onto the fovea. This series of refixations, required to realign the fovea to a peripheral target, are called *saccadic steps*. Aslin and Salapatek (1975) found that it often took about three or four equal-amplitude saccadic steps for 1- and 2-month old infants to fixate a peripheral target. In adults, a saccadic eye movement is complete in about $\frac{1}{5}$ second (range, $\frac{1}{8}-\frac{1}{3}$ second) after a change in target position. In 1- and 2-month-old infants, the first saccadic step may not occur until $\frac{1}{2}$ second after the introduction of the peripheral target. The subsequent series of saccades has similar latency. This means it may take up to 2 seconds to complete a saccade in infants under 2 months of age.

As the infant gets older, saccadic eye movements become more accurate. After the second month, large single saccades are used more often to change gaze. Children older than 1 year and adults produce saccades that are at least 90 per cent of the target distance; a second (and occasionally a third) corrective saccade is required until the line of sight is accurately aligned on the target (Jacobs et al., 1992).

It is interesting that although saccadic responses to the introduction of peripheral targets are immature in young infants, adult-like saccades can be made at other times. For example, if infants of 14 days are shown a stationary visual display, their scanning eye movements contain saccades that are as fast as those found in adults (see Hainline, 1988). Possible explanations for these differences between the immature refixation saccade and the 'mature' scanning saccade can be found in Hainline (1993). Hainline suggests that although anatomical structures may be functional early in life, increased latencies to peripheral targets and poorly formed saccades might result from a number of other factors. These include poor attention, reduced arousal, other cognitive factors, and perhaps a relatively noisy neural activity in the peripheral retina of infants than in that of adults.

VERGENCE EYE MOVEMENTS

Vergence eye movements are disjunctive eye movements that occur when a person changes fixation from a distant to a closer object (see Figure 12.1), or vice versa. When we look into the distance, the visual axes of the eyes are parallel; however, when we look at a close object, the visual axes converge so that the image of an object of interest is maintained on the fovea of each eye.

The state of vergence of the eyes depends on several factors: tonic innervation to the extra-ocular muscles, accommodation, the perceived distance of the object of interest, and retinal disparity.

Tonic innervation. In deep sleep, under anaesthesia, or immediately after death, the visual axes are in a divergent, anatomical resting position (Owens and Leibowitz, 1983). In awake, conscious individuals, the eyes are less divergent; this position is called the physiological position of rest. *Tonic vergence* is the innervation that converges the eyes from the anatomical to the physiological position of rest. The physiological position of rest, the distance phoria (Chapter 9), is usually 1–2 prism dioptres of exophoria (see Schor, 1990).

Accommodative state. Blur is the stimulus to refocus. For distance fixation, the ciliary muscles in the eye adjust the focus of the lens so that the object of interest is clear. If the object of interest (a) is replaced by a second object (b) positioned closer to the eyes, the retinal image of object b at first will be blurred. Approximately $\frac{1}{3}$ second later, the lens of the eye refocuses; that is, the accommodation has changed in response to the blur. Linked to the change in accommodation is a change in vergence acting to bring the lines of sight of the two eyes more in line with the near object. This *accommodative vergence* can be isolated from binocularly induced vergence by measuring the change in accommodation and vergence resulting from a stimulus to accommodate presented to one eye. The amount of change in accommodative vergence per unit change in accommodation is the AC/A ratio (Chapter 9). The normal range of the AC/A ratio is between 3 and 5. Excessive accommodative vergence occurs when the AC/A ratio exceeds 5 (von Noordon, 1990, p. 92).

Perceived distance. 'Knowledge of nearness' also results in a converging of the visual axes; this has been called proximal vergence. If retinal disparity information is removed, then proximal vergence contributes significantly the near vergence response (see Hokoda and Cuiffreda, 1983).

Retinal disparity. Disparity vergence, or *fusional vergence,* results from retinal image disparity. Zero retinal disparity is said to occur when corresponding points on the left and right retinae receive identical images. This happens when the lines of sight of the left and right eyes are directed towards a point target. If the target is replaced by a second target, in front or behind the point of intersection of the visual axes, each eye's retinal image now falls on non-corresponding (disparate) points (Chapter 9). After about $\frac{1}{6}$ second, a disparity vergence eye movement is evoked. This results in redirecting the lines of sight towards the new object. Retinal image disparity is the stimulus that is essential for refining binocular alignment (Rashbass and Westheimer, 1961).

In a normal visual environment (rather than in a laboratory setting), we use a combination of proximal vergence, accommodative vergence, and fusional vergence to adjust our binocular fixation to objects at different distances from our eyes. The combination of these responses makes up the *near response*. Schor and co-workers (1992) have recently described a model that explains the contributions of the different component mechanisms. Large errors arising from perceived distance are sampled at the beginning of the near response; these errors result in accommodative and vergence changes that initiate the response. Retinal blur and disparity are sampled continuously throughout the near response. Small retinal errors arising from blur and disparity are the stimuli for the refinement of the response. The completion of the near response is therefore dependent on proximal, accommodative, and vergence mechanisms.

Errors in vergence angle (strabismus)

Heterotropia, strabismus, or 'squint' is simply a misalignment of the visual axes (Chapter 9). The eyes are not aligned, and the foveas of the two eyes do not simultaneously receive the image of an object of interest. These errors in vergence are detected by the cover test (Chapter 9).

Development of vergence eye movements

At birth the eyes appear aligned; newborn infants are able to perform vergence eye movements in the appropriate direction, although with poor accuracy (Slater and Findlay, 1975; Aslin, 1977). By 1 month of age, infants are able to converge and diverge in response to targets moving along the midline. By 2–3 months of age, the vergence responses are faster and more accurate (Aslin, 1977). At this age there is more chance that some form of binocular fusion is present. Although most infants do not appear to have manifest strabismus, it is thought that bi-foveal fixation does not occur much before 2 or 3 months of age. The infant vergence system is probably not comparable to the adult system until at least 3 months of age. Before this age the vergence system is slower, less consistent, and less accurate (Salapatek and Banks, 1978).

The precise stimuli to evoke the infant vergence responses is unknown, with tonic, accommodative, proximal and disparity vergence helping the infant maintain eye alignment. It is probable that vergence responses not dependent on retinal feedback (i.e. tonic, accommodative and proximal) are present at birth, but that disparity vergence develops postnatally. Schor (1990) suggests that before 3–4 months of age, exotropic errors found when measuring binocular fixation in infants may result from the lack of fusional disparity vergence. Accommodative vergence is operating by the second week of life; an accommodative stimulus presented to one eye results in a reliable convergence response of the covered eye (Aslin and Jackson, 1979). During development, accommodative accuracy to near objects improves, and accommodative vergence begins to emerge as a major component of the composite vergence response (Schor, 1990).

Disparity vergence develops later. Using the 10-dioptre prism test (similar to the 4-dioptre base-out test described in Chapter 9), Aslin

(1981) assessed the development of disparity vergence in infants. Disparity vergence was deemed to be present if infants were able to make refixation eye movements to overcome disparity induced by 10 prism dioptres, base out, placed before the preferred eye during binocular fixation of a distance target. A positive response was found in 72% of 6-month-old infants and 13% of 4 month olds. Few 3-month-old infants demonstrated the refixation response at all. Disparity vergence responses emerge at about the same time as stereopsis. Some gross, possibly peripheral, disparity vergence movements probably occur before this time, producing the apparent binocular alignment during the first 4 months of life. In summary, accommodation and proximal convergence may maintain gross alignment in early infancy; by 3–4 months of age, the binocular disparity vergence system is developing.

CLINICAL MEASUREMENT OF EYE MOVEMENTS

One part of ophthalmologic, optometric and orthoptic examinations involves assessing a child's ability to maintain fixation on a target, and to be able to follow the target as it is moved in horizontal, vertical and oblique directions. Fixation should be steady, and pursuit movements smooth. The ability to fixate and follow demonstrates functioning of both sensory and motor systems. Sensory information must be adequate for the child to see the target, and motor functioning must be sufficient to allow the child to make the appropriate fixational and following eye movements.

Fixation and following

Method for binocular testing (Figure 12.8)
To test a child for fixation and following, follow these steps.

1. Hold a penlight (or a brightly coloured toy, for less attentive children) in the midline of the infant's or child's vision, about $\frac{1}{3}$ m away, and encourage the child to look at the light.
2. Note the child's ability to fix the light. Observe the child's eyes and the position of the light reflex with respect to the pupil, if a penlight is used as the target. Note whether the fixation is steady or unsteady, and if there is an obvious strabismus, which results in the shifting of the light reflex in the non-fixating eye (Chapter 9).
3. Move the penlight to the right, and encourage the child to follow it with her or his eyes. (Ensure that the child's head remains still.) Move the target so that the child's eye movements reach the farthest position to the right. Note whether both the child's eyes are able to follow the target, with an equal and appropriate amount of movement, or if there is an underaction or overaction of one eye.
4. Repeat the procedure for movements of the target to the left and in the two vertical and four oblique directions of gaze – up and down to the right, and up and down to the left.

Fig. 12.8
Eye movement testing in children.
The child is asked to follow the
movement of a small, brightly
coloured, toy.

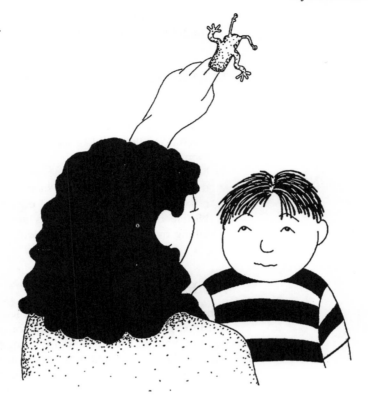

If the child is able to make appropriate following eye movements, then both sensory visual input and motor functioning of extra-ocular muscles have been demonstrated.

However, the ability to follow does not necessarily equate to good visual acuity. Older children with visual acuities between 6/60 and 6/120 are able to demonstrate good fixation and following (Day, 1990).

Clinically, infants older than 4 months should be able to pursue a hand-held moving object. Failure to do so indicates a visual or oculomotor abnormality (Schor, 1990).

Method for monocular testing
Repeat the protocol above monocularly. Use a patch to occlude one eye if the child will tolerate this; if not, you may choose to place a thumb over one eye. With the penlight or toy in the central position, observe if fixation is central, steady, and maintained (see Day, 1990). Central fixation is assumed if the light reflex is in, or very close to the centre of the pupil. *Central fixation* reflects the ability of the child to fixate with foveal vision. *Steady fixation* means that there is no nystagmus or unsteady eye movements when viewing the target. *Maintained fixation* is the ability to maintain central fixation of the

target during a cover test. Then test the ability of each eye to follow the target in the eight additional positions of gaze.

Method for saccadic testing

1. Hold two brightly coloured toys at approximately 30 degrees to the right and left of the mid-line.
2. Encourage the child to look first at toy 1, and then at toy 2, and then back at toy 1, etc.
3. Notice if the fixations are accurate, i.e. that her or his gaze falls on the appropriate toy. The saccades are classed as inaccurate if refixation eye movements are obvious.
4. Notice if the eye movements are rapid or slow (with the child taking over a second to complete the saccade).

Method for OKN testing

A brightly coloured striped scarf, at least 8 in wide and approximately 2 ft long provides a good stimulus for clinical OKN testing. Hold the scarf in front of the child, and then move it slowly to the right and to the left. Look for optokinetic nystagmus (Figure 12.9).

If optokinetic eye movements can be seen in both directions of motion, it is assumed that the sensory system is adequate for the visual stimulus, and that OKN motor pathways are intact. An inability to perform OKN may mean that the child has a severe visual

Fig. 12.9
How to test OKN in the clinic. The examiner slowly moves the scarf horizontally while the child looks at it.

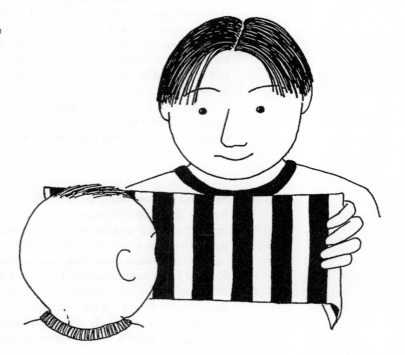

impairment. An inability to perform OKN for one direction of motion only may imply a hemispheric visual loss.

Monocular OKN should be tested as well. As well as observing whether OKN is present or absent, note whether the response is asymmetric, i.e. if each eye's slow-phase eye movement for monocular movement in the temporal-to-nasal direction is of a higher frequency than OKN in the opposite, nasal-to-temporal direction.

Method for VOR testing

If an infant is thought to have very poor vision, the VOR test may provide useful information (Day, 1990). In a normally illuminated room, hold the infant at arm's length. Spin a few rotations, inducing vestibular ocular nystagmus, then stop. If the visual pathways are intact, you will see one or two beats of afternystagmus in the child's eyes. In an infant with severe visual impairment or severe cerebellar disease, afternystagmus will be prolonged.

ABNORMAL EYE MOVEMENTS IN INFANTS AND YOUNG CHILDREN

No fixation and following

A number of visual and/or oculomotor disorders result in an absence or reduction of fixation and following.

Delayed visual maturation

Delayed visual maturation may be the diagnosis when no neurological abnormality is noted, visual evoked potentials (VEPs) and electro-retinograms (ERGs – Chapter 13) are normal (demonstrating normal functioning of the retina and visual pathways – Lambert, Kriss and Taylor, 1989), and the ophthalmological examination is normal except for an absence of fixation and following. Jacobs and associates (1992) described this scenario in a 5-month-old infant. In addition to an absence of fixation and following responses, a marked monocular OKN asymmetry was noted; saccadic eye movements were immature, with the child making multiple hypometric saccades. It was decided that there was a delay in oculomotor development, as part of delayed visual maturation. In infants with isolated delayed visual maturation, general and neurological development are normal. Children with delayed visual maturation show improvements in visual function usually before 6 months of age (Taylor, 1990a).

Congenital ocular motor apraxia

In this condition, ability to generate voluntary saccades is impaired (Leigh and Zee, 1991, p. 114). Children with ocular motor apraxia are able to make random saccades and quick phases of saccadic eye movements; but because they do not appear to fixate, they are sometimes thought to be blind. Apraxia is defined as the lack of voluntary saccadic eye movements despite an intact neurophysiological substrate for performing such movements (Leigh and Zee, 1991, p. 249). Within a few months of birth, children with this condition develop characteristic thrusting, horizontal head movements (Leigh and Zee, 1991, p. 249), which allow them to fixate objects in their periphery. Consistent among children with ocular motor apraxia is 'locking up' of the eyes during OKN and VOR testing (Jacobs et al., 1992). This means that the eyes become temporarily fixed in an extreme right or left gaze.

Congenital ocular motor apraxia usually improves with age. Patients become better at directing their eyes voluntarily, and their head movements become less noticeable (Leigh and Zee, 1991, p. 249).

Cerebellar Disease
Cerebellar disease is one of the conditions that may be associated with inappropriate saccades (Leigh and Zee, 1991, pp. 424–428). Fixation may be disrupted by 'square-wave jerks' – very small involuntary saccades that take the eyes off-target, followed by a second corrective saccade bringing the eyes back. Square-wave jerks are made during fixation and following eye movements (Leigh and Zee, 1991, p. 114).

Hemispheric lesion
Abnormal eye movements arising from a lesion to one side of the visual cortex are well represented by a case discussed by Jacobs et al. (1992). They described a 5-month-old infant, born prematurely at 27 weeks' gestation, who was not fixing and following. The eyes of this child had a tendency to deviate to the left. Pursuit eye movements were good to the left, but following eye movements were made up of saccadic eye movements for rightward movements of the target. A bias in OKN to a binocular stimulus was noted, with reduced OKN for target movement towards the right. A VOR bias was also found – poorer for slow phases toward the right. These eye-movement biases suggested a right-hemispheric lesion. Ultrasound demonstrated a right-hemispheric cyst; the left hemisphere was normal.

Nystagmus
Nystagmus is a rhythmic oscillation of the eyes which is usually bilateral, affecting the two eyes equally, and is usually involuntary (Taylor, 1990b). Nystagmus that occurs before the age of 6 months (early-onset nystagmus) occurs in 1 of 1000 males and in 1 of 2800 females (Forssman and Ringner, 1971).

Nystagmus may be idiopathic, that is, not associated with any accompanying ocular or neurological defect. This type of nystagmus is called congenital idiopathic nystagmus or motor nystagmus. More often, nystagmus is associated with ocular or neurological defects (Casteels al., 1992). When the nystagmus is greater in one eye than the other, or occurs only in one eye, a neurological disease should be suspected (Casteels et al., 1992).

Sensory-defect nystagmus is the most common form of early-onset nystagmus. It is usually associated with disorders of the anterior visual pathways, including cataracts, corneal opacities, optic disc atrophy or hypoplasia, and retinal disorders (Casteels et al., 1992). Some of these retinal disorders are associated with visible abnormalities of the retina (for example, albinism, retinopathy of prematurity and coloboma); but many are associated with normal-appearing fundi, such as achromatopsia, or subtle pigmentary abnormalities. If there is the slightest suspicion of an underlying retinal defect, then the child should be referred for an ERG (Chapter 13).

Blindness

Blindness resulting from a lesion in the visual cortex (cortical blindness) or from disease of the retina or the visual pathways from the retina to the visual cortex would result in a lack of fixation and following eye movements because of an inability to see the target. Visual evoked potentials and electroretinography (Chapter 13) are most useful in identifying children with cortical blindness and retinal disease, respectively. Nystagmus is an indication of damage to the anterior visual pathways. Infants and young children with cortical blindness are less likely to develop nystagmus.

Roving eye movements

Roving eye movements are large-amplitude, relatively low-frequency, multidirectional movements seen in children who are born blind, who become blind in the first few years of life, or who have severe visual impairment. In acquired conditions, these unsteady eye movements may become apparent before the vision has failed.

LABORATORY ASSESSMENT OF EYE MOVEMENTS

Electro-oculography

Electro-oculography (EOG) is a common method of recording horizontal and vertical eye movements in infants and children. It depends on a potential (voltage) difference between the retina and cornea. The cornea is 0.4–1 mV positive with respect to the retina; this voltage difference makes the eyes behave like two dipoles (batteries). As the eyes rotate, the 'battery' rotates, and changing voltages can be picked up by skin electrodes placed on either side of the two eyes.

Method for EOG recording (Figure 12.10)

1. Clean the skin on the temporal edge of the right and left eyes of the child with abrasive paste (e.g. Nuprep, D.O. Weaver and Co., Aurora, CO).
2. Place skin electrodes (gold-plated disc electrodes or silver/silver chloride electrodes, such as those from Neuromedical Supplies, Inc., Herndon, VA, USA.) on the skin, with an appropriate electrode paste or gel on the inner surface of the electrode.

Fig. 12.10
EOG recording. Child with two electrodes placed lateral to the eyes, with a third electrode on forehead.

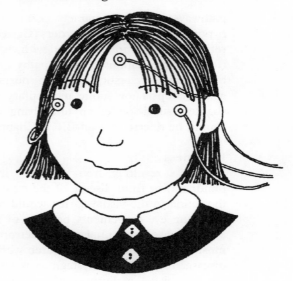

    a. If simultaneous right-and left-eye recording is required, then place electrodes on the nasal edges of each eye, as well.

    b. If vertical eye movements are required, then place additional electrodes above and below the eye to be tested.

3. Position a ground (earth) electrode on the child's forehead or attach it to an ear with an ear-clip electrode.

4. Feed the electrode signals to a differential preamplifier (e.g. a Grass AC/DC micro-electrode preamplifier, model p16; Grass Instrument Company, Quincy, MA, USA). For recordings of slow eye movements (pursuit, nystagmus slow-phase, vergence), you need a DC rather than an AC output from the preamplifier.

Electro-oculography is usable for eye movements up to ± 70 degrees, although recorded eye movements > 30 degrees relate less well to actual eye movements (that is, the linearity lessens). EOG is accurate to ± 2 degrees (Young and Sheena, 1975).

Artefacts from EOG recording result from muscle artefacts, lid movements, and non-linearity associated with large eye movements. Another important source of variability comes from changes in background illumination. If a subject is tested in a dark room after being in a well-lit environment, the recorded voltage per unit eye movement lessens significantly. It is important to minimize changes in room illumination when using EOG to record eye movements.

Toddlers sometimes pull electrodes off, even though they are relatively non-intrusive.

Corneal reflection

The front surface of the cornea approximates part of a sphere, and as such reflects bright objects in the same way as a convex mirror. The position of the corneal reflection changes with eye position (Young and Sheena, 1975). Hainline (1981) describes a television-based system, which can be modified for infant testing, that records eye movements via corneal reflections, using a commercially available infrared video eye-movement monitoring system, e.g. ASL (Applied Science Laboratories, Bedford, MA, USA). Parallel light from an infra-red light source enters the infant's eye. The light reflected by the retina is picked up by a television camera. An image of a back-lit bright pupil is seen with the television monitor. Light is also reflected by the front surface of the cornea, and appears on the monitor as a small image superimposed on the pupil. Movements of the eye relative to the head result in movements of the corneal reflection relative to the pupil image. Small movements of the whole head result in parallel movement of the corneal reflection and the pupil.

Method for corneal reflection recording

Hainline (1981) described a technique to record eye movements successfully in infants. She suggests holding the infant over a shoulder, while stabilizing the infant's head. The infant can then be positioned such that she or he can view the moving visual target while the experimenter ensures that the infant's eyes are aligned for recording. The experimenter achieves this by viewing two monitors, one of the child's face and the other of the enlarged image of the child's eye. The ASL system allows a small amount of head movement. This makes this system useful for infant testing, although a fair degree of restraint of the infant's head is still required for successful recording.

The accuracy of the system is at least ± 0.5 degrees in adults, although this varies among infants. An advantage of the corneal reflection television-based system is that horizontal, vertical and oblique eye movements can be recorded. A disadvantage is the greater head stability required for correct alignment of the infant's eyes. ASL model 4000 is appropriate to adapt for infant testing.

Limbus tracking

The iris is normally visible and distinguishable from the sclera at the iris–scleral boundary: the limbus. If light-emitting diodes are positioned in front of the eye (often using infra-red illumination), then the sclera and iris will reflect different amounts of illumination. The ratio between the dark iris and the light sclera is measured with a photosensor. This ratio is related to the horizontal position of the eye (Young and Sheena, 1975).

Method for limbus tracking recording

Glasses incorporating light-emitting diodes are placed on the child. (Some degree of co-operation is required for the child to keep the glasses on.) The interpupillary distance of the glasses needs to be adjusted to centre the diodes with respect to the scleral–iris border.

The ASL model 210 system can be adapted for children. Ober2 (Permobil Meditech AB, Timrå, Sweden) supplies glasses appropriate for testing children; the accuracy of this system is 1 degree for horizontal eye movements, with a range of ± 20 degrees. Infrared emission and detector components form the basis of the Ober2 eye-movement and blink recording system.

Limbal tracking systems are successful for recording horizontal eye movements, but are less accurate for vertical movements.

CONCLUSION

We began this chapter with a brief explanation of the different types of eye movements, which are essential for normal vision and outlined their development in infancy. The ability of a child to both fixate on a stationary target and to follow a moving target demonstrates functioning of both sensory and motor systems. We have described some methods for both routine clinical and laboratory assessment of eye movements in children. Abnormalities may be indicative of ocular or neurological impairments.

REFERENCES

Alpern, M. (1971). Effector mechanisms in vision. In J.W. King and L.A. Riggs (eds), *Woodworth and Schlosberg's Experimental Psychology*, 3rd edn. New York, Holt, Reinhart and Winston, pp. 369–94.

Aslin, R.N. (1977). Development of binocular fixation in human infants. *Journal of Experimental Child Psychology*, **23**, 133–50.

Aslin, R.N. (1981). Development of smooth pursuit in human infants. In D.F. Fisher, R.A. Monty and J.W. Senders (eds), *Eye Movements: Cognition and Visual Perception*. Hillsdale, NJ, Erlbaum, pp. 31–51.

Aslin, R.N. (1987). Motor aspects of visual development in infancy. In P. Salapatek and L. Cohen (eds), *Handbook of Infant Perception, Volume 1, From Sensation to Perception*. Orlando, FL, Academic Press, Harcourt Brace Jovanovich. pp. 43–113.

Aslin, R.N. and Jackson, R.W. (1979). Accommodative convergence in young infants: development of a synergistic sensory-motor system. *Canadian Journal of Psychology*, **33**, 222–231.

Aslin, R.N. and Salapatek, P. (1975). Saccadic localization of visual targets by the very young human infant. *Percept. Psychophys.*, **17**, 293–302.

Atkinson, J. and Braddick, O. (1981). Development of optokinetic nystagmus in infants. In D.F. Fisher, R.A. Monty and J.W. Senders (eds), *Eye Movements: Cognition and Visual Perception*. Hillsdale, NJ, Erlbaum, pp. 53–64.

Casteels, I., Harris C.M., Shawkat F. and Taylor D. (1992). Nystagmus in infancy. *British Journal of Ophthalmology*, **76**, 434–437.

Day, S. (1990). History, examination and further investigation. In D. Taylor (ed.), *Pediatric Ophthalmology*. Boston, Blackwell Scientific Publications, pp. 47–64.

Forssman, B. and Ringner, B. (1971). Prevalence and inheritance of congenital nystagmus in a Swedish population. *Annals of Human Genetics*, **35**, 139–147.

Hainline, L. (1981). An automated eye-movement recording system for use with human infants. *Behav. Res. Methods Instrum.*, **13**, 20–24.

Hainline, L. (1985). Oculomotor control in human infants. In R. Groner, G. McKonkie, and C. Menz (eds), *Eye Movements and Human Information Processing*. *Proceedings of the XXIII International Congress of Psychology of the International Union of Psychological Science (IUPsyS), Acapulco, Mexico, September 2–7, 1984*. Oxford, Elsevier, pp. 71–84.

Hainline, L. (1988). Normal lifespan developmental changes in saccadic and pursuit eye movements. In C.W. Johnston and F.J. Pirozzolo (eds), *Neuropsychology of Eye Movements*. Hillsdale, NJ, Erlbaum, pp. 31–64.

Hainline, L. (1993). Conjugate eye movements of infants. In K. Simons (ed.), *Early Visual Development, Normal and Abnormal*. Oxford, Oxford University Press. pp. 47–49.

Hokoda, S.C. and Cuiffreda, K.J. (1983). Theoretical and clinical importance of proximal vergence and accommodation. In C.M. Schor, K.J. Cuiffreda (eds), *Vergence Eye Movements: Basic and Clinical Aspects*. Boston, Butterworths, pp. 75–97.

Howard, I.P. (1982). *Human Visual Orientation*. New York, Wiley.

Jacobs, M., Harris, C., Shawkat, F. and Taylor, D. (1992). The objective assessment of abnormal eye movements in infants and young children. *Australian and New Zealand Journal of Ophthalmology*, **20**, 185–195.

Kremenitzer, J.P., Vaughan, Jr, H.G., Kurtzberg, D. and Dowling, K. (1979). Smooth-pursuit eye movements in the newborn infant. *Child Development*, **50**, 442–448.

Lambert, S.R., Kriss, A. and Taylor, D. (1989). Delayed visual maturation, a longitudinal clinical and electrophysiological assessment. *Ophthalmology*, **96**, 524–529.

Leigh, R.J. and Zee, D.S. (1991). *The Neurology of Eye Movements*, 2nd edn. Contemporary Neurology Series. Philadelphia, Davis.

Lewis, T.L., Maurer, D. and Brent, H.P. (1985). Optokinetic nystagmus in children treated for bilateral cataracts. In R. Groner, G. McConkie and C. Menz (eds), *Eye Movements and Human Information Processing. Proceedings of the XXIII International Congress of Psychology of the International Union of Psychological Science (IUPsyS), Acapulco, Mexico, September 2–7, 1984*. Elsevier pp. 85–105.

Maurer, D., Lewis, T.L. and Brent, H.P. (1983). Peripheral vision and optokinetic nystagmus in children with unilateral congenital cataract. *Behav. Brain Res.*, **10**, 151–161.

Mein, J. (1983). The OKN response and binocular vision in early onset strabismus. *Australian Orthoptic Journal*, **20**, 13–17.

Naegele, J.R. and Held, R. (1982). The postnatal development of monocular optokinetic nystagmus in infants. *Vision Research*, **22**, 341–346.

Owens, D.A. and Leibowitz, H. (1983). Perceptual and motor consequences of tonic vergence. In C.M. Schor and K.J. Cuiffreda (eds), *Vergence Eye Movements: Basic and Clinical Aspects*. Boston, Butterworths pp. 25–74.

Preston, K.L. and Finocchio, D.V. (1993). Development of vestibulo-ocular reflexes and optokinetic reflexes. In K. Simons (ed.), *Early Visual Development, Normal and Abnormal*. Oxford, Oxford University Press, pp. 80–88.

Rashbass, C. and Westheimer, G. (1961). Disjunctive eye movement. *Journal of Physiology (London)*, **159**, 339–360.

Roucoux, A., Culee, C. and Roucoux, M. (1983). Development of fixation and pursuit eye movements in human infants. *Behav. Brain Res.*, **10**, 133–9.

Salapatek, P. and Banks, M.S. (1978). Infant sensory assessment: Vision. In F.D. Minifie and L.L. Lloyd, (eds) *Communicative and Cognitive Abilities: Early Behavioural Assessment*. Baltimore, University Park Press.

Schor, C.M. (1990). Visuomotor development. In A.A. Rosenbloom and M.W. Morgan (eds), *Principles and Practice of Pediatric Optometry*. New York, Lippincott. pp. 66–90.

Schor, C.M., Alexander, J., Cormack, L. and Stevenson, S. (1992). Negative feedback control model of proximal convergence and accommodation. *Ophthalmic and Physiological Optics*, **12**, 307–318.

Schor, C.M., Fusaro, R.E., Wilson, N. and McKee, S.P. (1997). Prediction of early-onset esotropia from components of the infantile squint syndrome. *Investigative Ophthalmology and Visual Science*, **38**, 719–740.

Schor, C.M. and Levi, D.M. (1980). Disturbances of small field horizontal and vertical optokinetic nystagmus in amblyopia. *Investigative Ophthalmology & Visual Science*, **19**, 668–683.

Sherman, K.R. and Keller, E.L. (1983). Vestibulo-ocular reflexes of adventitiously and congenitally blind adults. *Investigative Ophthalmology & Visual Science*, **27**, 1154–1159.

Slater, A.M. and Findlay, J.M. (1975). Binocular fixation in the newborn baby. *Journal of Experimental Child Psychology*, **20**, 248–273.

Taylor D. (1990a). Delayed visual maturation. In D. Taylor (ed.), *Pediatric Ophthalmology*. Boston, Blackwell Scientific Publications. pp. 21–27.

Taylor D. (1990b). Nystagmus. In D. Taylor (ed.), *Pediatric Ophthalmology*. Boston, Blackwell Scientific Publications. pp. 595–602.

Tychsen, L., Hurtig, R.R. and Scott, W.E. (1985). Pursuit is impaired but the vestibulo-ocular reflex is normal in infantile strabismus. *Archives of Ophthalmology*, **103**, 536–539.

Westall, C.A. and Schor, C.M. (1985). Asymmetries of optokinetic nystagmus in amblyopia: the effect of selected retinal stimulation. *Vision Research*, **25**, 1431–1438.

Westall, C.A., Eizenman, M., Kraft, S.P., Panton, C.M., Chatterjee, S. and Sigesmund, D. (1998). Binocularity and optokinetic asymmetry in esotropia. *Investigative Ophthalmology and Visual Science* (in press).

Westall, C.A. and Shute, R.H. (1992). OKN asymmetries in orthoptic patients: contributing factors and effect of treatment. *Behav. Brain Res.*, **49**, 77–84.

Yarbus, A.L. (1967). *Eye Movements in Vision*. New York, Plenum.

Young, L. and Sheena, D. (1975). Survey of eye movement recording methods. *Behav. Res. Methods Instrum.*, **7**, 397–429.

Appendix 12.1

Eye-movement recording systems

Ober2, Permobil Meditech AB, Box 120, S-86100 Timrå, Sweden. Tel. 060-59 59 00. E-mail: itgroup@world.std.com.
Applied Science Laboratories (ASL), 175 Middlesex Turnpike, Bedford, MA 01730, USA. Tel. 1-617-275-4000. E-mail: (r)HYPERLINK mailto:asl@a-s-l.com.

Preamplifiers for EOG recording; Grass Instruments Astromed Grass, 600 East Greenwich Ave., West Warwick, Rhode Island, USA. Tel. (US) 1-800-349-4039; (from Canada) 1-800-565-2216; (from UK) 01 628 668836.

Silver-silver chloride electrodes; Neuromedical Supplies, Inc., 790 Station Street, Suite 210, Herndon, VA 22070-4606, USA. Tel. 1-703-471-6888. E-mail: (r)HYPERLINK mailto:Neuromed-@Neuro.com.

13

Electrophysiological testing

INTRODUCTION

Electrophysiology is the measurement of small electrical signals that occur in the body. We are interested here in such signals which occur in the visual system in response to visual stimulation. This chapter discusses *visual evoked potentials* (VEPs), the *electroretinogram* (ERG), and the *electro-oculogram* (EOG). The VEP may be used as an objective technique to help define visual function or diagnose a visual problem; the ERG and EOG are diagnostic tests of retinal function.

Many eye care practitioners and other people working with and caring for children with visual impairments are familiar with types of electrophysiological testing. This familiarity might arise from seeing electrophysiological reports, or from children (or their parents) discussing their personal experiences. The purpose of this chapter is to familiarize eye care givers with some of the electrophysiological terminology, the reasons electrophysiological tests are used, and what the results mean. In addition, technical specifications and protocols are described for the benefit of the future electrophysiologist. Detailed information about electrophysiological testing can be found in Heckenlively and Arden (1991).

The voltage changes with which we are concerned vary with time and can be plotted as a waveform. We will use the terms *implicit time* and *amplitude* to describe the timing and size, respectively, of the peaks that make up complex electrophysiological waveforms. Positive voltage changes will be referred to as positive peaks and negative voltage changes as negative peaks (referred to as troughs by some authors). In this chapter, in all figures depicting electrophysiological waveforms, the direction of the positive electrical changes is upwards. Implicit time is the time from the stimulus presentation to the highest point of a positive peak (or to the lowest point of a negative peak). The amplitude of a specific peak is usually measured from the preceding peak. The exception is the ERG a-wave amplitude: it is measured from the baseline at stimulus onset to the peak of the a-wave. The reader should be aware that some authors may describe the time to specific VEP peaks as the *latency* of the response; therefore, it is always important to determine the terminology used by each author when describing the electrophysiological waveform.

VISUAL EVOKED POTENTIALS

VEPs are sometimes known as visual evoked responses (VERs) or visual evoked cortical potentials (VECPs). These are simply different names for the same measure. The VEP is a response evoked from the visual cortex by a change in a visual stimulus, i.e. a change in luminance, contrast, or colour. The electrical activity contributing to a VEP is recorded from electrodes placed on the surface of the scalp, in much the same way as heart activity is measured by ECG electrodes. The VEP is a small-amplitude response measured in microvolts (1–20 μV) and embedded in the background brain activity of the electroencephalograms (EEG). The EEG is a record of the continuously changing electrical activity of the brain, which can be monitored through external electrodes attached to the scalp; it is made up of a number of changing potentials, including the alpha rhythm, beta activity, and theta activity. EEG amplitudes range between 60 and 100 μV.

The small-amplitude VEPs (1–20 μV) are submerged in the larger-amplitude EEG activity (60–100 μV). To extract the VEP from the 'noise', repeated responses must be averaged. The VEP is time-locked to the stimulus, which means that the change in the electrical activity of the visual cortex occurs at a constant time after each stimulus presentation. When a number of responses are averaged, responses that are not constant (that is, EEG activity or other sources of electrical noise) are cancelled to a certain extent, and the VEP waveform can emerge (Figure 13.1).

It is important to note that VEPs are dominated by cone activity and reflect the central 6–10 degrees of the retina (Sokol, 1986). This is a result of two factors: first, the foveal projection to the primary

Fig. 13.1
Example of visual evoked potential (VEP) embedded in EEG activity. In this, and in subsequent figures, the arrow (lower left) identifies the time of stimulus presentation. The number of responses increases from 2 to 4 to 8 to 16 to 40, from the topmost to the lowermost trace. It can be seen how the VEP waveform emerges through the averaging of increasing numbers of responses. The vertical bar (right) indicates an amplitude of + 12.0 μV, the horizontal bar (right) represents 20 milliseconds.

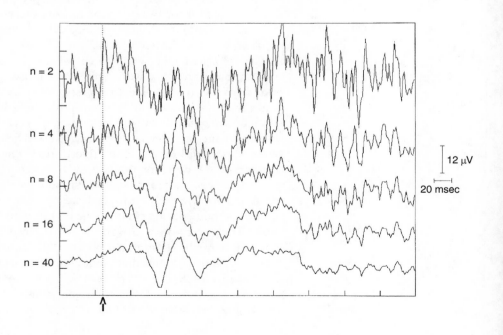

visual cortex (visual area I) terminates on the surface of the occipital cortex, while the peripheral retinal projection terminates in deeper tissue less accessible by surface recording. Second, a greater amount of cortex is devoted to receiving foveal input than peripheral retinal input.

Visual stimuli

The conventional stimuli used for the clinical measurement of VEPs are the flash, checkerboard, and grating stimuli.

A *flash stimulus* might be generated by a photostimulator (e.g. as manufactured by Grass Instruments). The stimulus should subtend at least 20 degrees at the eye, and should have a luminance approximating 3 $cd.s.m^{-2}$ (candela-seconds per square metre; Harding et al., 1996). The luminance of the photostimulator will vary if the child is not perfectly still, sitting directly in front of the photostimulator lamp. Therefore any measurement of luminance gives only a very rough idea of the level that actually falls on the eyes of the child. We recommend the use of a Grass Photostimulator, intensity setting 4, held 40 cm from the eye. Alternatively, a photostimulator, can be used to illuminate the inside of a Ganzfeld (a dome, approximately two feet in diameter, with a white, reflecting internal surface). The stimulus strength should be between 1.5 and 3 $cd.s.m^{-2}$ (Marmor and Zrenner, 1995). A Ganzfeld stimulus provides even illumination across the retina. The person sits with his or her chin on a chinrest, so that his or her eyes are positioned at the entrance to the dome.

A *checkerboard stimulus* comprises equal-sized black and white squares like a chessboard. The size of the checks can be adjusted in order to test for visual cortical responses to different element sizes. For investigating the integrity of the visual system, Kooijman and colleagues (1986) recommended a check size of 50 minutes of arc. To measure visual acuity, the check sizes might vary from 240 to 5 minutes of arc.

Two types of checkerboard targets are used. The first is called the *alternating checkerboard stimulus,* also known as pattern reversing. Checks are always visible, but they simultaneously alternate between light and dark; in other words, the white squares are replaced by black squares, and vice versa. This means that the overall luminance remains the same, so that the cortical response arises from changes at the contours of the checkerboard and not from any overall change in luminance.

The second type of checkerboard is the *pattern onset-offset stimulus,* sometimes known as the appearance-disappearance checkerboard. In this stimulus a checkerboard pattern is replaced by an unpatterned diffuse field of the same mean luminance. Again, this ensures that the VEP results from the checkerboard and not from any overall luminance change. The International Society for Clinical Electro-physiology of Vision (ISCEV) VEP standards recommend that the pattern appears for 200 ms (pattern onset), followed by the diffuse background for 400 ms (pattern offset). Apkarian (1993) suggests that a pattern onset of 40 ms followed by a 460 ms offset is more appropriate for paediatric testing.

The checkerboard stimulus is defined in terms of the visual angle subtended by the width of a single check, in minutes of arc. A high-contrast checkerboard (black/white checks), with the checks varying in size from trial to trial, is used for acuity assessment. A checkerboard in which the checks maintain the same size from trial to trial, but in which the contrast between the dark and light checks changes, is used to assess contrast sensitivity (see Chapter 8). Equiluminant checks changing in chromaticity from trial to trial are used to assess colour vision.

A *grating stimulus* consists of either horizontal or vertical stripes. The stripes might be in the form of a sine wave or a square wave. The specifications of a grating are reported in cycles per degree (cpd), with one white stripe and one black stripe constituting a single cycle (Chapters 1 and 7).

The VEP waveform

Transient visual evoked potentials

The transient VEP has a complex, multi-peak waveform. The transient VEP is the averaged response to a stimulus sufficiently sporadic to allow brain responses to return to pre-stimulus activity before the next stimulus presentation. The usual rate of stimulus presentation for a transient response is 2 presentations per second (1 Hz). The implicit times reported for the waveform will vary according to the stimulus type, the amplifier type and the amplifier settings.

An example of a transient VEP to flash stimulus (the flash VEP, or FVEP) is shown in Figure 13.2. The FVEP is made up of a complex series of negative and positive peaks, beginning with a negative peak (N_1) at approximately 30 ms. The first positive peak (P_1) occurs at about 50 ms, although this peak is not always seen in young children. A second negative peak (N_2), which occurs at about 75 ms, is followed by a second positive peak (P_2) at about 100 ms. In infants, the positive and negative peaks occur later than these values. When reporting FVEPs it is usual to report on the implicit time to P_2 and the N_2–P_2 amplitude.

A transient VEP waveform in response to an *alternating checkerboard* is shown in Figure 13.3. The adult response shows a typical negative peak at 70–95 ms (N_1) and a prominent positive peak at 90–120 ms (P_1, sometimes called P_{100}). There is a second negative peak at 120–160 ms (N_2) and a second positive peak at approximately 200 ms (P_2). In infants, the positive and negative peaks appear later. The VEP is quantified by the measurement of the implicit time of P_1, and the amplitude between the P_1 positive peak and the preceding N_1 negative peak. In Figure 13.3 the implicit time is 94 ms and the amplitude 36 mV.

A transient VEP waveform response to an *onset checkerboard* (the appearance of a checkerboard stimulus) is shown in Figure 13.4. The

Fig. 13.2
A transient flash visual evoked
potential, showing negative and
positive components. The timing
of the components varies in
children. The vertical and
horizontal bars (right) indicate 4 μV
and 20 milliseconds respectively.

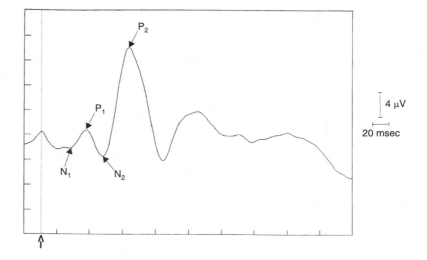

VEP response to pattern onset consists of three peaks of alternating
polarity, called C_1, C_2, and C_3. At around 75 ms there is a positive
peak (C_1); this is followed by a negative peak at around 100–125 ms
(C_2); then a second positive response occurs around 150 ms (C_3).
The VEP is quantified by the measurement of implicit time to C_1, C_2,
and C_3, and by the amplitude between C_1 and C_2.

A VEP is deemed to be present if it is recognizable, repeatable, and
falls within the range of implicit times normal for the child's age. The
VEP is recognizable if the appropriate peaks are present. The
waveform is said to be repeatable if, for repeated checkerboard
presentations (for same-size checks), the peaks occur within 5 ms of
each other. The waveform falls within normal limits if the reported

Fig. 13.3
A transient visual evoked potential
to an alternating stimulus. The
implicit time of the P_1 peak is at
94 ms in this example. The
amplitude is higher than usual, at
about 36 μV. The vertical and
horizontal bars (right) indicate 4 μV
and 20 milliseconds respectively.

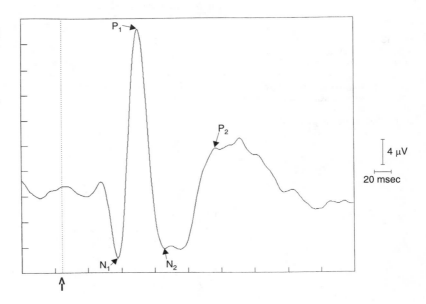

peak (or peaks) appear within a predetermined range of the expected time for the patient's age.

Steady-state visual evoked potentials

When the stimulus alternation rate is faster than 8 alternations per second (4 Hz), there is insufficient time for a complete VEP waveform. The shape of the waveform begins to resemble a series of sine waves (Figure 13.5a): the brain response has reached a steady state. The predominant sine wave will be at twice the frequency of the stimulus. Higher-frequency sine waves may be seen to be super-imposed on this dominant frequency, at two times, three times, and possibly four times the frequency of the dominant response. The VEP is best assessed with Fourier analysis, with which VEPs can be converted to a power spectral-density array (Figure 13.5b). The VEP amplitude is defined in terms of power of the response (equals the square of the amplitude) at specific frequencies; the time character-istics of the response are defined by the phase (Moskowitz and Sokol, 1980).

Recording visual evoked potentials

Electrode placement

The International Society for Clinical Electrophysiology of Vision (ISCEV) (Harding et al., 1996) and the Working Group, Physical Methods in Ophthalmology (Kooijman et al., 1986) recommend standards for clinical VEP assessment. Complying with such standards helps reduce variability in testing protocols between different laboratories. The standards have been formulated more for testing adults and older children. In paediatric testing, we comply with the standards, but with certain modifications aimed at increasing the success rates of testing young children.

Fig. 13.4
A transient visual evoked potential in response to pattern onset. The C_1, C_2, and C_3 components are quite variable between children. The vertical and horizontal bars (right) indicate 4 μV and 20 milliseconds respectively.

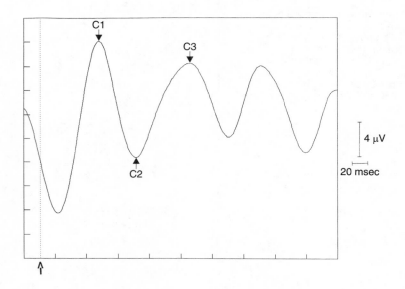

Fig. 13.5
(a) A steady-state visual evoked response (VEP) to a 4 Hz stimulus, displayed as a function of time. The vertical and horizontal bars (right) indicate 4 μV and 20 milliseconds respectively. (b) The same steady-state VEP displayed as a function of frequency. The predominant frequency component of the VEP is at 8 Hz, twice the stimulus frequency. The vertical and horizontal bars (right) indicate 1 μV and 2 Hz respectively.

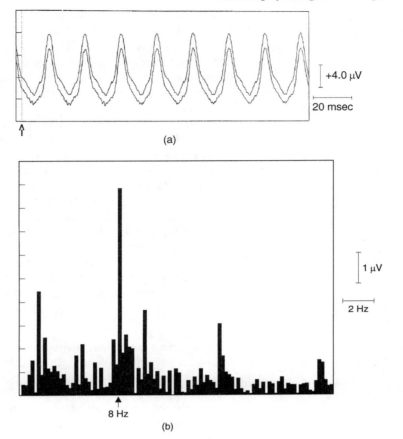

(a)

(b)

ISCEV standards for VEP testing recommend that electrode placement follow the 10–20 system (Harding et al., 1996). The active recording electrodes are placed over the active source, which for visual evoked potentials is the visual (occipital) cortex. A reference electrode is placed over an area unresponsive to visual stimuli, and a ground (earth) electrode connects a second inactive area to the ground terminal of the equipment.

The 10–20 system defines electrode placement according to certain bony landmarks of the skull. For visual evoked potentials, important landmarks are the inion and the nasion. The inion is the posterior horizontal ridge just above the base of the skull. The nasion is the dip at the top of the nose, below the bony protuberance of the brow. The visual (occipital) cortex lies beneath the skull a few centimetres above the inion. The two-character designations for active electrodes over the occipital cortex begin with the letter O; electrodes along the midline have z as a following subscript.

An electrode is placed on the midline just above the inion, at 10% of the distance between the inion and the nasion. This active electrode position is labelled O_Z. Other electrodes can be placed on either side of O_Z, the distance from O_Z being calculated as a percentage of the measured lateral distance between the nasion and inion. Electrode positions of active electrodes O_1 and O_2 are placed to the left and right, respectively, of O_Z, at a distance equal to 5% of the lateral head circumference; similarly, the positions of active electrodes O_3 and O_4 are 10% of that distance to the left and right of O_Z (Figure 13.6). This percentage system results in consistent electrode placement on heads of different sizes.

ISCEV VEP standards recommend that the reference electrode should be placed at F_Z, along the midline above the nasion, at 30% of the distance between the nasion and inion. Kooijman and colleagues (1986) recommend that the reference electrode be placed at F_Z, at the earlobe, or at the mastoid. A second alternative for the reference electrode is to link the two electrodes together, one on the right and one on the left ear (Apkarian, van Veenendaal and Spekreijse, 1986). A third possibility for the reference electrode is a clip electrode attached to either ear.

The ISCEV standards recommend that the ground electrode be placed at C_Z, halfway between the nasion and inion (the vertex of the skull). Kooijman and associates (1986) recommend a clip electrode attached to either ear to serve as the ground.

Measuring electrical impedance

Before testing begins, the potential for electrical activity to pass from the skin to the electrode must be tested. An impedance meter measures how well an electrode is likely to transmit electrical signals; with the electrodes attached, the impedance is measured using the active electrodes and the reference electrode. If the impedance meter reads less than 5 kilohms for all electrodes, then the impedance of the active electrode and the ground electrode is measured. Again the impedance must be less than 5 kilohms. If the impedance meter reads more than 5 kilohms, then the electrodes affected must be reattached.

Fig. 13.6
A schematic of electrode placement. (Reprinted from Harding, G.A., Odom, J.V., Spileers, W. and Spekreisjse, H. (1996). Standard for visual evoked potentials. *Vision Research*, **36**, 3569. © 1995. With kind permission of Elsevier Science Ltd.)

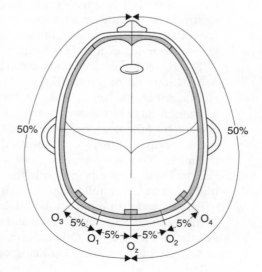

Data acquisition and amplification

During testing cortical signals are fed into the differential amplifier (low pass, 200 Hz; gain, 20 000 Hz), and to a computer through an analogue-to-digital interface. At The Hospital for Sick Children in Toronto, we use the Neuroscan Inc. (El Paso, TX, USA) evoked potential hardware and Neuroscan Scan/Stim/Stats software packages. The computer receives an electrical signal from the stimulus generator every time the stimulus pattern changes (i.e. at every flash, pattern reversal, or onset of a pattern appearance). An artefact-rejection mode is available in the software that eliminates voltages over 100 μV that might arise from head or body movements. For each stimulus condition, two records should be obtained, each containing an average of approximately 50 sweeps (range, 30–70 sweeps).

The electrical signals are transmitted to a differential amplifier which is electronically isolated from the child being tested. The amplifier measures the difference in electrical potential between each active electrode and the reference electrode. The purpose of the differential amplifier is to eliminate (non-visual) electrical activity common to both active and reference electrodes. When the electrical activity at the active electrodes is the same as that at the reference, then the differential amplifier does not relay the signal arising from the non-visual source. The signal being transmitted from the differential amplifier is therefore from the cortical response to the visual stimulus alone. If a reference electrode is placed over a visually unresponsive area, then differential amplification provides a response uncontaminated by non-visual activity.

Unfortunately, no reference electrode is truly inactive (Regan, 1989, p. 13). In fact, there are problems with any location. The ear location has been found to be within the potential field of the VEP; F_Z is contaminated by a signal of opposite polarity to the positive peak of the transient VEP (Harding, 1991); and the linked-ear configuration may reduce one's ability to detect hemispheric asymmetry (Regan, 1989, p. 15). In paediatric testing, the optimum choice of reference electrode position is that which is minimally affected by the visual signal and best tolerated by the child. In our paediatric patient population we choose one ear for the position of the reference electrode and the other ear as the position for the ground electrode (Figure 13.7). More detailed information about electrode placement can be found in Harding (1991) and Regan (1989, pp. 11–13). For more details relating to technical specifications, refer to the ISCEV standards for visual evoked potentials (Harding et al., 1996).

Paediatric VEP assessment

Use of VEPs to assess the integrity of the visual pathways

The VEP reflects the activity of the visual pathway from the retina to the striate cortex (and extrastriate cortex, depending on electrode placement). Therefore, abnormalities of the retina, optic nerve, optic chiasm, optic radiations or visual cortex may result in abnormal

VEPs. The extent and type of the abnormality, as well as the choice of visual stimulus, determine the VEP response. Retinal disease, especially that affecting the macula, may result in abnormal VEPs (Smith et al., 1990). Optic nerve disease often results in increased implicit times of the VEP. The VEP is very sensitive in detecting interocular acuity differences found in amblyopia (Sokol, 1990; Geer and Westall, 1996). Misrouting of optic nerve fibres at the optic chiasm results in characteristic VEP findings in albinism (see later discussion), and conditions that affect cortical vision usually result in abnormal VEPs. A discussion of clinical conditions that affect VEPs in both adults and children can be found in Sokol (1990) and in Taylor and McCulloch (1992).

If a child appears to be blind, measuring VEPs can provide valuable information. The VEP has been found to be an important prognostic tool in acute-onset cortical blindness in the absence of prior neurological abnormalities (following surgery, trauma, infectious disease, hypoxia, or other insults). If flash VEPs are present during the acute stage of the blindness, then recovery can be predicted (Taylor and McCulloch, 1991). However, if a neurological defect is present, then an initial abnormal VEP is not a good predictor of the later visual outcome (Granet et al., 1993). In perinatal asphyxia, flash and pattern VEPs recorded during the postnatal period have been found to be good predictors of visual outcome, that is, normal VEP responses (compared with age-matched controls) predict good visual outcomes, while poor responses predict poor outcomes (McCulloch, Taylor and Whyte, 1991).

When an infant appears to be blind, yet the ocular exam is normal and there does not seem to be any abnormality of the central nervous system, it may be that the visual pathways are simply slow to develop – a condition called delayed visual maturation. In this condition, VEPs to flash and checkerboard patterns may or may not be present. In some cases, the VEPs might fall within the normal limits of amplitude and implicit time for the infant's age (Lambert, Kriss and Taylor, 1989). In other cases, the VEP may not be recordable. This does not

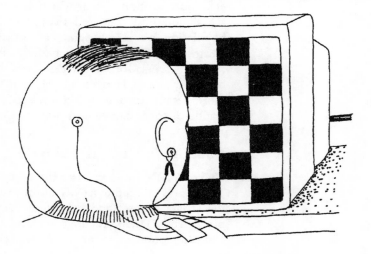

Fig. 13.7
A child with clip ear electrodes plus an electrode at O_z, sitting in front of a checkerboard stimulus.

mean that these infants cannot or will not see (Skarf, 1989; Granet et al., 1993); it may merely be another manifestation of delayed visual maturation. Subsequent VEPs would show an improvement in the case of delayed visual maturation, but not in the case of cortical blindness.

Use of VEPs to assess visual acuity

Smallest check size technique. Children are often referred to electrophysiology units for VEP testing to help determine the child's level of visual acuity. Marg and associates (1976) derived visual acuity, using square-wave pattern onset-offset gratings, by determining the highest spatial frequency (cycles per degree) that elicits a VEP definable from the recorded response to defocused stripes. Using this technique to study the development of visual acuity, these investigators found that visual acuity was adultlike at an age between 4 and 6 months. A similar finding has since been made for pattern onset-offset targets (Orel-Bixler and Norcia, 1986). Using square-wave checks, McCulloch and Skarf (1994) defined the minimum check size necessary to generate a reproducible VEP recording as the threshold check. Apkarian (1993) converted the threshold check to a VEP acuity: in a population where Snellen acuity could reliably be measured, she determined the minimum pattern size to give a reliable pattern-onset VEP response. She then calculated the correction factor to equate Snellen acuity (represented as minimum angle of resolution) with the smallest check to give rise to a VEP. Her data demonstrated that a reliable pattern-onset VEP to a check size of 3 minutes of arc corresponded to a Snellen acuity of 20/20 (6/6) or 1 minute of arc. Therefore, the threshold check is divided by 3 to give a VEP acuity in minutes of arc; for example, if the minimum recordable pattern size is 9 minutes of arc, then the VEP acuity is actually 3 minutes of arc.

Extrapolation technique. Another technique used to assess visual acuity has been to plot VEP amplitude against check size, and then to extrapolate the response to determine the check size that corresponds to zero amplitude or a baseline noise amplitude (Figure 13.8) (Sokol, 1978; Tyler et al., 1979; Regan, 1980; Sokol and Moskowitz, 1985; Apkarian, van Veenendaal and Spekreijse, 1986; Orel-Bixler, Haegerstrom-Portnoy and Hall, 1989; Orel-Bixler and Norcia, 1986). VEP extrapolation is usually used with steady state VEPs. For transient VEPs, extrapolation of amplitude versus check size to determine visual acuity may give inaccurate results (Apkarian, van Veenendaal and Spekreijse, 1986; McCulloch and Skarf, 1991). The use of extrapolation to determine visual acuity in clinic patients may be limited by the length of time required (Sokol, 1986), during which the child may change her or his behavioural state, which in turn may dramatically change the VEP amplitude, waveform, and implicit time (Apkarian, Mirmiran and Tijssey, 1991).

Sweep VEPs technique. VEP extrapolation is usually used for steady-state VEPs, where the recording time is much quicker and changes in

Fig. 13.8
Extrapolation of VEP amplitude vs. check size in an 8-week-old child. The stimulus was a 4 Hz checkerboard stimulus. The VEP acuity by extrapolation to a noise level of 2 mV is 4 min arc.

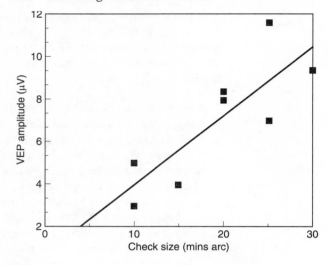

behavioural states would have less opportunity to affect the responses to different check sizes. VEP extrapolation techniques form the basis of the sweep VEP. The steady-state VEP is recorded continuously while *sweeping* stimulus parameters, i.e. while they steadily and rapidly change (Regan, 1973). For acuity assessment, a grating is swept through a set of increasing spatial frequencies, to beyond the acuity limit. Tyler et al. (1979) recorded the sweep VEP using a sine-wave grating reversing in contrast 24 times per second. In adults subjected to various amounts of visual blur, they found very good correlations between psychophysical acuity and the extrapolated VEP acuity. Development of visual acuity has been recorded by sweep VEP using a 6 Hz stimulus. Norcia and Tyler (1985) recorded sweep VEPs in 197 infants using vertical sine-wave gratings reversing in contrast. They found visual acuity to be 4.5 cycles per degree in the first month, reaching a plateau of 20 cycles per degree between 8 and 12 months of age.

Problems with using VEPs to estimate visual acuity
The previous paragraphs demonstrate the variety of methods used by different laboratories to determine VEP acuity. One technique is no more correct than the next, as long as the VEP acuity is relative to normal limits set by age using the same technique.

Successful VEP recording is dependent on attention and co-operation by the subject. Any measure of VEP degrades during states of poor attention, such as when a child is fussy or becomes bored. Using transient VEPs to determine visual acuity is greatly affected by changing attentional states. The time taken to record transient VEPs to a series of check sizes is often too long for a young child to tolerate. The development of the sweep VEP has alleviated this problem, by cutting the time taken for a determination of visual acuity down to 10–20 seconds (Apkarian et al., 1986).

Unfortunately, some problems remain. Although early reports showed equivalent acuity estimates for different temporal frequencies of the stimulus (Tyler, Apkarian and Nakayama, 1978; Tyler et al., 1981), Apkarian and colleagues (1986) demonstrated that different acuity estimates were found at different temporal frequencies in a 12-week-old baby. Although the sweep technique cannot be assumed to be 100% accurate, many vision researchers have found the sweep technique to be a valuable method of measuring visual acuity and contrast sensitivity in the developing infant visual system (Tyler, 1991).

In paediatric clinical testing, many other problems exist when VEPs are used to assess visual acuity. The presence of neurological problems, seizures, visual cortical insults, electrolytic abnormality, or nystagmus all affect VEPs, meaning that visual function can not be accurately evaluated (Hoyt, 1984). Since VEPs depend on behavioural state, periods of inattention or variable behaviour prevent reliable recording (Apkarian, Mirmiran and Tijssen, 1991). When checkerboard stimuli are used, horizontal nystagmus grossly degrades VEPs, and sometimes results in falsely delayed responses (Smith, 1984; Sokol, 1986). A more accurate assessment of acuity can be recorded in the presence of horizontal nystagmus if horizontal stripes (Rosenberg and Jabbari, 1987) or pattern onset-offset (Apkarian, 1993) stimuli are used for VEP recording. VEP abnormalities in developmental delay may result from gross disorganization of the brainwaves of the EEG rather than from gross abnormalities of visual function (Smith, 1984). Abnormal VEPs may also result from poor accommodation rather than from pathology of the visual pathway (Smith, 1984).

Comparisons between VEP acuity and behavioural acuity in a clinical population

The primary shortfall of using VEPs to assess visual acuity can be seen from studies comparing behavioural acuity with VEP acuity in children with varying degrees of visual loss or neurological impairment. Behavioural acuity measurement includes the use of acuity cards or forced-choice preferential looking (Chapter 7). In the following paragraphs, acuity is considered in terms of spatial frequency (cycles per degree – see Chapter 7); therefore, lower spatial frequency relates to poorer visual acuity. Although there is some correlation between behavioural acuity estimates (Teller acuity cards, Cardiff cards) and VEP acuity (vertical bars), the relationship is inconsistent. Mackie et al. (1995) found the range in acuity difference between the two techniques spans up to 7 octaves. Since 1 octave equals a halving or doubling of acuity, 7 octaves represents a difference between the two estimates of 132 times. Most data fell between 0 and 4 octaves of difference between the two techniques (i.e. ranging from no difference to a factor of 16 times different). In most cases, they found that acuities achieved with VEPs were worse than those found using acuity cards, with the greatest difference being for children with poorer visual acuity.

Orel-Bixler and colleagues (1989) used sweep VEPs (gratings) to determine VEP acuities, and compared them with acuities found using grating acuity cards. They found the results of the two techniques agreed within 1 octave for 66% of their clinical population. In contrast to the study by Mackie and associates, they found acuities to be worse when measured with acuity cards than with sweep VEPs, with the greatest difference being for children with poorer visual acuity. The difference between the two techniques ranged from no difference up to a factor of seven times different.

In a study comparing acuities measured with forced-choice preferential looking (FPL) (projected grating) and VEP extrapolation (checkerboard reversing at 3.8 alternations per second), Bane and Birch (1992) found acuity differences of up to 4.62 octaves in children with visual impairment (a difference of over 16 times between the two techniques). They found FPL acuities to be better than VEP acuities in children with visual impairment.

These studies demonstrate the large differences in estimated acuity that result when VEP techniques are compared with behavioural testing techniques. In our own laboratory we compared VEP and Teller acuity in 175 children with a range of neurological and ophthalmological disorders. Acuity levels in children with optic nerve disorders were lower when measured with VEPs than with Teller cards, whereas in patients with neurological disorders resulting in severe cognitive defects acuity levels were lower with Teller acuity cards than with VEPs.

In summary the accuracy of visual acuity measurement using visual evoked potentials depends on: (1) the level of the child's visual function; (2) the presence of nystagmus; and (3) the presence of optic nerve disorders. Whether behavioural or VEP testing gives better acuity estimates also depends on the VEP technique used.

Acuity levels obtained with either behavioural or VEP techniques are influenced by many factors. Reports including acuities estimated with both techniques would provide a closer approximation to the true level of the child's visual function.

Development of visual evoked potentials

Development of the VEP waveform (transient VEP)

The implicit time of all components of the pattern-reversal VEP decreases with increasing age. A number of studies (Moskowitz and Sokol, 1983; McCulloch and Skarf, 1991) have demonstrated the decrease in P_1 implicit time with development. At 1 month of age, the VEP response to large checks consists of a prominent positive peak (P_1) – a simpler waveform than that of an older child or adult (Figure 13.9). Moskowitz and Sokol (1983) found the mean implicit time of the P_1 response to large checks (48 and 60 min) to be 220.5 ms (SD, 32.5 ms) for a 1-month-old infant. At 2 months of age, the VEP response to large checks consists of negative peaks (N_1 and N_2) preceding and following the large positive peaks (P_1 mean, 178 ms; SD, 23.8 ms). At 3 months, the P_1 implicit time has been reduced to

Fig. 13.9
Visual evoked potential (VEP)
waveforms to an alternating
checkerboard (120 minute) in a $3\frac{1}{2}$-
year-old child (top) and a 5-week-
old infant (lower). Note the timing
of the P_1 peak in the infant, and
how the shape of the infant VEP is
spread out compared with the
older child's VEP. The vertical and
horizontal bars (right) indicate 8 μV
and 20 milliseconds respectively.

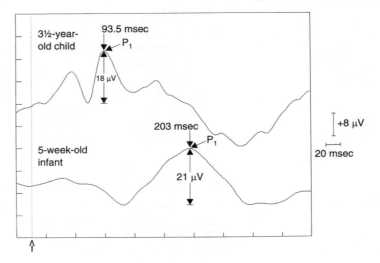

140 ms (SD, 18.1 ms), and a late positive response (P_3) has emerged.
By 4 months, the mean of the P_1 implicit time is 119 ms (SD,
7.3 ms). By 4 years of age, the P_1 implicit time is 108 ms (SD,
6.1 ms), and VEP records are very similar to those obtained from
adults (Moskowitz and Sokol, 1983; Sokol, 1986).

Such numbers depend on the analogue amplifier settings of the
laboratory where the data are collected; therefore, each lab must
collect normal control data from infants with normally developed
visual systems for correct interpretation of VEPs in an infant clinical
population.

Development of temporal tuning (steady-state VEP)
As well as being selectively sensitive to different spatial frequencies
(Chapter 8, Contrast Sensitivity), the human visual system is selectively sensitive to different temporal frequencies, i.e. different rates
of stimulus alternation. Thus the visual system has a temporal as well
as a spatial tuning characteristic. In addition, the peak of the temporal
sensitivity curve is dependent on the spatial frequency of the stimulus;
and both spatial frequency and temporal frequency tuning change
with age.

It is essential to know the development of these processes if steady-
state VEPs or sweep VEPs are to be used for infant acuity assessment.
Moskowitz and Sokol (1980) recorded VEP responses in infants 7–26
weeks of age to checkerboards (check sizes of 48, 24 and 12 min of
arc) alternating at different temporal frequencies. For the 48 min of
arc check size, they found the peak of the temporal frequency curve to
be 4 alternations per second for the 7–10-week age group. By 11–14
weeks of age, the peak was broad, spanning 4–10 alternations per
second, with the major peak having shifted to 8 alternations per
second; and by 15–22 weeks, the function still peaked between 8 and
12 alternations per second, but became more sharply tuned. For the
24-minute check sizes, all ages showed a peak response at 10–12

alternations per second, with the 19–26-week-old infants also showing a smaller peak at 4 alternations per second. The 12-minute check size gave a major peak at 12 alternations per second; a secondary peak was evident at 4 alternations per second for all age groups, being more prominent for infants over 19 weeks of age.

Moskowitz and Sokol (1980) suggest that the optimum stimulus presentation for studies of high spatial-frequency mechanisms in infants over 4 months of age would be 4 alternations per second.

Clinical protocols for paediatric VEP testing

Clinical protocols vary between laboratories (Fulton, Hartmann and Hansen, 1989; Sokol, 1990; Apkarian, 1993). The procedure used at The Hospital for Sick Children, Toronto, Visual Electrophysiology Unit, is as follows:

1. Choose electrode placements according to the 10–20 system.
2. Prepare the skin at each position by rubbing with a cotton-tipped swab (e.g. a Q-tip) and an abrasive saline jelly such as Nuprep (D.O. Weaver and Co., Aurora, CO).
3. Fill gold disc electrodes with conductive electrode paste (e.g. EC2, Grass Instruments) and tape them to the back of the child's head at O_Z and at the other desired active electrode positions.
4. Attach an electrode to one ear as a reference. The other ear serves for the ground.
5. Measure the electrode impedance. If impedance is more than 5 kilohms remove electrode, re-do skin preparation and re-attach the electrode.
6. Once the electrodes are attached, seat the child 50 cm from the visual stimulus pattern, alone or on the parent's lap (depending on the child), in a darkened room.
7. Collect at least 40 repetitions for each stimulus parameter for each eye.

Stimulus: pattern VEPs

Transient pattern alternation (Sokol, 1990), transient pattern onset (Apkarian, 1993), and steady-state (4 Hz) pattern alternation (Fulton, Hartmann and Hansen, 1989) are the stimuli typically used for recording pattern VEPs in children.

An observer, hidden from view, stands behind the computer and monitors the child's fixation at all times. The observer accepts data (by means of a remote switch) only when the child is looking towards the computer monitor. If necessary, the observer sings, jiggles keys, or presents small toys in front of the computer screen to maintain the child's attention and direct her or his interest toward the screen.

1. Choose at least three pattern-check sizes, according to the child's age (see Fulton, Hartmann and Hansen, 1989; Sokol, 1990) and apparent visual capability.

2. For visually alert children, begin the testing with a 60-minute check size; otherwise, start with a 120-minute check size.
3. If responses are repeatable, decrease the check size in octaves.
4. If repeatable responses are not obtained, then increase the check size.

For young infants and children with visual or neurological disorders, we test with both eyes to obtain an estimate of VEP acuity, and then proceed to monocular testing if the child's co-operation allows. For children with obvious monocular visual deficits, we record the VEP of each eye in turn.

Although the smallest check size giving rise to a repeatable VEP gives a useful assessment of monocular acuity difference, Sokol (1990) suggests that this may be too time-consuming. He suggests that the difference in amplitude between the two eyes, in response to a single check size, gives a good indication of interocular acuity difference.

The VEP implicit times obtained are compared with our normal control data to determine if the response is normal or delayed. If no repeatable pattern response is obtained, we proceed to recording the VEP with a flash stimulus.

Stimulus: flash VEPs

Fulton, Hartmann and Hansen (1989) use a full-field Ganzfeld illuminated by a Grass strobe, flashing at 2 times per second, with a flash intensity of Grass setting 2 or more. The child is supine, with each eye alternately occluded by an adhesive patch. At The Hospital for Sick Children, Toronto, we record flash VEPs to a Grass photostimulator at intensity setting 4, held 40 cm from the child's eyes. For monocular testing, we use two adhesive patches plus a black cloth patch to ensure that no light leaks into the occluded eye.

VEPs in albinism

Oculocutaneous albinism is associated with hypopigmentation of the eyes, skin, and hair, whereas *ocular* albinism predominantly affects the eyes. The ocular manifestations of albinism include decreased visual acuity, macular hypoplasia, nystagmus, translucent irides, photophobia, strabismus, and hypopigmentation of the fundus. In addition, there is an abnormal decussation of retinal ganglion cell axons at the chiasm (Guillery, 1974). Normally, the majority of temporal retinal fibres (approximately 45%) remain uncrossed; in the presence of albinism a greater percentage cross to the contralateral hemisphere. This misrouting can be detected with VEPs: upon monocular stimulation, VEP waveforms from the ipsilateral cortex are inverted compared with those from the contralateral cortex (Guo et al., 1989; Apkarian, 1992).

Different laboratories have used a range of techniques to determine optic-nerve misrouting in albinism (e.g. Apkarian, 1992; Kriss et al., 1992; Fitzgerald and Cibis, 1994). We have compared the various techniques for assessing multi-channel VEPs in children with albinism (Soong, unpublished data). This included a comparison between 5 channel (O_1, O_2, O_3, O_4 and O_z) and 3 channel recording (O_1, O_2 and O_z), as well as comparisons between analysis techniques. We recommend the method of Fitzgerald and Cibis (1994), which involves recording monocular VEPs using three channel VEPs (O_1, O_2 and O_z). For each eye the response at O_2 is subtracted from the response at O_1. Comparison of these inter-hemispheric difference potentials demonstrate the presence or absence of optic-nerve misrouting. Figure 13.10 shows a child ready for 3 channel VEP recording.

Clinical protocol for multi-channel VEP recording (The Hospital for Sick Children, Toronto) method

1. Place three gold disc electrodes over the left, midline and right occiput (O_1, O_z, O_2, respectively).
2. Use the child's ears for the reference and ground electrodes.
3. Record VEPs in response to a monocularly presented 1 Hz flash stimulus (Grass photostimulator, intensity setting 4) held 40 cm in front of the child.
4. For children over 6 years, record VEP responses to a pattern-onset checkerboard stimulus (60-minute checks) as well.

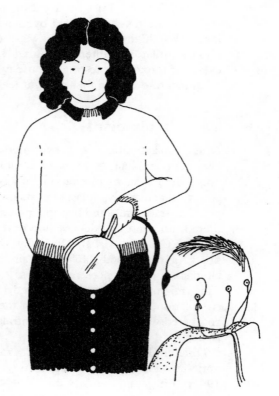

Fig. 13.10
A child prepared for multi-channel VEP recording. Two of the three active electrodes are visible. The stimulus is delivered from a Grass photostimulator held 40 cm in front of the child.

5. Collect 80 repetitions for each eye. Split the VEPs into two averages, each of 40 responses, to test for repeatability and reproducibility.
6. For each eye, subtract the left occiput (O_1) VEP from the right occiput (O_2) VEP.
7. Compare the right-eye and left-eye occipital ($O_2 - O_1$) difference potentials. Similar $R - L$ occipital difference potentials suggest the absence of albinism, whereas a reversal of the $R - L$ occipital difference indicates the abnormal crossing of fibres at the chiasm that is suggestive of albinism.

Reporting VEPs (Table 13.1)

Table 13.1   Reporting paediatric visual evoked potentials

Age
   – Note age of child at testing
Symptoms
   – List parent's perceptions, e.g. visually attentive/inattentive, problems with bright lights, seems to see better to one side (right or left) etc.
Clinical question
   – Is this VEP for acuity assessment, or for investigation of the visual pathways?
Existing conditions
   – List known ophthalmological conditions in the patient
   – List medical conditions
Degree of co-operation during testing
   – Indicate as Good, Fair, or Poor
Refractive error
   – Note refractive error and if glasses were worn during testing
Stimulus
   – Identify stimulus type (flash, pattern alternating, pattern onset)
   – Indicate size of stimulus field, contrast of pattern, intensity of flash, rate of presentation
Interpretation
   – Identify each pattern element tested (e.g. check size)
   – Indicate whether each eye's response is present, and with an implicit time within normal values for the child's age
Acuity Assessment
   – Indicate method: e.g. threshold check size, extrapolation.
   – Use appropriate units: checks – minutes of arc, grating – cycles per degree
   – Specify whether acuity is within range expected for age. Otherwise specify amount reduced from median of normal age range (log units reduction)
Were ISCEV standards followed?

THE ELECTRORETINOGRAM

The ERG is an electrophysiological test that assesses the aggregate response of the retina. An electrode at the front of the eye picks up electrical activity from the retina. Carefully chosen testing conditions and stimulus parameters make it possible to isolate the cone and rod responses from the retina.

The ERG recording has two major components, the negative a-wave and the positive b-wave. Measurements are made of the amplitude of the components and of the time taken from flash onset to reach the peak of each component.

ISCEV standards for electroretinography (Marmor and Zrenner, 1989, 1995) recommend that ERGs be recorded for five response types:

- the rod-response ERG to a very dim flash (maximal response attenuated by 2.5 log units) stimulating a dark-adapted retina
- the maximal response in reaction to a bright flash (between 1.5 and 3 cd.s.m^{-2}) – the rod-cone response of the dark-adapted eye
- the oscillatory potentials
- the cone response, recorded from the light-adapted eye, in the presence of a rod-suppressing background (17–34 cd.m^{-2}); and
- the flicker response, also recorded from the light-adapted eye.

Figure 13.11 shows examples of these five ERG response types.

Origins of the electroretinogram

The a-wave has a negative potential when measured at the cornea. The onset of light causes the intracellular electrical potential of the photoreceptors to become more negative by decreasing sodium current going into the photoreceptor outer segments (Fishman, 1990). The negative change in potential (known as hyperpolarization) at the photoreceptor is responsible for the negative a-wave.

The b-wave has a positive potential when measured at the cornea. The hyperpolarization of the photoreceptors causes a decrease in chemical neurotransmitter at the junction of the photoreceptors and bipolar cells. This changes the polarization of the bipolar cells, with many becoming depolarized (a positive change in intracellular potential). As a result of the depolarization of bipolar cells, there is an increase in extracellular potassium, causing a depolarization of Mueller cells. The transretinal current flow along the length of the Mueller cells is largely responsible for the positive b-wave of the ERG measured at the cornea (Fishman, 1990).

Oscillatory potentials are the series of wavelets (largely) super-imposed on the ascending limb of the b-wave. These wavelets have a frequency of between 100 and 160 Hz, and are formed by both rod and cone systems. It is thought that cells of the inner retina, possibly amacrine or interplexiform cells, generate the oscillatory potentials (Fishman, 1990).

Clinical use of electroretinograms in children

A number of retinal and choroidal diseases can affect ERGs, some in a very specific manner. ERGs can be used to distinguish between rod and cone defects, and between defects of the receptors and the deeper (middle) retinal layers. This means that ERGs are very useful in the diagnosis of several retinal conditions. Some of the retinal diseases that give abnormal ERG results are Leber's congenital amaurosis, achromatopsia, congenital stationary night blindness, cone dystrophies, cone-rod dystrophies, retinitis pigmentosa, and choroideraemia.

Retinal disease may be accompanied by nystagmus (e.g. rod monochromatism, cone dystrophy) or roving eye movements (e.g. Leber's congenital amaurosis). If the child has problems seeing in dim light, this signals an abnormality of the rod system (retinitis pigmentosa, congenital stationary night blindness). If the cone system is affected, the child may have problems with photophobia; this happens in rod monochromatism and in cone dystrophies. If cone activity is reduced, then visual acuity is likely to be affected. At The Hospital for Sick Children, Toronto, we receive ERG referrals for children with nystagmus, unexplained visual loss, night blindness and photophobia.

Clinical protocols for paediatric ERG testing

The protocol used in The Hospital for Sick Children, Toronto, Visual Electrophysiology Unit follows that recommended by the International Society for Clinical Electrophysiology of Vision (Marmor and

Fig. 13.11
The five response types of the ERG. From the topmost to the bottom most trace: rod response, mixed rod-cone (maximal) response, cone response, oscillatory potentials (from the mixed rod-cone response), flicker response. For the first three response types two responses are shown to demonstrate repeatability. The vertical and horizontal bars indicate the amplitude and time scales, respectively.

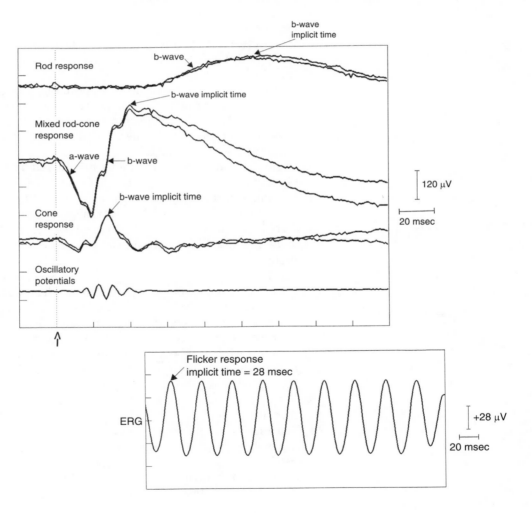

Zrenner, 1989, 1995). ISCEV makes allowances for the fact that some differences in protocol may be required for paediatric testing. Readers should refer to the ISCEV standards for a more complete guide to ERG testing.

1. Dilate the child's pupils with a solution of 1% cyclopentolate and 2.5% phenylephrine hydrochloride (0.5% cyclopentolate, in infants under 3 months old).
2. Dark adapt the child for 30 minutes.
3. Apply 1 drop of 0.5% proparacaine hydrochloride to anaesthetize the cornea.
4. Choose a contact-lens electrode (e.g. a Burian–Allen electrode, Hansen Ophthalmic Development Laboratory, Iowa City, IA, USA) of a size chosen to be appropriate for the child's age and eye size.
5. Place a drop of artificial tears (e.g. Tears naturale II, Alcon Canada Inc., Mississauga, ON, Canada) into the lens to protect the cornea.
6. Insert the electrode.
7. Use a central forehead electrode as a ground.
8. Use a Ganzfeld (LKC Technologies, Gaithersberg, MD, USA) illuminated by a Grass photostimulator, intensity 8, as the visual stimulus.
9. Seat the child with her or his head positioned at the opening of the Ganzfeld stimulator, either alone or held on a parent's lap (Figure 13.12). Infants lie supine on a stretcher; the Ganzfeld is lowered over the infant's head so that he or she is correctly positioned at the opening.
10. Begin the testing with very dim flash, achieved by attenuating the Grass flash by 3 log units (the LKC filter is set at 3.0). Save a minimum of three repeatable, artefact-free ERG responses.
11. Increase the intensity in 0.3 log unit steps. Repeat the testing until there is no attenuation, i.e. the last of the series of ERG responses to be measured is the maximal ERG response to the standard flash, which should have a luminance between 1.5 and 3 $cd.s.m^{-2}$.
12. Record the cone response after the child is light-adapted: turn on the background light of the Ganzfeld with the child's head held in the opening of the Ganzfeld for 3 minutes. Set the luminance to between 17 and 34 $cd.m^{-2}$. (ISCEV standards recommend 10 minutes; we have chosen a shorter time for paediatric testing.) Record the cone response using a background light to suppress the rod response.
13. Measure the child's cone flicker response to a 30 Hz flicker stimulus.
14. Separate the oscillatory potentials superimposed on the ascending limb of the b-wave from the b-wave by digitally filtering the ERG (high pass, 100 Hz). Separate dark- and light-adapted oscillatory potentials from the maximal response ERG and cone response, respectively.

Fig. 13.12
Infant with Burian–Allen electrode
sitting at a Ganzfeld.

Electrical signals from the retina in response to the flash are led to pre-amplifiers with a bandwidth of 1–300 Hz and then to a microprocessor for analysis. Software analysis allows us to reject data

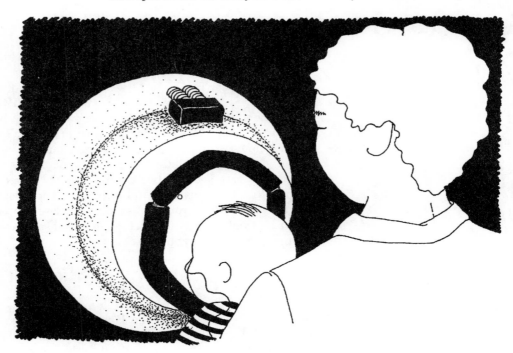

contaminated by blinks and eye movements. ERG waveforms in response to different flash intensities are averaged after testing; the implicit time and amplitude of each waveform are then compared with age-matched normal responses.

Calibration of the Ganzfeld flash

It is important to measure the luminance of the flashes of different light intensities to ensure that abnormally low ERG amplitudes are a result of retinal abnormality and not due to reduced luminance of the flash. The DR-2000 radiometer/photometer (Gamma Scientific, San Diego, CA, USA) is capable of recording the luminance to very brief flashes.

Other types of recording electrodes

Some visual electrophysiology laboratories prefer to use electrodes other than contact-lens electrodes. The silver-impregnated fibre electrode (Coupland, 1991) is less invasive than the contact-lens electrode; the length of fibre can be draped in the lower fornix (conjunctival fold) of the eye. A second type of electrode used by some laboratories are skin electrodes. A skin electrode can be a gold disc electrode attached just under the lower lid, with the reference electrode at the outer canthus. Both thread and skin-type electrodes are tolerated better by young children. However, ISCEV standards do not recommend skin electrodes because they give smaller, more variable responses that may be harder to discern from electrical noise or movement artefact.

Development of ERG waveforms

ERG waveforms show dramatic development within the first 6 months of life (Fulton and Hansen, 1985). Figure 13.13 compares the maximal response ERG in a 13-week-old infant and an adult. At the Hospital for Sick Children, Toronto, we recorded ERGs from infancy to adulthood in 90 subjects with no known retinal disease (Westall, unpublished data). Between 3 and 5 years of age ERG amplitudes and implicit times, from the ISCEV recommended response types, fall within normal adult limits. For paediatric ERG recording, it is essential to have age-matched control data for correct interpretation of the ERG. It is important to understand that, relative to the adult control data, ERGs are diminished and delayed in ocularly normal infants; it would be easy to falsely assume that such results, normal for infants, were due to retinal disease.

ERG AND VEP RECORDING

Some visual electrophysiology laboratories advocate simultaneous ERG-VEP recording. The ERG electrodes used must be of a type that does not interfere with the clarity of the visual stimulus; therefore fibre or skin electrodes would serve this purpose. Other labs record ERGs

Fig. 13.13
Mixed rod-cone response of a 13-week-old infant (top), compared with that of an adult (bottom). Note the reduction in the b-wave amplitude and increase in b-wave implicit time in the infant ERG compared with that of the adult.

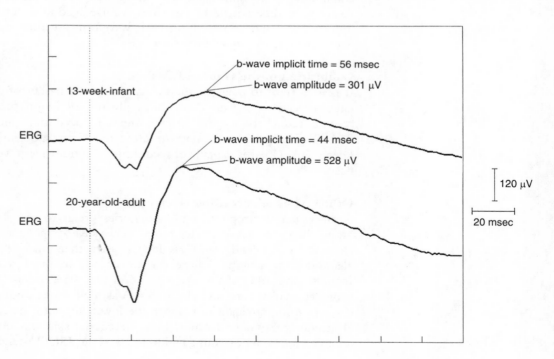

Reporting electroretinograms (Table 13.2)

Table 13.2   Reporting paediatric electroretinograms

Age
  – Age of child at testing
Clinical question
  – Identify reason for referral, to rule out retinal disease, to help identify medical condition or to test for carrier status of retinal disease
Symptoms
  – List child's or parent's perceptions, e.g. night-blindness, photophobia, poor vision?
History
  – Family history of retinal disease
Existing conditions
  – Ophthalmological
  – Medical
Medications
  – List medications (some medications affect the ERG)
Pupil diameter
  – Note dilated pupil diameter in mm
Visual acuity
  – What is the visual acuity and is it within normal range expected by age?
Sedation
  – Note if ERG testing was done with the child sedated or under general anaesthetic.
Degree of co-operation
  – Indicate as good, fair, or poor
Refractive error
  – Note refractive error
Interpretation
  – Indicate each stimulus parameter (rod responses, rod-cone responses, cone responses, flicker responses, oscillatory potentials). For each parameter specify luminance of response, as well as background luminance for cone-mediated responses
  – Indicate whether each eye's response is normal, diminished or delayed (compared with age-matched control data), or non-recordable
Were ISCEV standards followed?

---

and VEPs in the same children on separate occasions. There are advantages and disadvantages to either protocol.

The human retina has many more rods than cones (20:1); therefore, the flash ERG is dominated by rod activity. In contrast, VEPs are dominated by cone activity and reflect the central 6–10 degrees of arc of the retina (Sokol, 1986). Simultaneous ERG-VEP recordings therefore help distinguish between cone and rod abnormalities. Pathology that affects the mid- and far-peripheral retina, e.g. retinitis pigmentosa, has a greater effect on the ERG than the VEP, whereas abnormalities of foveal function, e.g. maculopathy, exhibit VEP rather than ERG abnormalities (Sokol, 1986).

If an infant is unable to fix or follow, or if the child has nystagmus or roving eye movements, ERG and VEP recordings will help determine whether the problem is retinal or cortical. Abnormal ERGs are found in conditions such as Leber's congenital amaurosis, congenital stationary night blindness, and rod monochromatism. If the ERG is normal but VEPs are abnormal, then the lack of visual responses result from pathology of the visual pathways or visual cortex (Sokol, 1986).

THE ELECTRO-OCULOGRAM

A description of the EOG, its measurement, and its use in retinal disease can be found in Fishman (1990). The EOG measures indirectly the electrical difference that exists between the cornea and the retina, called the *resting* or *standard potential* of the eye. The cornea is approximately 6 mV positive with respect to the retina, which changes with changing retinal illumination. The standing potential of the eye is generated mainly by the transepithelial potential across the pigmented epithelium of the retina.

The EOG changes under light-adapted and dark-adapted states; therefore, clinical measurements of the EOG are made using these two conditions of retinal illumination. Skin electrodes, either side of the eyes, record electrical changes induced by constant amplitude saccadic eye movements. Recorded EOG voltages decrease with dark adaptation, reaching a trough after about 12 minutes (the dark trough); then, after a period of light adaptation, the EOG increases to reach a peak (the light peak). One of the ways of evaluating the EOG is to record the ratio of the light peak to the dark trough; this is called the Arden ratio. For an alternative method, see Marmor and Zrenner (1993).

Clinical use of electro-oculograms in children

EOGs are most appropriate when testing for the possibility of diseases that affect the retinal pigment epithelium. Fishman (1990) outlines those dystrophies of the pigment epithelium that may give rise to EOG abnormalities.

The only disease that is consistently associated with abnormal EOGs, however, is Best's (vitelliform) macular dystrophy. Best's disease is an autosomal-dominant macular degeneration that may be congenital or may have an onset of up to 7 years of age. Early on, the macula is often described as having a 'sunny-side-up egg' appearance. Later in the disease's progress, the yolk-like material is absorbed, leaving an atrophic, disoriented, pigmented macula (Sheie and Albert, 1977). In the later stages, visual acuity drops, and the fundus may resemble that in other types of macular disease. The Arden ratio is reduced, even in those who are in the early stages of Best's disease or in those who carry the gene yet do not manifest any fundus changes (studies quoted by Fishman, 1990).

Recording the electro-oculogram

The EOG is measured indirectly, by surface electrodes placed on either side of the eye. Figure 12.10 shows the position of the outer electrodes. For EOG recording of each eye independently it is important that electrodes are placed close to the outer and inner canthi of the right and left eyes. Saccadic eye movements are made between two fixation lights. The eye acts as a dipole; as it moves towards one recording electrode or the other, the changing electrical signal is detected.

ISCEV has recently recommended a standard method of EOG assessment (Marmor and Zrenner, 1993). The purpose of a standardized recording protocol is to facilitate comparison of EOG responses throughout the world.

The stimulus should be a full-field Ganzfeld, providing even illumination across the retina. At the back of the dome, fixation lights – red light-emitting diodes (LEDs) that act as fixation targets for saccadic eye movements – are horizontally separated by 30 degrees of visual angle. At The Hospital for Sick Children in Toronto, we use the LKC system, which allows the operator to extinguish one diode while the other remains illuminated.

Clinical protocol for EOG testing

The following protocol, taken partially from the Standard for Clinical Electrooculography (Marmor and Zrenner, 1993), and partially from The Hospital for Sick Children, Toronto, protocol, can be used with children as young as 5 years (Buffa, unpublished data).

1. Before testing, make sure the child has been in ordinary room light levels (35–70 lux) for at least 15 minutes. Strong light (e.g. ophthalmoscopy, bright sunlight) should be avoided for at least 60 minutes prior to testing.
2. Choose electrode sites: one site on both sides of each eye, as close to the eye as possible, and a fifth location on the forehead for the ground electrode.
3. Clean the skin with alcohol swabs or an abrasive skin preparation (e.g. Nuprep) at the electrode sites. (Children sometimes complain that the alcohol irritates their eyes; therefore, we prefer to use an abrasive skin preparation.)
4. We use skin electrodes (silver-silver chloride) with a self-adhesive collar and with a small amount of conductive gel placed on the surface of the electrode.
5. Check that the impedance between the electrodes is less than 10 kilohms.
6. With the Ganzfeld off, seat the child with her or his head positioned at the Ganzfeld opening; use a chinrest and headrest to help stabilize the head.
7. Turn off the room lights.
8. About once a minute, alternate the LEDs 10 times. Ask the child to keep her or his head still and to look toward the red light, which will be seen to bounce from right to left. The resulting eye movements are saccadic eye movements in response to the alternating LEDs.
9. Record the EOG continuously.
10. After at least 10 repetitive saccades, turn the LEDs off.

11. Repeat this process once per minute for 15 minutes. The minimum amplitude of the EOG during this period, designated as the dark trough, occurs at approximately 11 to 12 minutes.

12. Turn the background light on the Ganzfeld on. The stimulus intensity should be between 400 and 600 cd.m^{-2} when the child's pupils have not been dilated. (The value chosen should be fixed for each laboratory.)

13. Once a minute, illuminate the right and left LEDs alternately as was done in the dark phase. The EOG amplitude will increase and, after about 12 minutes, start decreasing again. The maximum EOG amplitude, designated the light peak, occurs approximately 12 minutes after the background light has been turned on.

14. If no increase in EOG amplitude is seen, continue recording for at least 20 minutes after the background light is presented.

15. Calculate the Arden ratio (i.e. the ratio of light peak to dark trough).

Paediatric protocol

Fulton and colleagues (1989) outlined the protocol for EOG testing in infants and young children; additional details can be found in Hansen and Fulton (1983).

1. Apply two electrodes at the outer canthi; a third ground electrode can be placed over the mastoid or on the centre of the forehead.

2. Seat the child's parent on a chair in the testing room that is capable of horizontal clockwise and anti-clockwise oscillation; seat the child on the parent's lap.

3. Turn the lights out.

4. Hold an illuminated toy in the midline to act as a fixation marker for the child. Encourage the child to watch the toy.

5. Rock (turn) the chair between two points 22 degrees to the right and left of the midline. As the chair rocks, the vestibulo-ocular reflex (Chapter 8) causes the child's eyes to remain stable with respect to the world. That is, when the chair moves to the right, the eyes will move by the opposite amount to the left. The fixation toy, which is held in the same position in the midline, helps encourage the child's fixation.

6. Repeat the rocking of the chair for several cycles, once per minute for 15 minutes.

7. The eye movement amplitude to the rocking is between 30 and 50 degrees (Fulton, Hartmann and Hansen, 1989). As the process is being repeated in the dark, measure the dark trough of the EOG.

8. Turn the lights on.

9. Repeat the rocking EOG for a further 15 minutes while recording the light peak.

10. Calculate the light peak/dark trough ratio.

Reporting the electro-oculogram (Table 13.3)

Table 13.3   Reporting paediatric electro-oculograms

Age
  – Age of child at testing
Clinical question
  – Identify reason for referral
Symptoms
  – List child's or parents' perceptions, e.g. photophobia, poor vision
History
  – Family history of retinal disease
Existing conditions
  – Ophthalmological
  – Medical
Medications
  – List medications (some medications affect the ERG)
Visual acuity
  – What is the visual acuity and is it within normal range expected by age?
EOG ratio
  – Specify EOG ratio and identify if the Arden ratio was used
Age matched control data
  – Specify the range of normal EOG ratios for the child's age
Time to peak
  – Identify the time between the onset of the light phase and the peak of the light response
Amplitude of dark trough
  – Specify the amplitude of the dark trough in microvolts
Were ISCEV standards followed?

INFECTION CONTROL

The infections most likely to be transmitted during electrophysiological testing are respiratory infections and the common cold. It is therefore important that people working in electrophysiology laboratories wash their hands frequently. It is important to wash hands before testing the first patient of the day, between patients and after the last patient of the day. If someone has a bad cold or infection then it may be appropriate for that person (whether patient or examiner) to wear a face mask.

Disc electrodes used for visual evoked potentials and electro-oculography do not pierce the skin, therefore the risk of transmitting infection is minimal. The electrodes can be soaked in water with a mild detergent for a few hours and then cleaned with a soft toothbrush.

However, there is more chance of transmitting infection with ERG electrodes. The electrodes have been in contact with the patient's tear film, and therefore there is a chance of transmitting hepatitis or HIV. After every patient ERG electrodes need to be sterilized. Each person should know the procedures required by their own organization. The Hospital for Sick Children, Toronto, protocol requires that Burian–Allen electrodes are soaked for 10 minutes in hydrogen peroxide after which they are rinsed in water and dried carefully.

CONCLUSION

Much of this book has been concerned with the use of psychophysical techniques for assessing the vision of infants and children. However, there are situations in which objective assessment, through the use of electrophysiological testing, will be indicated. For example, VEPs can provide valuable information when a child appears to be blind, while ERGs or EOGs are useful when diagnostic information about retinal function is required. In this chapter we have provided an introduction to the electrophysiological assessment of children's vision, including clinical protocols and guidelines for writing reports. We believe that this information will be of use not only to those who are about to undertake such clinical work themselves, but to other eye care practitioners who may need to understand clinical reports and research papers based on electrophysiological techniques and to communicate with parents and other professionals about electro-physiological assessments of children under their care.

REFERENCES

Apkarian P. (1992). A practical approach to albino diagnosis – VEP misrouting across the age span. *Ophthalmic Paediatr. Genet.*, **13**, 77–88.

Apkarian, P. (1993). VEP assessment of visual function in pediatric neuro-ophthalmology. In D.M. Albert and F. A. Jakobiec (eds.), *Principles and Practice of Ophthalmology.* Philadelphia, Saunders, pp. 622–647.

Apkarian, P., Mirmiran, M. and Tijssen, R. (1991). Effect of behavioural state on visual processing in neonates. *Neuropediatrics*, **22**, 85–91.

Apkarian, P., van Veenendaal, W. and Spekreijse, H. (1986). Measurement of visual acuity in infants and young children by visual evoked potentials. In B. Jay (ed.), *Detection and Measurement of Visual Impairment in Pre-verbal Children.* The Hague, Junk, Publishers. pp. 168–189.

Bane, M.C. and Birch, E.E. (1992). VEP acuity, FPL acuity and visual behavior of visually impaired children. *Journal of Pediatric Ophthalmology and Strabismus*, **29**, 202–209.

Coupland, S.G. (1991). Electrodes for clinical electrophysiological testing: basic recording. In J.R. Heckenlively and G.B. Arden (eds.), *Principles and Practice of Clinical Electrophysiology of Vision.* St Louis, Mosby Year Book, pp. 177–182.

Fishman, G.A. (1990). The electro-oculogram in retinal disorders. In G.A. Fishman and S. Sokol (eds), *Electrophysiologic Testing in Disorders of the Retina, Optic Nerve and Visual Pathway*, Ophthalmology Monographs, San Francisco, American Academy of Ophthalmology, pp. 91–99.

Fitzgerald, K. and Cibis, G.W. (1994). The value of flash visual evoked potentials in albinism. *Journal of Pediatric Ophthalmology and Strabismus*, **31**, 18–25.

Fulton, A.B. and Hansen, R.M. (1985). Electroretinography: application to clinical studies of infants. *Journal of Pediatric Ophthalmology and Strabismus*, **22**, 251–255.

Fulton, A.B., Hartmann, E.E. and Hansen, R.M. (1989). Electrophysiologic testing techniques for children. *Documenta Ophthalmologica*, **71**, 341–354.

Geer, I. and Westall, C.A. (1996). A comparison of tests to determine acuity deficits in children with amblyopia. *Ophthalmic & Physiological Optics*, **16**, 367–374.

Granet, D.B., Hertle, R.W., Quinn, G.E. and Breton, M.E. (1993). The visual-evoked response in infants with central visual impairment. *American Journal of Ophthalmology*, **116**, 437–443.

Guillery, R.W. (1974). Visual pathways in albinos. *Scientific American*, **230**, 44–54.

Guo, S., Reinecke, R.D., Fendick, M. and Calhoun, J.H. (1989). Visual pathway abnormalities in albinism and infantile nystagmus: VECPs and stereoacuity measurements. *Journal of Pediatric Ophthalmology and Strabismus*, **26**, 97–104.

Hansen, R.M. and Fulton, A.B. (1983). Corneoretinal potentials in human infants. *Doc. Ophthalmol. Proc. Series*, **37**, 81–86.

Harding, G.F.A. (1991). Visual evoked cortical potentials: basic recording. In J.R. Heckenlively and G.B. Arden (eds.), *Principles and Practice of Clinical Electrophysiology of Vision*. St Louis, Mosby Year Book, pp. 399–407.

Harding, G.F.A., Odom, J.V., Spileers, W., and Spekreijse, H. (on behalf of the International Society for Clinical Electrophysiology of Vision) (1996). Standard for visual evoked potential. *Vision Research*, **36**, 3567–3572.

Heckenlively, J.R. and Arden, G.B. (eds) (1991). *Principles and Practice of Clinical Electrophysiology of Vision*. St Louis, Mosby Year Book.

Hoyt, C.S. (1984). Controversies in pediatric ophthalmology – the clinical usefulness of the visual evoked potential. *Journal of Pediatric Ophthalmology and Strabismus*, **21**, 231–234.

Kooijman, A.C., van Norren, D., de Sera, P., Thijssen, J.M. et al. (Working Group, Physical Methods in Ophthalmology) (1986). Minimum procedures for visual electrodiagnostic testing. *Documenta Ophthalmologica*, **63**, 13–18.

Kriss, A., Russell-Eggitt, I., Harris, C.M. et al. (1992). Aspects of albinism. *Ophthalmic Pediatr. Genet.*, **13**, 89–100.

Lambert, S.R., Kriss, A. and Taylor, D. (1989). Delayed visual maturation: A longitudinal clinical and electrophysiological assessment. *Ophthalmology*, **96**, 524–528.

Mackie, R.T., McCulloch, D.L., Saunders, K.J. et al. (1995). Comparison of visual assessment tests in multiply handicapped children. *Eye*, **9**, 136–141.

Marg, E., Freeman, D.N., Peltzman, P. and Goldstein, P.J. (1976). Visual acuity development in human infants: evoked potential measurements. *Investigative Ophthalmology & Visual Science*, **15**, 150–153.

Marmor, M.F. and Zrenner, E., for the International Society for Clinical Electrophysiology of Vision (1989). Standard for clinical electro-retinography. *Archives of Ophthalmology*, **107**, 816–819.

Marmor, M.F. and Zrenner, E., for the International Society for Clinical Electrophysiology of Vision (1993). Standard for clinical electro-oculography. *Documenta Ophthalmologica*, **85**, 115–124.

Marmor, M.F. and Zrenner, E., for the International Society for Clinical Electrophysiology of Vision (1995). Standard for clinical electro-retinography, 1994 update. *Documenta Ophthalmologica*, **89**, 199–210.

McCulloch, D.L. and Skarf, B. (1991). Development of the human visual system: monocular and binocular pattern VEP latency. *Investigative Ophthalmology & Visual Science*, **32**, 2372–2381.

McCulloch, D.L. and Skarf, B. (1994). Pattern reversal visual evoked potentials following early treatment of unilateral, congenital cataract. *Archives of Ophthalmology*, **112**, 510–518.

McCulloch, D.L., Taylor, M.J. and Whyte, H.E. (1991). Visual evoked potentials and visual prognosis following perinatal asphyxia. *Archives of Ophthalmology*, **109**, 229–233.

Moskowitz, A. and Sokol, S. (1980). Spatial and temporal interaction of pattern-evoked cortical potentials in human infants. *Vision Research*, **30**, 699–707.

Moskowitz, A. and Sokol, S. (1983). Developmental changes in the human visual system as reflected by the latency of the pattern reversal VEP. *Electroencephalography and Clinical Neurophysiology*, **56**, 1–15.

Norcia, A.M. and Tyler, C.W. (1985). Spatial frequency sweep VEP: visual acuity in the first year of life. *Vision Research*, **25**, 1399–1408.

Orel-Bixler., D., Haegerstrom-Portnoy, G. and Hall, A. (1989). Visual assessment of the multiply handicapped patient. *Optometry and Vision Science*, **66**, 530–536.

Orel-Bixler, D. and Norcia, A.M. (1986). Differential growth in acuity for pattern reversal and pattern onset-offset targets. *Clinical Vision Science*, **2**, 1–9.

Regan, D. (1973). Rapid objective refraction using evoked brain potentials. *Investigative Ophthalmology* **12**, 669–703.

Regan, D. (1980). Speedy evoked potential methods for assessing vision in normal and amblyopic eyes. *Vision Research*, **20**, 265–269.

Regan, D. (1989). *Human Brain Electrophysiology*. Amsterdam, Elsevier, pp. 1–167.

Rosenberg, M.L. and Jabbari, B. (1987). Nystagmus and visual evoked potentials. *Neuro-Ophthalmology*, **7**, 133–136.

Sheie, H.G. and Albert, D.M. (1977). *Textbook of Ophthalmology*, 9th edn, chapter 13. Philadelphia, Saunders, p. 307.

Skarf, B. (1989). Discussion of: Lambert, S.R., Kriss, A. and Taylor, D. (1989), Delayed visual maturation, a longitudinal clinical and electrophysiological assessment. *Ophthalmology*, **96**, 529.

Smith, D.N. (1984). Controversies in pediatric ophthalmology – the clinical usefulness of the visual evoked potential. *Journal of Pediatric Ophthalmology and Strabismus*, **21**, 235–236.

Smith, R.G., Brimlow, G.M., Lea, S.J. and Galloway, N.R. (1990). Evoked responses in patients with macular holes. *Documenta Ophthalmologica*, **75**, 135–144.

Sokol, S. (1978). Measurement of infant visual acuity from pattern reversal evoked potentials. *Vision Research* **18**, 33–39.

Sokol, S. (1986). Clinical applications of the ERG and VEP in the pediatric age group. In R.Q. Cracco and I. Bodis-Wollner (eds), *Evoked Potentials*. New York, Alan R. Liss, pp. 447–454.

Sokol, S. (1990). The visual evoked cortical potential in optic nerve and visual pathway disorders. In G.A. Fishman and S. Sokol (eds), *Electrophysiologic Testing in Disorders of the Retina, Optic Nerve and Visual Pathway*. Ophthalmology Monographs, San Francisco, American Academy of Ophthalmology, pp. 105–141.

Sokol, S. and Moskowitz, A. (1985). Comparison of pattern VEPs and preferential looking behaviour in three-month-old infants. *Investigative Ophthalmology & Visual Science*, **26**, 359–365.

Taylor, M.J. and McCulloch, D.L. (1991). Prognostic values of VEPs in young children with acute onset of cortical blindness. *Pediatric Neurology*, **7**, 111–115.

Taylor M.J. and McCulloch, D.L. (1992). Visual evoked potentials in infants and children. *Journal of Clinical Neurophysiology*, **9**, 357–372.

Tyler, C.W. (1991). Visual acuity estimation in infants by visual evoked cortical potentials. In J.R. Heckenlively and G.B. Arden (eds), *Principles and Practice of Clinical Electrophysiology of Vision*. Philadelphia, Mosby, pp. 408–416.

Tyler, C.W., Apkarian, P., Levi, D.M. and Nakayama, K. (1979). Rapid assessment of visual function: an electronic sweep technique for the pattern visual evoked potential. *Investigative Ophthalmology & Visual Science*, **18**, 703–713.

Tyler, C.W., Apkarian, P. and Nakayama, K. (1978). Multiple spatial frequency tuning of electrical responses from human visual cortex. *Experimental Brain Research*, **33**, 535–550.

Tyler, C.W., Nakayama, K., Apkarian, P. and Levi, D.M. (1981). VEP assessment of visual function. *Vision Research*, **21**, 607–609.

Appendix 13.1

Companies dealing with electrophysiology hardware and software

Grass Instruments Astromed Grass, 600 East Grenwich Ave., West Warwick, Rhode Island, USA. Tel. (US) 1-800-343-4039. Tel. (from Canada) 1-800-565-2216, (from UK) 01-628-668836.

Neuroscan Inc., 790 Station Street, Suite 210, Herndon, VA 22070, USA. Tel. 703-787-7575.

Nicolet Biomedical Instruments, 5225 Verona Road, Madison, WI 53711-4495, USA. Tel. 608-273-5000.

LKC technologies, 2 Professional Drive, Suite 222, Gaithersburg, MD 20879, USA. Tel. 301-840-1992.

Electrodes

In Vivo Metric, P.O. Box 249, Healdsburg, CA 95448, USA. Tel. 707-433-4819.

Neuromedical Supplies, Inc., 790 Station Street, Suite 210, Herndon, VA 22070-4606, USA. Tel. 703-471-6888.

14

Taking action

INTRODUCTION

The previous chapters have given detailed information about the range of assessment methods available for gathering information about a young child's eyes and visual system, within the context of his or her overall development. For clarity, we have left the bringing together and utilization of this information to the end of the book. This final chapter deals with the construction of a treatment or management plan and includes guidelines for prescribing refractive corrections and for managing ocular deviations, reading difficulties, accommodation anomalies and low vision. We also cover the verbal communication of test results, prognosis and management plan to parents and children as well as the writing of reports for parents, care workers and other relevant professionals. Finally, ethical and legal issues in child vision care are discussed. Much of this chapter should be of interest to our broader readership, although the section on legal issues is directed more specifically at the optometrist.

PRESCRIBING REFRACTIVE CORRECTIONS WHEN THERE IS NO STRABISMUS

The decision to give a child a prescription for glasses will depend on a number of factors which must be taken into account both separately and in association. These are age, refractive error, presence of strabismus or high phoria, visual acuity, signs and symptoms and ocular health. In this section we consider cases in which there is a refractive error, but no strabismus. We discuss factors that need to be considered when prescribing for children below 5 years of age and 5 years and over, respectively, then provide some summary guidelines for prescription followed by a brief section on contact lenses. A later section on ocular deviations will consider spectacle correction as part of the overall management of children with strabismus.

Factors to consider when prescribing for 0–4 year olds

It is difficult to give a definitive list of occasions which require that a prescription be given. Although there are a few indicators, it is impossible to give a list of rules which encompasses every potential

344

situation. There are a number of factors to be taken into consideration and balanced against one another in prescribing for this young age group and each eye care practioner must ultimately develop his or her own criteria for making clinical decisions.

Readers are directed towards papers describing the infant vision screening programmes in Cambridge and Bristol (England) for information relating to the outcome of prescribing for hyperopic refractive errors (Atkinson, 1993; Atkinson et al., 1996). These papers describe the refractive and acuity development of over 9000 infants from 9 months to 5 years of age. Infants with hyperopia were randomly assigned to two groups: one group received a partial correction at 9 months of age while the other received no correction. The studies showed that the development of visual acuity is delayed in the first four years in children with uncorrected hyperopia in comparison with those who received a partial correction and those with no significant refractive error. By 5 years of age there was less difference in visual acuity between the children with uncorrected hyperopia and those with corrected hyperopia or minimal hyperopia. Atkinson (1993) comments that the investigators do not know if the delay in visual acuity persists into the early school years.

Based on the studies to date, there are circumstances which indicate a more vigorous approach to prescribing spectacles for young children and others which indicate that we should be more conservative, as discussed below.

Factors indicating a more vigorous approach

1. High and medium refractive errors are risk factors for amblyopia and should be corrected. Uncorrected persistent anisometropia, astigmatism and hyperopia have been shown to give rise to either binocular or monocular amblyopia (see Chapters 2 and 5).
2. If unaided vision is reduced when the child is examined and can be improved with spectacle lenses, a prescription should be given.
3. The Cambridge study (Atkinson et al., 1996) showed that the prevalence of accommodative esotropia was lower in the group who received a partial spectacle correction when compared with the group who received no correction. This suggests that, in some cases, the eye care practitioner may prevent esotropia by prescribing a hyperopic correction.
4. Hyperopia should be corrected in children with esophoria, especially if the AC/A ratio is high (Chapter 9). The purpose of this is to minimize accommodative vergence which may in turn prevent the onset of esotropia.
5. Children with uncorrected hyperopia may have more difficulties in reading skills than children without hyperopia. Some investigators believe that this may be related to eye strain. Children with uncorrected hyperopia have been shown to have poorer perceptual skills (Rosner and Gruber, 1985), defined as 'the ability to view spatially organized information in an analytical manner, for example, to identify task-pertinent features of an array such as

the length and orientation of lines' (Rosner and Rosner, 1987). Although there is much debate about the relationship between visual, perceptual and reading problems, there is some evidence that correction of moderate amounts of hyperopia before the age of 4 years prevents a lag of visual perceptual skills development and may reduce some forms of reading difficulties. A prescription should be given for significant hyperopia in these early years. Reading problems are discussed later in the chapter.

Factors indicating a conservative approach

1. In Chapter 5 we showed that refractive errors are more common in infants than in the adult population and are short lived. The range of refractive errors is far greater than in adults, with a greater prevalence of astigmatism and anisometropia. Hyperopia tends to be greater and myopia is not uncommon, particularly in the first six months. We do not recommend prescribing for refractive errors if they fall within the normal range for the child's age if there are no indications to suggest otherwise. The eye care practitioner must therefore be aware of these normal ranges (Chapter 5).
2. Gwiazda, Thorn, Bauer and Held's (1993) study suggests that 12 months is a good age for routine examination of infants with no observed ocular or visual problems. If significant astigmatism (up to 2 D) or anisometropia (up to 2 D) is found, we recommend follow-up over the next 6–12 months, rather than prescribing straight away. Higher amounts of these refractive errors would lead to more concern and probably a prescription.
3. Emmetropization may still be continuing up to the age of 6 years (Gwiazda et al., 1993) and, clearly, it is undesirable to interrupt this process. A full spectacle prescription may halt the process, as the residual refractive error – perhaps the stimulus to emmetropization – is no longer present. However the evidence is still equivocal. Atkinson et al. (1996) found that partial correction of infants with high hyperopia had no effect on the progression towards emmetropia while Ingram et al. (1990, 1991) found that children with high hyperopia who consistently wore a partial prescription maintained more hyperopia, but had better visual acuity, than those who did not. Thus it is unclear how much uncorrected refractive error is necessary for emmetropization to proceed optimally. Generally, it is agreed that most infants should be undercorrected so that some residual refractive error will act as a stimulus for emmetropization.

Ingram et al. (1990) observed a lower prevalence of strabismus (and better visual acuity) in children who demonstrated some emmetropization than in those whose ametropia did not reduce. This is a chicken and egg situation: does the predisposition to strabismus also affect the emmetropization mechanism or does poorer emmetropization (and, consequently, higher hyperopia) result in strabismus? Similarly, it has been suggested that good acuity is required for the feedback mechanism for emmetropization, and this poses another question: is poorer acuity the result or the cause of poorer emmetropization?

In the absence of clear answers to these questions, and based on our awareness of the emmetropization process, the risk factors for amblyopia and strabismus and the possible link with some learning difficulties, we have attempted to generate a list of circumstances in which glasses would be prescribed. These are summarized after our discussion of considerations in the 4–15-year-old group.

Factors to consider when prescribing for 5–15 year olds

By the age of 4 years astigmatism and anisometropia have generally reduced to more adult-like levels, therefore persistence of these refractive errors at this age should warrant concern and probably a prescription.

After the age of 6 years, there is a gradually increasing prevalence of myopia (Chapter 5). A child who is found to be emmetropic at this age is likely to become myopic (hyperopia of approximately 1 D is the norm). These children should be followed up in 1 year. The average rate of progression towards myopia is 0.5 D per year in children who become myopic. Once a child has become more than 0.5 D myopic, especially at the ages when board work is more a part of their schooling, a prescription should be considered as they are likely to have difficulty at school.

Myopia

There have been volumes written and many theories and strategies advocated about the prevention and correction of myopia (Woo & Wilson, 1990). Surgical treatments on the cornea (e.g. keratomileusis, keratophakia, epikeratoplasty, radial keratotomy and the more recent photorefractive keratectomy) have met with varying degrees of success and there are complications with all these methods. Few practitioners would advocate these procedures for children in whom myopia is still likely to progress and before a child can make an informed choice for themselves about a surgical procedure which may have permanent consequences on vision. The exceptional case when lens removal might be suggested would be in high myopia with the presence of a partial cataract. (The presence of a mature cataract would be an indication for surgical removal whatever the refractive error). Other surgical treatments (scleral reinforcement, scleral plication and stromectomy) are even more invasive with worse potential complications.

The use of drugs (atropine to reduce accommodation in the belief that active accommodation increases myopia) has been attempted. Myopia may be controlled temporarily while the drug is in use, but appears to progress on discontinuation. Other difficulties are adherence, side-effects of the drug and potential toxicity (atropine is a potentially dangerous drug to be lying around in anyone's house).

It has been suggested that wearing corneal hard contact lenses may reduce the progression of myopia (Stone, 1976), but this does not appear to be confirmed by other studies (Baldwin et al., 1969). Bier and Lowther (1986) found no significant difference in myopia progression whether fitted with rigid or hydrogel contact lenses. The deliberate fitting of a rigid contact lens (to change the shape of the cornea, thus reducing myopia) is known as orthokeratology. This has been undertaken with some transient success, i.e. there is some reduction of myopia, allowing the person to go uncorrected temporarily, but intermittent wearing of the contact lens is required to maintain the flattening. Side-effects are corneal oedema, abrasions, fluctuation of vision, irregular astigmatism, and keratoconic changes. This treatment is no longer recommended by most contact lens practitioners.

Variations in the spectacle prescription have been advocated, including full prescription, partial prescription, over-correction, full or part-time wear, and bifocals. Others have suggested full-time wear from the beginning in order to develop a new and correct association between accommodation and convergence. Again there has been inconsistency between studies on the efficacy of these approaches (Woo and Wilson, 1990), so that we have to conclude that there is no evidence that the spectacle prescription influences the rate of myopia progression. Thus we are free to prescribe what is optimal for functional vision for each child.

The most common practice, therefore, is to prescribe spectacles for occasional distance vision until the myopia has reached approximately 2 D, when full-time wear would be recommended. Follow-up should be every 6 months.

Hyperopia

Traditionally, we have been conservative in our correction of hyperopia, waiting until obvious symptoms of asthenopia (eyestrain) or some other clear signs of 'need' are evident, assuming that accommodation in children is sufficient to overcome moderate degrees of hyperopia. These assumptions need to be challenged, as we may have been underserving this population. Therefore, we are now more willing to prescribe for medium and high hyperopia in order to aid these children's school work. If a child with hyperopia is having reading difficulties or other learning difficulties at school, a prescription should be considered. Even a small prescription may make a difference to school performance in some cases.

Summary – guidelines for prescribing when there is no strabismus (0–15 years)

We would *consider* prescribing glasses in the following circumstances:

- Persisting astigmatism (over 2 D after 1.5 years of age; over 1.5 D after 3 years of age). Some would suggest a partial correction of the astigmatism, others a full correction with partial correction of associated hyperopia.
- Persisting anisometropia (over 2 D after 1.5 year of age; over 1.5 D after 3 years of age).
- High and medium hyperopia (greater than or equal to 3.5 D of hyperopia at 1 year of age or greater than 2 D at 4 years). For these children a partial prescription is suggested (unless strabismic – see below), leaving them 1 D undercorrected.
- Myopia greater than 2 D up to the age of 1 year (or when the child is walking) or greater than 1 D between 1 and 4 years – give a reduced correction. More than 0.5 D in school children – give a full correction.
- Unaided or corrected visual acuity is reduced (compared with the normal range) in one or both eyes in a way which is consistent with the refractive error findings, i.e. the reduction appears to be refractive in origin. In the case that reduced acuity is not refractive in origin, the cause must be determined and managed accordingly.
- Hyperopia in the presence of esophoria, especially with a high AC/A ratio. For esophoria at near with little hyperopia, consider a bifocal reading add.
- Learning difficulties or asthenopic symptoms; any refractive error, even smaller amounts of hyperopia, astigmatism or anisometropia.

We would *definitely* prescribe when there is:

- High ametropia of any type.
- Aphakia (this should be overcorrected by +3 D in the first year, reducing to +1–+1.5 D overcorrection by 1 year of age; contact lenses are the preferred mode of correction).

Whenever a prescription is given, a full explanation should be given to the parents about why glasses have been prescribed, with advice regarding how often the child should wear the spectacles. Generally, when glasses are prescribed for children, follow-up should be after 6 months (unless there is reason to see them sooner than this). The refractive error of a child can change rapidly and therefore fairly frequent follow-up is required. If, after a period of time, the refractive error is no longer outside the normal range, e.g. if anisometropia has diminished, the spectacle wear should be discontinued.

Contact lens corrections in children

We have already discussed the use of contact lenses as a treatment for the progression of myopia. Contact lenses may be requested for cosmetic reasons by some children (or by their parents) with moderate myopia. The use of contact lenses is also desirable, and sometimes necessary, for the treatment of certain ocular conditions, including high myopia, anisometropia, keratoconus, irregular astigmatism, aphakia following removal of dislocated lenses, and cataracts (traumatic, developmental or congenital) (Brent, 1983). Some of these cases may require the fitting of contact lenses in young infants, in which case the initial fitting and over-refraction is best achieved under general anaesthesia. On the basis of extensive experience at the Hospital for Sick Children in Toronto, Brent reports that many children over the age of 4 can be fitted with lenses in the clinic without too much difficulty.

The use of contact lenses for younger children and infants is a situation where parental involvement is paramount, and lens use may be impossible if two adults are unavailable (at least initially) for insertion and removal, if the parents have low vision, if there is poor hygiene or if the parents cannot cope with the child's initial distress. Parents need a great deal of demonstration, information and support. Brent (1983) is a good source of information on matters such as the use of hard and soft lenses, fitting procedures, keratometry, refraction, instructions for parents and follow-up. Further information about contact lenses may also be found in Gasson and Morris (1997).

OCULAR DEVIATIONS

As discussed in Chapter 9, an esodeviation is the latent (esophoria) or manifest (esotropia) convergent misalignment of the visual axes.

Infantile (early onset) strabismus

A quote from von Noorden (1996, p. 315) gives optometrists, orthoptists and physicians a very clear message: 'We insist that every child whose eyes are not aligned by 3 months of age be given a complete ophthalmological examination.'

Von Noorden strongly advocates early surgical correction for early onset strabismus and more ophthalmologists are now taking the same course. This is a change from previous treatment strategies. There are several reasons for this: first, there is increasing evidence that surgical correction of esotropia in the first two years of life will result in increased chance of sensory binocular vision (Ing, 1983). Deller (1988) suggests that the only delay in surgery would be for preoperative treatment of any amblyopia. Second, delay in surgical correction of strabismus results in strabismus-induced changes to the extra-ocular muscles which interfere with later surgical correction (von Noorden, 1996, p. 317). A further reason for the trend towards early surgical treatment is that the risks of anaesthesia are much less than they used to be (American Academy of Ophthalmology, 1994, p. 290).

It is important to detect and treat amblyopia in infants with early onset esotropia. Von Noorden (1996, p. 311) quotes a number of studies that suggest that amblyopia is commonly associated with infantile esotropia. He warns the reader that amblyopia not treated early will inhibit the return of binocular functions.

Sometimes infantile convergent esotropia is accommodative, although this is not typical. Hyperopic refractive errors need to be fully corrected as soon as possible. If surgery is to be performed, then refractive correction should be done before surgery because correction of high hyperopia may alter the angle of strabismus and therefore the angle for surgical correction. The acceptable outcome of surgical or refractive strabismus treatment is an angle of strabismus less than 10 prism dioptres (American Academy of Ophthalmology, 1994, p. 291). A good outcome is microtropia. It is important to explain to the parents the necessity for follow-up and regular examinations after surgery. This can easily be neglected as the child's eyes now look straight, but a small angle strabismus may still be present and amblyopia may develop.

Acquired esotropia

The most common type of acquired esotropia is accommodative esotropia (Chapter 9). It is important to fully correct any hyperopia as soon as possible. If detected and treated early before amblyopia has developed, the prognosis is good. In the case of intermittent esotropia which is treated early with spectacles, the prognosis for full normal binocular vision is high. If the refractive correction is delayed, or the child does not comply with wearing the glasses, then the esodeviation may not respond to subsequent reduction in accommodation (American Academy of Ophthalmology, 1994, p. 292) and deeper amblyopia is likely, which in turn may lead to reduced adherence to the treatment (as discussed below).

Treatment for acquired refractive accommodative esotropia is the correction of the refractive error and the treatment of amblyopia (see following pages). The full cycloplegic hyperopic correction should be prescribed for children under 6 years with constant refractive esotropia. Intermittent esotropia may be controlled by prescribing for the majority of the hyperopia. After 2 months of wearing glasses the visual acuities and refractive error should be rechecked. Cycloplegic refraction should be done at regular intervals and the prescription updated accordingly. The successful outcome is when the angle of esotropia is less than 10 prism dioptres. Over 6 years of age children should be prescribed the maximum hyperopic correction that they can tolerate. Children with accommodative esotropia should be tested at least twice a year. The hyperopia may increase until 5–7 years of age, and updated prescriptions need to be given.

Sometimes a reading addition of up to $+4\,D$ may reduce an accommodative esodeviation to acceptable limits. This is a particularly good form of treatment when there is distance binocular fusion, but a near esotropia. The reading addition can be incorporated into a pair of bifocals glasses. Base out prism can also be used to eliminate a small residual angle. The required reading addition can be calculated from a determination of the AC/A ratio, or the addition can be tried over the distance prescription and the cover test used to determine what addition is required to eliminate (or reduce) the angle of strabismus.

Acquired exotropia

Any significant refractive error should be corrected, with the following exception. Von Noorden (1996, p. 350) suggests that hyperopic refractive errors less than +2.00 D should not be corrected in children with exodeviations: the resulting accommodative effort required may help alleviate the exodeviation. Some children have a high AC/A ratio and minus lenses may then be used to stimulate accommodative convergence. Either of these scenarios – the non-prescribing of plus lenses or the over-prescribing of minus lenses – may create too much accommodative effort for the older child, when eye strain from real or induced hyperopic error may ensue. Prolonged treatment using these methods should therefore be avoided.

If the increased accommodative effort does not help reduce the exodeviation, or if the child is over 6 years of age then another way of treating exodeviations is the prescription of base in prism. Ravault, Bongrand and Bonamour (1972) propose treatment with prisms as an alternative to surgical correction in some cases. They propose full prismatic correction of the angle of deviation, followed by a gradual reduction in the strength of the prism to stimulate fusional vergence. In addition to spectacle treatments some orthoptic treatments could be very valuable.

As mentioned in Chapter 9, one of the theories of the cause of exotropia is that suppression leads to the breakdown of binocular fusion. There are a number of orthoptic treatments for suppression. The orthoptist or other eye care practitioner may use a major amblyoscope for anti-suppression treatment. Alternatively, red filter treatment is a useful anti-suppression therapy: a red filter is worn over the dominant eye and the child draws with a red pen; the eye with the filter will not see the red drawing if the colour of the pen matches the filter. This treatment is forcing the image from the suppressed retina back into consciousness.

Convergence insufficiency

Although not necessarily an exodeviation, convergence insufficiency is one of the most common causes of eyestrain, ocular discomfort and reading problems which become apparent in the teenage years. Convergence insufficiency is diagnosed when the near point of convergence is significantly greater than the normal range (10–11 cm). In convergence insufficiency the child may not be able to converge closer than 20 cm. In addition the near fusional amplitudes are poor and there may be an exophoria at near. Orthoptic treatment has been found to be quite successful (von Noorden, 1996, p. 470).

Orthoptic exercises include anti-suppression treatment, convergence exercises and awareness of physiological diplopia. For example the child is asked to look at a near object, while being made aware of the doubling of a distant target in physiological diplopia. The presence of physiological diplopia indicates that suppression has not occurred. The near object is removed and the child tries to maintain convergence of his or her eyes, which is signalled by the continuing diplopia of the distant object. The child tries to increase the time periods of successful voluntary convergence (von Noorden, 1996, pp. 510–512). Some people with convergence insufficiency may also have reduced accommodation. In these cases reading glasses may be required in addition to orthoptic exercises.

Amblyopia treatment

Monocular amblyopia results from strabismus or anisometropia. Bilateral amblyopia results from large, equal, uncorrected refractive errors. Deprivation amblyopia, which is usually caused by congenital or early acquired media opacities is the least common, but most damaging and difficult to treat, form of amblyopia.

It is important to refer a child with any obstacle to vision such as a cataract or other media opacity for ophthalmological assessment. After the obstacle to vision has been removed then glasses are prescribed and treatment for amblyopia is initiated.

First, the refractive error should be corrected. Contact lenses are the preferred form of correction for unilateral or bilateral aphakia in infants and young children. Contact lenses minimize the retinal image size difference between the eyes in a unilateral correction and allow a less distorted peripheral vision for unilateral and bilateral aphakia. In aphakia the refractive error needs to be corrected immediately, and patching treatment started. Studies at the Hospital for Sick Children in Toronto have shown that remarkable improvements in visual function can be achieved with a promptly initiated, vigorous patching regime (Lewis, Maurer and Brent, 1995).

In cases of amblyopia resulting from esotropia, anisometropia and hyperopia the full cycloplegic refraction is prescribed for children under 6 years, and the maximum tolerated prescription is given for older children. A spectacle correction worn for 2–3 months often in itself causes considerable improvement in both anisometropic and bilateral amblyopia.

After determining the improvement resulting from spectacle correction, patching treatment may be required. Patching the better eye forces the child to use the poorer eye. Each eye care practitioner may have a preferred patching regime and the following is simply a guideline for those who require more information. Part-time patching is often preferred by the child, parent and teacher over full-time patching. Indeed, full-time occlusion is definitely contra-indicated in cases where there is binocular vision, i.e. in intermittent strabismus or anisometropic amblyopia. The patching might be for half a day, or for periods of 1–2 hours throughout the day. The amount of time per day when the child wears a patch should reflect the degree of amblyopia. Moderate to severe amblyopia needs half-time occlusion.

Some children do not comply with patching. Parents often report that the child will pull the patch off soon after each treatment session has started. In the very young child techniques such as attaching splints to the child's arms have been used to ensure that the child will be unable to remove the patch for a specific time period each day. We would advise less controversial patching techniques: the child may hurt himself or herself if the practitioner is not trained in this technique which may, in turn, lead to a suit for malpractice. Other methods of treatment are available. One method for babies is to patch his or her eye before the baby wakes. An alternative is to degrade the image to the good eye to a point at which the child prefers to use the amblyopic eye; this is often called penalization and there are several ways it can be achieved. Pharmaceutical penalization, using cyclo-plegic agents, is one method, although each optometrist needs to examine the legality of this procedure in the jurisdiction where she or he practices. Atropine drops or ointment (0.5% or 1%) are given to the better eye, which is then unable to accommodate for near viewing, forcing the amblyopic eye to be used for near work.

Alternative methods that avoid the use of pharmaceutical agents and their possible harmful side-effects are the use of a diffusing filter over the spectacle lens of the dominant eye, or the provision of a spherical lens to promote the use of the amblyopic eye for close work; for this optical penalization, the amblyopic eye is given an add sufficient to cause the child to use it for close work. The power of the lens or the density of the diffusing filter is established such that the good eye becomes inferior to the amblyopic eye at the distance at which the child will be performing vision tasks. For any type of patching or penalization therapy, close monitoring of the visual acuity in each eye is required, because over-treatment can lead to amblyopia of the better eye. The eye care practitioner should ask parents to watch out for a switch in fixation preference from the previous 'good eye' to the previous 'poor eye' when both eyes are open. For this reason regular follow-up appointments are necessary to monitor progress. Again, each eye care practitioner will have their preferred schedule, but we would recommend appointments every 3 months for children under 3 years of age and every 6 months for older children.

The desired endpoint of amblyopia treatment in the case of strabismus is free spontaneous alternation of fixation, although one eye may still be used more frequently, and/or linear Snellen acuity that differs no more than one line.

Patching treatment is also being found to be successful in toddlers and young children with regressed tumour scars after treatment for retinoblastoma, when the visual acuity in one eye is poorer than in the other eye. Visual acuity of the poorer eye improves, demonstrating that visual loss occurred as a result of deprivation in a still developing eye, as well as from the localized retinal damage (Geer, unpublished data).

Sometimes children are unresponsive to treatment, especially if they are over 5 years old when treatment is initiated. The refractive error should be rechecked. Also, the optic nerve should be investigated. If neither of these investigations can account for the visual acuity deficit then it might be decided that the child has intractable amblyopia. In such cases, and in any case where there is significantly reduced acuity in one eye compared with the other, safety glasses should be considered regardless of whether there is any significant refractive error. We suggest that safety glasses should be considered in the following scenarios:

1. Acuity in the poorer eye is less than the driving standard (6/12 in Canada). In the case of accidental loss of vision to the better eye, the child would be barred from driving when he or she became an adult and this can be a serious social and economic handicap (see Shute and Woodhouse, 1990, for a discussion of visual problems and ability to drive).
2. The poorer eye has acuity such that it would be classed as having low vision. This is commonly taken to be 6/18 or worse. In this case the loss of the good eye would result in the child requiring low vision aids. The implications of vision loss are greater in this case than above.
3. A three-line difference of Snellen acuity exists, in the case of a child who already has reduced acuity in both eyes. If vision is lost in the better eye, there will be a significant loss of visual functioning (factor of $2\times$) between the two eyes.

These guidelines for safety glasses apply to any child who is at the walking stage or beyond. Of course, this does not negate the need to recommend safety glasses for any child with normal acuity in both eyes who is engaged in activities where there is significant risk, such as in the case of ball sports such as tennis, squash or cricket.

Amblyopia treatment should always be attempted and it usually does result in an improvement in visual acuity. There may be some improvement even in the teenage years. The child should be kept as visually active as possible during periods of patching. For example, hand eye co-ordination games are good, as are computer games which demand much concentration. In fact, allowing computer games during the times of patching is a good way to improve compliance; for example, the child is encouraged to play games to see how well the amblyopic eye can score.

Once treatment has been discontinued 50% of the children will show some degree of recurrence of their previous amblyopia. In these cases there should be some renewed patching treatment, for example 1–3 hours per day to maintain acuity (American Academy of Ophthalmology, 1994, p. 265).

Summary – prescribing glasses for children with strabismus

- Infantile esotropia. Hyperopic refractive errors need to be fully corrected as soon as possible. Consider prisms for residual deviation or bifocals for residual deviation at near.
- Accommodative esotropia. Full cycloplegic refractive error. Consider bifocals for residual deviation at near.
- Amblyopia resulting from esotropia, anisometropia and hyperopia. Prescribe the full cycloplegic refraction for children under 6 years, and the maximum tolerated prescription for older children.
- Exodeviations. Hyperopic refractive errors less than $+2.00$ D should NOT be corrected in children with exodeviations, but other refractive errors should be corrected. Undercorrect hyperopia greater than 2 D.
- Persisting amblyopia worse than the driving standard in the amblyopic eye or three lines difference between the eyes. Consider safety glasses.

READING DIFFICULTIES

Sometimes a parent will bring a child for a visual assessment because of difficulties in school, most commonly because of reading problems. In some cases, the child will have been formally assessed by a psychologist as having a reading disability or dyslexia. In other cases this possibility will have been suggested (for example, by a teacher), while in still other cases a parent may believe the child has such a reading problem whether or not other involved professionals agree with this. Sometimes a parent makes a specific request for some treatment which they have heard to be successful, such as the use of tinted lenses.

The area of learning difficulties is a complicated one and is controversial amongst those who specialize in the field (Prior, 1996). Definitions vary, but a reading disability is frequently assessed in relation to IQ: a child may be considered to have a reading disability if he or she is performing significantly below age norms despite adequate intellectual ability; assessment therefore requires specialized skills and must be done by an educational or clinical child psychologist. Although optometrists and ophthalmologists do not have the appropriate professional background to assess a reading disability, their expertise in the eyes and visual function may nevertheless play a useful role. It is possible that a refractive error (especially hyperopia or anisometropia), inadequate accommodation, convergence insufficiency or an oculomotor imbalance could contribute to reading difficulties. In these cases appropriate eye glasses and/or eye exercises should be of help, although if the child has fallen significantly behind at school additional tuition will be required also.

Thus the prime responsibility of the eye care practitioner is to provide a thorough eye examination. This should include a careful examination of binocular functioning (fusional reserves, fixation disparity, eye movements and aniseikonia if anisometropia is present) and accommodation (amplitude, lag with dynamic retinoscopy and accommodation facility) and the appropriate treatment of any anomalies. A report of visual functioning should also be provided for parents and teachers (and for the psychologist, if one is involved).

Some eye care practitioners provide alternative treatments for reading difficulties based on a number of published and unpublished studies. For example, there is evidence, albeit controversial, that some children with a reading disability (dyslexia) have poor vergence control and poor stereopsis and that six months of monocular occlusion for reading and close work may help to improve vergence control and reading (Stein and Fowler, 1985, discussed by Shute, 1991a).

Perhaps the best-known alternative treatment is the provision of tinted lenses, an intervention based on unpublished research by Irlen, an American psychologist, who coined the phrase 'scotopic sensitivity syndrome' for visually-based reading problems. A review of the evidence propounded by Irlen and others during the 1980s came to the conclusion that there is no evidence to support the existence of 'scotopic sensitivity syndrome' and that most of the research in the area was of very poor quality. Any improvements that were demonstrated, either in reading itself or relief of eyestrain symptoms, may be attributable to placebo effects and/or the reduction of glare coming from the page (Shute, 1991b). It was suggested that, since Irlen's own testing and prescription procedures were unvalidated, a simple and cheap alternative would be to try coloured overlays on the page. Some recent studies have shown that tinted lenses can result in fewer headaches and reduced eye strain in children selected on the basis of poor reading and/or eye-strain symptoms, perceptual distortions of reading or headaches (Wilkins et al., 1994). More information for vision care practitioners on selecting coloured overlays and suggestions on how to determine the colour that provides the most relief of symptoms is described by Wilkins (1994). Further consideration of this issue can be found in Evans et al. (1996) and Evans (1997).

Later in this chapter there is a discussion about how to deal with requests for therapies which you consider are not substantiated by the available research evidence.

ACCOMMODATION ANOMALIES

The dynamic retinoscopy technique for measuring accommodational response was described in Chapter 4. Children with Down syndrome and cerebral palsy often have reduced accommodational response to such an extent they may be seriously disadvantaged in their school work. (Children with low vision may also have reduced accommodation; this group is considered further below.) Children with multiple impairments are very likely also to have a high refractive error, either hyperopia or myopia with astigmatism. Other considerations are the amount and type of close work performed, the degree of individual supervision received, the child's cognitive potential and the level of visual functioning. With some severely challenged children, the level of their education is simple self-awareness or stimulation tasks, which may not require fine near acuity. In addition they may not be able to change their spectacles themselves. With some of these severely challenged children, a general purpose prescription (e.g. under-correction of myopia) may be a better practical solution than bifocals or single vision reading glasses.

Possible situations and courses of action are:

1. If reduced accommodation is detected in a child with hyperopia which is currently under- or un-corrected, the first step is to give a full correction for the hyperopia and review the child in a few months. If accommodation is still reduced at that time, consider a reading prescription.

2. If reduced accommodation is detected in a child with myopia, consider under-correcting the myopia enough to bring the accommodative response into the normal range. If a full distance prescription is recommended, let the child wear the prescription for a few months before re-measuring accommodation response and considering reading glasses. Our findings indicate that the accommodative response immediately after changing the distance prescription is influenced by that change, i.e. accommodation will be further reduced if increased minus lenses are placed before the eyes than are habitually worn.

3. If accommodation is clearly outside the normal range for the age, the addition can be determined by dynamic retinoscopy. Our current clinical experience indicates that the minimum addition to bring the neutral point within the normal range should be prescribed. If it is possible this addition can be provided for a trial period (by means of loaned glasses). With some children a subjective response to the addition can be determined as they look at print, a picture book with fine detail or even the dynamic retinoscope target. With other children a measurement of near acuity can be determined with and without the addition, in order to confirm the need for the addition and to demonstrate the need to parents/carers. The addition can be considered in either bifocal or single vision reader form. Factors which will determine this decision are as follows:

   i.   Whether the child can understand and use bifocals.
   ii. Head posture.
   iii. Null point of nystagmus or direction of better eye movement control.

    iv. The level of supervision of the child – will someone be present to change their glasses?

    v. The attention span of the child (single vision readers may improve attention span for near assignments, because it limits clear vision to the task in hand).

    The optometrist must also bear in mind that teachers are already required to cope with the many and varied requirements of special needs children, therefore one pair of glasses which can be used for all tasks may be better in practice than reading glasses which are not used.

4. Duckman (1984) suggests a training programme for improving accommodation in children with cerebral palsy. He instituted training with ± 2.00 D 'flippers'. These are trial lens spheres mounted such that the binocular minus lenses are held over the child's own spectacles and can be quickly exchanged for binocular plus lenses, and the child has to 'clear' their vision each time the lenses are flipped from minus to plus and vice versa. After training with this he found that accommodation was improved in 57% of children with CP. However, his measurements of accommodation both before and after the training were subjective in nature and no indication was given of how long this training remained effective.

CHILDREN WITH LOW VISION

Infants

Information about the condition and its prognosis
It is important to give the parents time to ask questions which may have come to mind during the examination. Many conditions affecting infants are congenital malformations and are stable: the parents need to know that the condition will not progress, but neither will there be great improvement. In the case that an eye condition may cause decreased acuity, we need to be able to convey this information honestly to parents in an empathetic manner (see section below on 'Breaking bad news').

Parents are most concerned about receiving a functional visual assessment and the potential for the child to be visual at school and to learn to read print (albeit with visual aids). The parents may have been told that their baby is 'blind' or 'legally blind'. An ophthalmologist may have said that there is no treatment and registered the child as legally blind and the parents' minds will be reeling with the implications. Most parents will ask, 'How much can my child see?' or 'How does my child see things?' if they are aware that the infant has some visual ability.

Giving the results of functional assessment
Giving information about functional vision is very valuable to the parents. This will normally include information about visual acuity,

binocular vision, ocular motility and tracking ability, visual fields and null point of nystagmus. Giving the information to parents that their baby can see certain sized targets at certain distances is extremely important, so that they can use appropriately sized toys, pictures and so on. A word of caution is required here regarding grating acuity and Snellen acuity. In low vision, acuity for gratings is better than for optotypes, particularly in foveal or macular disease and amblyopia. The difference can be significant and increases as acuity decreases. Mayer, Fulton and Rodier (1984) found that the median difference was a factor of $4\times$ for children with acuities 6/60 or poorer, although there is also a large amount of variability between children. We must keep this in mind when counselling parents, when acuity has been measured by preferential looking for gratings.

Basic information which can be used to help the child with everyday functioning should be given. Also, information regarding parent support groups and other supports which are available through national organizations should be given so that rehabilitation can start early.

Refractive correction

Infants with low vision frequently have medium to high refractive errors. Whether a correction is given depends on the relative refractive error compared with visual acuity. However, these children deserve a clear retinal image, in order to give optimum opportunity for the development of visual acuity. It must be remembered that VA is developing and that the visual system is still plastic, as with normally sighted children. We therefore favour a vigorous approach in correcting refractive errors. A full correction is preferable in most cases, as fear of interference with emmetropization is less of an issue here. Children with high refractive errors are less likely to show emmetropization, as are children with low VA (Haegerstrom-Portnoy et al., 1996). Indeed, it has been suggested that their high refractive errors are a result of poor VA (Nathan et al., 1985), the poor retinal image interrupting the feedback loop which is thought to control emmetropization. We can therefore simply concentrate on giving optimum visual acuity.

The expected impact on later schooling

Even when their child is still in infancy, parents will be wondering what the future holds. Is it expected that their child will be able to learn to read print, with or without low vision aids (LVAs)? If LVAs will be required, where are they available and what are they? Is the child likely to be dependent on Braille or other sight-substitution methods? These are all questions to be addressed at some point. However, it must be added that it is not always possible to predict in these early years and in certain eye conditions what future visual performance will be. For example, in the case of cortical visual impairment in a multiply-challenged child there can be dramatic improvements in visual function in the first few years. However, a knowledge of the diagnosis in many cases will enable the low vision clinician to make a good prediction of future visual function; for example, children with albinism perform well visually with the help of LVAs, while those with Leber's congenital amaurosis are likely to need very high levels of magnification, electronic devices for school work and/or sight-substitution.

Vision stimulation

Leguire et al. (1992) and Tavernier (1993) suggest that the normal visual environment contains a wealth of visual information to the normal visual system (contours of low, medium and high contrast, objects containing fine, medium and coarse detail), but only provides very low contrast, blurred information to the impaired visual system, which is thus not maximally stimulated. Thus the visual pathways and cortex may remain underdeveloped. Barraga, Collins and Hollis (1977) suggest, therefore, that visual development, which occurs spontaneously with normally-sighted individuals, requires purposeful stimulation for optimum development in infants with low vision. Vision stimulation is the purposeful provision of high contrast, bright stimuli to encourage a visual response in children with low vision and then to train the utilization of existing visual and visual-motor abilities.

Barraga was one of the first to suggest visual stimulation in 1964 (Barraga, 1964), but little concrete proof has existed until recently as to its efficacy. Leguire et al. (1992) have described one of the few studies which provide objective evidence that visual stimulation is effective. They implemented a vision stimulation programme that involved a series of square wave gratings selected for different spatial frequency and orientation according to the channel theory of vision. Checkerboards at different orientations and faces were also included to maintain interest. All stimuli were high contrast and high luminance and were presented twice a day every day for a year. The aetiology of visual impairment ranged from cortical visual impairment, optic nerve hypoplasia, congential nystagmus, monocular cataract, optic atrophy and optic nerve coloboma. The latency of the pattern and flash VEPs decreased after one year, indicating a general improvement in visual function in the group receiving vision stimulation, while a similar control group who received no vision stimulation showed no change of VEP. These are some of the first objective data indicating that vision stimulation works. Furthermore, Groenendaal and van Hof-van Duin (1992) found improvements in several measures of visual function in children with severe perinatal hypoxia. Some had neurological defects and others had mental and physical impairments. Over a period of three years, improvements in visual function were found in some children even up to the age of 16 years. They suggest that the sensitive period may be delayed for children with brain damage due to hypoxia.

These findings indicate that vision stimulation should be attempted for children with multiple impairments due to neurological damage, not just in infancy, but even up to the age of 16 years. Those who may benefit most are those with cortical visual impairment. These children, who often have profound multiple impairments, display a different pattern from those with low vision due to an ocular disorder: they frequently have variable visual function, short visual attention span, compulsive light gazing and peripheral field loss, while the ocular examination, external appearance of the eyes and ocular motility are normal (Jan and Groenveld, 1993).

Barraga and Collins (1979) described the normal development of visual skills in 8 stages. These include such abilities as response to light, tracking, fixation, recognition, identification and discrimination of shapes, parts of shapes, faces, recognition of picture representations, copying and drawing, figure-ground differentiation, visual closure and identifying letters and words. Such visual skills (apart from reading) develop naturally and without formal teaching in children with normal visual and neuromotor systems in a reasonably supportive environment (Rosner and Rosner, 1990). Barraga and Collins suggest that it proceeds in the same order for both those with normal sight and those with visual impairments, but that the latter may get confined to the lower stages or not be able to complete some stages. Overbury et al. (1989) agree that there is a hierarchy of visual skills; performance at their two most complex categories, figure-ground and reading tasks were inter-correlated, and were more severely affected by adventitious vision loss in adults than the simpler tasks such as matching and copying.

We use ideas from the lower levels of Barraga's scale and these are outlined below. A printed sheet with ideas is given to parents/carers. Vision stimulation can be suggested for children with low vision from any cause, but we use it most frequently with children with multiple disabilities and low vision. It can be recommended even with children who have very minimal visual reponses. In some children with a history of seizures, an epileptic attack may be precipitated by flashing or bright lights, in which case those stimuli should be omitted (parents are usually aware if this is the case).

Below is a shortened version of the information given to parents/carers when vision stimulation is recommended.

1. Gaining visual attention using high contrast patterns and lights.
   Examples are Christmas tree lights in a darkened room, flashing lights, penlights with interchangeable filters or plastic translucent toys, metallic wrapping paper reflecting light from a flashlight (torch), high contrast stripes, circles, squares or simple faces, computer screen-savers, projected photographic slides, phosphorescent or fluorescent painted objects (e.g. a glove or sock with a painted face, mobiles with objects painted with phosphorescent or fluorescent paint (use a fan or hairdryer to move the objects), tinsel coated with phosphorescent paint, patterns with fluorescent felt tip pens (textas), an old umbrella (preferably dark) with phosphorescent glow stars attached or painted with phosphorescent or fluorescent shapes (twirl the umbrella to get a visual effect).

2. Tracking a moving light.
   Using the high contrast, high luminance objects listed above, teach

tracking by moving in all directions. Teach tracking with eye and head movements, then with only eye movements. Teach tracking with hand contact on the object. Move along the horizontal first, then in oblique and vertical directions. Finally, use circular motions. Teach following the target towards and away from the child. How far away can they follow it as it moves away? Use lights and then high contrast three-dimensional objects.

3. Reaching for a target.
   Encourage the child to reach towards the stimulus and touch it. Then teach him/her to reach and pick something up. Do this holding the object in different areas of the visual field (remember that there may be blind spots in some areas) or on a table covered by a plain cloth which contrasts with the target.

4. Giving meaning to visual experience, linking visual experience with tactile and auditory experience.
   Use brightly coloured, large objects such as toys, drinking mug, ball, fork etc. which would be used by the child day to day. Encourage the child to take the flashlight, shine it on things near by (still in the dark room), and turn it on and off. Let the child turn the room lights on and off. Use tactile stripes, i.e. with different texture for the black and the white areas. Encourage recognition of objects.

All these steps should be performed with high contrast/high luminance objects first, but as the child reponds, the contrast and luminance can be reduced, while maintaining a response.

Glare control

If an eye condition exists which is known to cause difficulty with glare, appropropriate tints should be prescribed, with or without an incorporated spectacle prescription, if necessary. Tints are prescribed subjectively in adults with low vision, that is, we simply demonstrate different selective transmission tints in sunlight, or indoors if glare is experienced there also. In the Centre for Sight Enhancement at the University of Waterloo, we stock some of the NoIR tints, the Corning CPF tints, Younger PLS tints or ordinary brown or grey spectacle tints. In adults with a variety of eye disorders, those with anterior eye disorders benefit from one of the CPF tints, as demonstrated by improved low contrast acuity (Leat, North and Bryson, 1990). However, those with retinal disorders often express subjective benefit from similar tints. Therefore, at present, there is no better method (for adults) than the person choosing which tint gives optimum comfort and contrast enhancement. With infants, tints can be tried objectively, and comfort is judged by how much the child opens the palpebral aperture rather than screwing up his or her eyes. The PLS and CPF lenses both significantly change the colour rendering of the visual scene (being dark red and reddish-brown tints), and therefore are used only if a definite advantage is gained from the selective transmission of the tint. Otherwise, if found to be equally effective in controlling light sensitivity, a grey or brown generic ophthalmic tint with a UV filter is used. The Corning lenses have the advantage of being photochromic (but are glass) while the Younger tints are plastic, but not photochromic. For a child with photophobia both indoors and outdoors, the new Transitions+ plastic photochromic lens is an option.

Some examples of tints for specific conditions are given below.

- Children with albinism have normal colour vision and therefore a lens which significantly alters the colour rendering is not indicated. They will require tints for outdoors and will benefit from a dark grey or brown spectacle tint with a UV filter (85% absorption). They may also benefit from lighter tints for indoors, therefore the Transitions+ is an option in these cases.
- Infants with achromatopsia will usually benefit from CPF or PLS tints, seen by the fact that they will then open their eye and lift up their heads when out of doors (in fact, this can be almost diagnostic for the condition if nystagmus, reduced acuity and photophobia are present). In achromatopsia, the lighter CPF or PLS tints should also be considered for indoor use and the darker CPF or PLS 550 for outdoors, They will also benefit from darkly tinted sideshields, especially for outdoor use. The optimum tint will depend on whether the achromatopsia is complete or incomplete: if complete, use red tints; if incomplete, use reddish-brown lenses.
- In case of cone dystrophies, the optimum tint will depend on the residual colour vision. If there is no colour vision, use red tints; if poor colour vision, use reddish-brown tints; if fairly good colour vision, use dark brown tints.

Some practitioners seem to be reluctant to prescribe such tints for young children, but we feel that this fear is unjustified. Normally-sighted adults wear sunglasses in the sun, yet let their children go without, despite obvious discomfort shown by screwing up their eyes. A child requires protection from UV light as much as (or more than) an adult. A child with a glare-producing eye disorder has even more need of tints and some children, such as those with albinism, have more need for protective UV filters.

Toddlers and preschoolers

Much which can be accomplished in infants is also applicable to this age group, particularly if the child is first seen as a toddler. The questions that parents are asking will be very similar. In addition, as the child grows older, more information and more accurate information can be gathered regarding functional vision. For example, visual fields can be measured more accurately and contrast sensitivity evaluated. This is true even of children with multiple impairments, who may not be able to respond to tests with greater accuracy as they get older. However, additional measures of visual functions help to confirm or disconfirm previous measures, which may have been difficult to estimate on previous occasions.

Vision stimulation can still be recommended at this age for those with multiple disabilities or low vision. After this, as the child grows older, and if there is some mastery of the types of tasks above, visual perceptual skills can be taught. This would be classified as visual training, rather than vision stimulation and involves more complex tasks such as sorting, matching and organizing tasks involving three-dimensional objects and two-dimensional shapes or line drawings, tracing of line drawings, recognition of objects and parts of objects, recognition of line drawings, matching of shapes or letters, copying a picture or pattern and figure-ground exercises. These are similar to the tasks suggested for normally-sighted children with visual perceptual problems and can be undertaken as part of a child's educational programme. Indeed, although such activities may already be in use as a part of the child's programme (as is common amongst neurologically impaired children), the vision care practitioner can give some printed suggestions to the parents. Rosner and Rosner (1990) give a more detailed description of tasks designed for children with visual perceptual skills deficits, which are very similar to the exercises suggested by Barraga (1970) specifically for visually-impaired children. The Rosners' tasks must be modified for children with visual impairment by assuring that the detail within the tasks is within the child's acuity limit (hence the need for giving parents clear information regarding acuity). Young children with visual impairment may perform some of the tasks with three-dimensional 'real' objects tactually, rather than visually. This may help them to understand the concepts of 'same' or 'different', but in order to train vision, tasks which can only be undertaken visually should be included and emphasized. Suffice it to say that many of the more complex tasks are similar to the drawing/word/puzzle-book games with which normally-sighted children grow up. Some of these tasks and games need to be intentionally taught to children with low vision and/or neurological deficits. Project IVEY (1983) also describes a formalized programme for children with visual impairments.

Orientation and mobility (O & M)

Within the context of low vision, orientation refers to the ability to use remaining vision and/or other senses to determine one's position within the environment. Mobility refers to the ability to use one's remaining vision and other senses to navigate from one position to another within the environment. O & M training refers to the teaching of safe, successful and efficient travel strategies which compensate for the loss of vision.

Early intervention with O & M training is advantageous. As discussed in Chapter 1, blind children lack an understanding of their own bodies and their reduced visual awareness of the environment decreases the incentive to move and explore, resulting in poorly developed posture and motor abilities. These skills must be deliberately fostered. The skills necessary for acquisition of spatial concepts should be taught through movement programmes early in life. Special physiotherapy programmes can be invaluable as soon as the child begins to crawl.

The young child can be taught simple O & M, such as orientating towards a window or other light source. Cane (or a simpler technique, precane) can also be taught as a method of protection of the lower body for the ambulatory preschooler with severe visual impairment. The long cane is the traditional long white one used by a person with visual impairment to tap the ground in front of them as they walk, thus checking for obstacles, steps, etc. The precane is a roughly rectangular tubular structure, sometimes with wheels, used by young severely visually impaired toddlers to give them confidence when beginning to walk. Young children are able to learn both these techniques (Clarke, Sainato and Ward, 1994), although there is some debate over whether the child should learn the long cane technique in preparation for the rest of life, or precane, which is easier and possibly more effective in younger years. O & M should also be considered for children who have other disabilities in addition to low vision.

Low vision aids (LVAs)

Simple LVAs such as stand magnifiers can be introduced at the developmental age of 2–3 years and may actually help a visually impaired child to use his or her unaided vision more efficiently (Ritchie, Sonksen and Gould, 1989), as well as accustoming the child to aids and allowing the viewing of detail otherwise denied them. They would not be used for reading at this stage, but rather for viewing small objects of interest such as insects and postage stamps, which otherwise would remain a blob despite the child using a very close working distance. A slightly older developmental level would be required for the use of distance aids such as telescopes, but these may also be introduced to some children before school. Binoculars with a wide field of view are probably easier to handle at this age than a monocular, even if the child does not have binocular vision.

School age children

As the child starts to learn to read, all the types of low vision aid which are available for adults can be used. The most commonly-used optical LVAs are bifocal additions, stand magnifiers (including dome magnifiers), spectacle microscopes, hand-held monocular telescopes and bioptic telescopes for board work and tints for glare control. Closed circuit televisions (CCTVs) are also commonly used in schools along with adapted computers (which, by means of software or hardware, enlarge the print on the screen) and other electronic aids. The only major difference in low vision aid assessment and provision between children and adults is the presence of accommodation in children. A full explanation of low vision aid assessment and rehabilitation as it refers to children is outside the scope of this text. The interested reader is referred to Faye (1984), amongst other text books on low vision.

Participation in appropriate sports should be encouraged to enhance physical development and strength and self-esteem. Some ideas in this area were presented in Chapter 2.

Children should be seen at least yearly, particularly as they go through the primary grades, until they are in secondary schooling around the age of 12 years. This is because, as they progress through the grades, the print size which they are required to read gets smaller, the volume of school work gets larger and their amplitude of accommodation decreases. It is quite usual for children to accept an increase to their reading addition yearly (Sloan and Habel 1973). Below, we provide a section on how to determine the reading addition in children, since we are not aware of any step-by-step methodologies described elsewhere (but see Bailey, 1980) for the optics of combining reading adds with active accommodation).

Prescribing near additions in children with low vision and with active accommodation

The only major difference in low vision aid assessment and provision between children and adults is the presence of accommodation in children (apart from children with aphakia). A child will obtain magnification by bringing the print close and using accommodation. A different approach to prescribing reading additions is therefore indicated. Despite having a large amplitude of accommodation, children may still experience accommodation stress from reading for extended periods at a close distance. A reading addition is indicated if the child is experiencing asthenopic symptoms or short attention span for reading, or if the child cannot read print small enough for their requirements. A target print for the child must be identified and will largely depend on the reading material used at the child's grade level (Table 14.1). For fluency in reading a reserve of acuity must be allowed (Whittaker and Lovie-Kitchin, 1993) and we recommend at least a reserve of $2\times$ for a child. Therefore, if most of the print is 2M (16N) aim for 1M at least. Children may need supplementary magnifiers for particular tasks such as map work in which the print is especially small and low contrast. The dome (paperweight) magnifiers work well as supplementary magnifiers which can be used at a close working distance in conjunction with a reading addition. See below for a description of how to prescribe bifocals for children.

Table 14.1 Print sizes at different grades and recommended target print size

Grade	Typical print size	Print size requirement
Kindergarten, grade 1		N12–N16 (1.5–2M)
Grades 2 and 3	N20 (2.5M)	N10 (1.25M)
Grades 3–6	N13 (1.6M)	N6 0.8M)

The following is a series of steps which can be followed to estimate the required reading addition for a child:

1. Measure the word reading or near acuity at the habitual reading distance (which may be as close as 10 cm). Charts with sentences or words are preferable to those with single letters (reduced Snellen charts). The ideal chart would be one with a logarithmic scale, large words, and in M print or N notation. It is also useful to have one which uses the simpler type face to which children are accustomed. The Lighthouse now produce a suitable low vision reading chart for children. If the child is not yet reading, then use letters or symbols (such as the LH symbols or near Ffooks symbols). The near acuity is recorded as the N or M print and the distance at which it was read.

2. Estimate the expected accommodation for the child's age. Assume that the child can use 1/2 of this amplitude for extended tasks; this is the available accommodation (Millodot and Millodot, 1989). This is the available accommodation used in the calculation below.

3. Calculate the estimated reading addition. As a starting point use the difference between this available accommodation (in dioptres, D) and their dioptric reading distance as an addition:

$$\text{reading add (D)} = \text{dioptric reading distance} - \text{available accommodation}$$

4. Remeasure near acuity with calculated add. Notice if the child brings the reading material closer or if she or he is able to read smaller type or to read more fluently. If the child does not bring the print closer it indicates either that accommodation has been relaxed by the amount of the add or that the child was not accommodating sufficiently beforehand and that therefore his or her accommodation was under stress. With older children ask if the print appears clearer. If the child is able to read sufficiently small print for age-related tasks (the target print), allowing for the reserve of acuity, prescribe this add. If the child does bring the print closer, a lower add may be indicated.

5. If the target print size is not obtained, it may be necessary to increase the add (by at least 1.25 × steps) and to ask him/her to hold the print closer. Estimate the magnification required (ratio of print obtained, with original add, to target print). Calculate the increased add by:

$$\text{new add (D)} = \text{estimated magnification} \times \text{original add (D)}$$

6. Measure near acuity with new add.

Do not be surprised if the final result indicates that the child is using less than half of the theoretical accommodation for his or her age. Children with low vision frequently seem to have reduced available accommodation. This is most likely due to decreased accommodation accuracy because of a blurred retinal image. The blurred image results in poorer stimulus for accurate accommodation as seen in nystagmus (Ciuffreda, 1991), amblyopic eyes (Hokada and Ciuffreda, 1982) and in people with normal vision whose vision is deliberately degraded (Ciuffreda, 1991). In these conditions there may be one or more of the following: fewer higher spatial components of the perceived image (image blur), increased retinal eccentricity, increased retinal image motion, or decreased contrast. All of these have been shown to have a deleterious effect on the accuracy of accommodation (Ciuffreda, 1991).

The alternative to reading additions is stand magnifiers. Children do well with these. A stand magnifier should be chosen which has a transverse magnification equal to estimated magnification and with a high emergent vergence. Children with accommodation require stand magnifiers with a considerable emergent vergence as they will exert proximal accommodation and will naturally hold magnifiers close to the eye.

These steps are a guide to determining the reading addition that would be prescribed. There is then the question of the form that this lens should take. Most frequently bifocals are used; children adapt to them more easily than do adults. Usually a straight top bifocal is recommended, but in the higher additions a round segment becomes necessary due to the availability of lenses. The bifocals are often set a little higher (1 mm above the lower lid line or bisecting the distance between the lower lid and the lower pupil margin) than in an adult, to ensure that the child uses the segment. Generally, multifocals are not used, since these reduce the reading area for the child and are not available in the higher adds that are frequently prescribed for children. Occasionally, separate reading glasses are recommended. This is usually in cases of nystagmus in which the null point is above, or far to one side of the primary position. In these cases acuity would be reduced if the child was forced to depress the eyes to view through a bifocal segment.

DECISIONS – INVOLVING CHILD AND PARENTS

We established in Chapter 3 the importance of involving both parents and child fully in the consultation, with the vision care practitioner acting as an expert consultant who is seeking to be sensitive to the belief system of the family. This is important not just for the sake of taking an effective history, but also for making decisions about what action is needed in the light of the visual assessment. We discussed the importance of parental involvement in any necessary rehabilitation programmes, and the fact that children are also more likely to follow advice if they have been fully involved in discussions. It is important, then, to avoid the tendency found in paediatric consultations to share information and discuss treatment plans with parents rather than the child (Pantell et al., 1982).

The giving of information and advice will probably occur at various points in the consultation, but it is at the end, following the examination, when this is particularly relevant. The optometrist will have information to get across to the family about the child's vision or perhaps general health. It will be necessary to try to account for any reported symptoms, and there may be certain instructions to follow: when to wear glasses, how to look after contact lenses, how to use a low vision aid, how best to present educational materials to a child with a visual impairment, that referral to a general practitioner or ophthalmologist is needed, and so on.

Promoting understanding

There is a great deal of evidence that even adults frequently fail to understand medical information. One reason is that clinicians often present information in too difficult a form. The second is that people bring in their own beliefs, and interpret what the practitioner says in the light of their own existing framework of understanding. Even simple, everyday words can be ambiguous in a medical context. Other problems can arise when the practitioner uses technical terms, such as 'dilated', 'fixate', 'meridian', 'periphery' and 'astigmatism' (Shute, 1991a).

Many misunderstandings could be cleared up if people asked questions, but there is plenty of evidence that they do not often do so (e.g. Klein, 1979). Establishing good rapport and using good communication skills (Chapter 3) will help to overcome such reluctance. Plenty of opportunity should be given for parents to ask questions in a supportive atmosphere, so that they do not feel foolish because of their ignorance. It is useful to have some simple explanations of various points ready, such as the description we gave earlier in the book of the astigmatic eye as being shaped more like a rugby ball than a soccer ball.

Helping parents to remember information

Even if people understand information, they may forget it once they leave your consulting rooms. There are a number of factors which influence remembering (Ley, 1988).

- The more information people are given, the more they are likely to forget, so it is important not to overload them with unnecessary information.
- People recall best what they consider to be the most important points, so clarify what those are.
- People remember best what they are told first, so give the most important information first.
- People remember best information which is repeated.
- Remembering is helped by categorizing the information under headings – for example, saying, 'I am going to tell you what the problem is, what treatment I suggest and what outcome I expect.'
- Remembering is reinforced by giving written information to take home.

Helping parents and older children to adhere to advice

Non-compliance with practitioner instructions and advice is a problem in health care professions. However, The word 'adherence' tends to be used more these days because it has a less judgemental quality. If you find that a person is not adhering to advice, there will be good reasons for that, such as those listed below:

- A friendly atmosphere was not established.
- The advice was irrelevant to the person's perceived problem.
- Perceived benefits of the action were outweighed by barriers.
- The advice was given in language the person did not understand.
- The information-giving was poorly structured.
- The person had to wait a long time to be seen.

So, looked at like this, adherence is not so much a matter of simply expecting or hoping that people will follow instructions, but it is something that the practitioner has a fair degree of control over through using good communication skills.

One example of non-adherence is that teenagers may refuse to use prescribed visual aids such as magnifiers and telescopes. This is often because they become self-conscious at this age about the appearance of such aids. Since developing a positive self-image and acceptance by peers are important developmental tasks for young people, their concerns are not to be dismissed lightly. Older children and teenagers are often more concerned with the social aspects of health issues than anything else, so they may refuse to use their aids regardless of the resultant problems in seeing. The low vision adviser must therefore be aware of the cosmetic implications of aids and discuss them with young clients (Faye et al., 1984). Alternatives such as CCTV and the use of taped notes may have to be used until the young person feels ready to use other methods again. A young person who refuses to use a low vision aid at school can still be encouraged to use it at home. This example illustrates the advantage of open discussion and flexibility to meet individuals' needs.

Breaking bad news

One possible outcome of visual assessment is that bad news will have to be broken, perhaps confirming that a child is visually impaired, or that a pre-existing condition is worsening. Alternatively, what seems to you to be a relatively mild problem may be taken very badly by the parents or child; this may relate to particular concerns they have, or it may be a 'last straw' phenomenon to a family already under stress. You will have gathered information during history-taking about what the family already knows, suspects or fears, so that your explanation can be couched within their framework (Davis, 1993). Information about the child's visual problem and its cause should be followed by information about the likely outcome and any therapies or other interventions that can be brought into play. It is never the case that nothing can be done – if 'cure' is not possible, then 'coping' should be emphasized.

Despite your best efforts, parents may not take bad news easily. There may initially be disbelief, often tinged with anger, fear and frustration. You should be prepared for the parent to argue with you, to dismiss your findings, and to want to shop around various professionals seeking a more acceptable diagnosis. Do not be offended by this, feeling that your professionalism has been insulted, but understand that such reactions are natural; acknowledge their desire to seek a second opinion, and leave the door open for them to come back at a later stage (Karnes and Teskla, 1980).

Davis (1993) has made some specific suggestions for dealing with an emotionally-charged bad news situation, as follows:

1. Be attentive to the person's behaviour to gauge their mood.
2. Respond appropriately. Match your mood with theirs. Do not rush.
3. Determine existing knowledge and beliefs.
4. Provide information accurately, simply, in line with the individual's beliefs. Give a balanced picture, neither falsely reassuring nor unduly negative.
5. Pause and allow reaction, whether anger, weeping or denial without criticism.
6. Check out feelings.
7. Comfort if necessary – it may be appropriate to touch the person.
8. Invite and/or answer questions honestly, admitting any uncertainty.
9. Be honest about own feelings. If you express real sadness, for example, people will value this and see you as a genuine and caring person.
10. Give warning of impending end of session.
11. Summarize information and check understanding.
12. Agree on general plan. For example, you may want to make a follow-up appointment. A person may be in a better position to ask questions and take in information once they've had time to digest the news.
13. Negotiate immediate action. Does the person want to wait in another room for a while, have a cup of tea, call up a relative?
14. Check out your own feelings. Do you need to talk to a colleague or take some time out? You may have to postpone this if you have another appointment immediately, but do not neglect your own needs. If you work in a high-stress practice, burnout is a possibility.
15. Liaise with other professionals about the case as necessary.

Parental requests for unsubstantiated therapies

Another difficult, yet common, situation, is one in which parents have brought along a child requesting some specific visual 'therapy' which they may have heard about through friends or the media, generally with the aim of solving their child's reading difficulties. Given that learning to read is a developmental task of central importance in childhood, and on which many future tasks, such as forging a career, depend, it is understandable that failure to learn to read causes great distress and some parents will be attracted to seemingly quick and simple (though often expensive) solutions. As discussed earlier, the evidence for such therapies is often slim or non-existent, and given the present state of knowledge the recommended role for the optometrist is to offer routine optometric services to correct any visual difficulties and to liaise with the child's school and any other relevant professionals such as the educational psychologist and special educator.

Miles (1988) has discussed how to deal with the situation where a parent insists on a therapy which the practitioner believes to be ineffective. First, review with the family the evidence for the proposed therapy – this means keeping up with developments and applying a sceptical scientific eye to reports of wonder therapies. Could results be easily explained by placebo effects or by conventional visual explanations? Convey your understanding of the situation to the family, being open about doubts but not totally discouraging. If the parent still insists on the therapy in question, convey the potential costs, including wasted time and money and disappointment. At this point you may decline to offer the therapy if you judge that more harm than good is likely to come from it. Alternative therapies could also be suggested, such as using coloured transparent overlays on the page for reading rather than buying expensive tinted lenses.

CO-OPERATION WITH OTHER PROFESSIONALS

It is frequently the case that a range of professionals other than optometrists will be involved with the child in various ways, e.g. general medical practitioners, orthoptists, ophthalmologists and teachers. In some cases, a true team-care approach is used, as described in the case of the Tomteboda Resource Centre for Visually Handicapped Children in Sweden, described by Lindstedt (1986). There, the optometrist works alongside an ophthalmologist, psychologist, special teacher and human factors engineer. The child's visual assessment is an integrated part of the total developmental assessment of the child, and helps in the formulation of a rehabilitation programme. Courses for parents are also offered at the Centre, which concentrates especially on the youngest children, in view of what is known about early visual development and the role of vision in early general development (Chapters 1 and 2). Multidisciplinary teamwork for the management of childhood visual impairment has also been discussed by Youngson-Reilly, Tobin and Fielder (1995).

It is, however, relatively unusual for an optometrist to work in this way as part of a team. It is more likely that a child will be referred, perhaps by the general medical practitioner, or as a result of a visual problem being detected during routine screening at school. It is important to ensure that relevant information reaches any other professionals who may be working with the child (see below). If the child has a visual impairment, then building collaborative relationships with other professionals, as well as with parents, is particularly important (Hill, 1987). As children reach school age, educational concerns come to the fore, and optometric input is useful in decision-making about whether braille, vision or a mixture of methods should be used, and in the provision of aids to maximize the visual capability that the child has. If a child is provided with a low vision aid but the teachers are not told about its use, and there is no follow-up, it is likely to remain unused.

There may be occasions, also, when information from other professionals will be valuable in terms of assessing a child, especially if that child has disabilities. A speech therapist's report, for instance, can aid in communicating with a child (in fact, the authors have sometimes assessed children with severe communication difficulties with the direct assistance of a speech therapist).

PROVIDING WRITTEN INFORMATION TO PARENTS AND OTHER PROFESSIONALS

It is important that information about the child's vision is disseminated to many people who would like, and indeed need, information, such as the doctor, the parent and the school. In some optometric situations this is an unfunded service. In addition, confidentiality must be respected. In the case of simple reports to parents, school, vision resource teachers etc, we have found it effective to allow a parent or carer to be responsible for information dissemination. Alternatively, a report can be written to one person and photocopies sent to the others, with the consent of parents. In most cases one letter addressed to the parents for the first visit is sufficient and provides the required information, with subsequent letters if the recommendations change. An additional method for report writing is to use a standard form with appropriate boxes for the requisite information (see Appendix). Somewhat different forms can be used for normally sighted children and those with visual impairment or other disabilities. In the case of a report to the child's GP, referring doctor or when a new referral is being made, the letter should be addressed directly to the doctor concerned and is considered part of the examination of the child, i.e. no fee should be charged. In this case, this letter could be copied to other professionals concerned (with the consent of the parents) and to the parents themselves.

Report-writing is particularly important in cases of children with low vision or multiple disabilities as the size of print which they can read both with and without their low vision aids, the need for high contrast, the optimum lighting and the best position for visual material are all vital pieces of information needed for the child's schooling. Frequently, this is the main reason for the child's being brought to the optometrist.

The following is a list of information that can be important to include in reports to parents or to be sent to the school.

1. Diagnosis and prognosis of any ocular pathology. Is the condition stable or non-stable? If eye pathology is not present, mention that the eyes are healthy.
2. Visual acuity (e.g. 6/30) and which test was used (e.g. preferential looking). Describe acuity in lay terms also (see below).
3. Is this acuity as expected for the child's age, i.e. within the normal limits or not?
4. Near reading acuity, the distance at which it was read, and the type of task, i.e. single or crowded, letters, symbols, or continuous text.
5. Visual fields and implications.
6. Contrast sensitivity and implications.
7. Colour vision.
8. Advice re. lighting, use of high contrast, types of writing utensil, reading stands etc.
9. What glasses/LVAs have been prescribed and when they should be used.
10. Advice re. nystagmus null point.
11. When is patching to be undertaken, of which eye and for how long.
12. What other assessments or referrals are recommended, e.g. referral to ophthalmologist, genetic counsellor, family doctor, augmentative communication assessment.
13. What other supports should be in place, e.g. vision resource teacher, orientation and mobility training.
14. Suggestions regarding programming, e.g. vision stimulation programme.
15. When the child will be seen again for follow-up.

An example of a form adapted from one used at the Centre for Sight Enhancement, Waterloo, is shown in Appendix 14.1. It includes an explanation of visual acuity and a table of type face equivalents. A copy of the report is kept in the child's file.

It is important to give information in understandable terms for lay persons. We suggest that, for children with low acuity, the actual clinical measurement is given and then an explanation, for example, 6/36 means that the child requires objects 6× larger or closer than an adult with normal vision. Parents almost always want to know this information, but what has more practical application is the print size that the child is able to see and at what distance or (if grating preferential looking has been used) the width of lines that were detected. A photocopy of the print size given to the parents can be helpful, but be aware that some photocopiers slightly reduce the print size when supposedly copying 1 to 1. Although the actual near acuity can be given it is also important to stress that for educational purposes and daily tasks, it is important for the visual detail to be larger than the acuity limit. This is to allow for a 'reserve of acuity'. For any person, reading at the acuity limit will be slow. Whittaker and Lovie-Kitchin (1993) suggest an acuity reserve of a factor of 3 for reading at normal speeds of 160 words per minute or more, that is, the print size used for education must be 3× the acuity limit for continuous text. Therefore, we recommend that the line thicknesses used for a child should be at least three times the acuity limit (see sample form).

A colour vision defect can be expected in 8% of normally-sighted boys and is likely in 75% of children with low vision (Kalloniatis and Johnston, 1990). When a colour defect is known to be present, advice is required regarding colour-coded information at school and with respect to career opportunities. In the case of a congenital colour defect (and normal visual acuity), very specific information can be given regarding which colours are likely to be confused (Chapter 11). In low vision, the colour defect may follow less easily defined patterns. There may be a classical colour defect or a more generalized loss of sensitivity to chroma, more difficulty in distinguishing adjacent hues, or loss of sensitivity for spectrally extreme hues. Knoblauch and Arditi (1994) give guidelines for colour usage for people with low vision which have been adapted as below. These principles can be applied to young visually impaired children or multiply challenged people who cannot respond to a colour vision test reliably.

1. Optimize the luminance contrast, i.e. use a light colour such as yellow with a dark colour such as dark red. We find that most people can understand this concept.
2. Choose dark colours from the spectral extremes (e.g. reds and blues) with light mid-spectral colours (e.g. green, yellow or orange).
3. Avoid white or grey against any colour of similar lightness.
4. Avoid colours from adjacent parts of the spectrum.
5. Avoid using pastel colours together (one pastel and one saturated colour may be acceptable).

A simple information sheet with some good and bad examples of colour contrast could be prepared and given to parents/teachers.

LEGAL AND ETHICAL ISSUES

It seemed to us to be important for this book to include some discussion of legal and ethical issues in optometric work with children. We have attempted to compile some general guidelines, although producing these has not been easy given our intended international readership (who will therefore be practising under various jurisdictions) and the sparsity of attention given to ethics in the optometric literature (Spafford and Strong, 1995). In fact, a literature search on legal and/or ethical issues with regard to children's optometric care revealed nothing. We have therefore drawn on other areas of professional practice such as medicine and psychology as well as material specific to optometry but with the adult population. We have included legal material from the USA and from Commonwealth countries, but it is not intended to provide an exhaustive coverage: rather, our intention is merely to raise an awareness of some relevant legal issues.

Ethics

Ethics is concerned with rules governing right and wrong conduct. It is usually distinguished from conduct determined by law, although professionals inevitably have to weigh up both ethical and legal issues in determining how to behave. Professional associations frequently draw up codes of practice for members and although these can be helpful it has also to be recognized that they may be drawn up in some ignorance of systems of ethics (McConkey, 1995). Absolute adherence to such a code may not always be right (Davidson, 1995) and a professional may find that the values encompassed in such a code may at times conflict with those held by society at large (Spafford and Strong, 1995) or by him or herself (Davidson, 1995). Furthermore, it is not always clear whether a particular professional code of conduct is binding or represents ideal standards to which members should aspire (Spafford and Strong, 1995), and particular issues of concern (such as working with children) may be omitted.

It is commonly thought that optometrists are increasingly likely to face ethical dilemmas. Some which may have occurred to readers at various points in this book are: How far do you push a child who objects to testing? Is it right to refuse services to those with intellectual impairments? If a parent is not patching a child who has amblyopia what is your obligation to the child? What do you do if you discover that a child has been given an inappropriate prescription by a colleague?

Rest (1983) has described four processes underlying ethical behaviour which may guide the professional faced with an ethical dilemma.

1. Be sensitive to the needs of others.
2. Engage in moral reasoning when a course of action is being contemplated.
3. Decide what values are most important in a moral dilemma.
4. Execute and implement a plan of action.

This approach stands independently of particular value systems, and it has been suggested that this is the way ethics should be taught, i.e. through a problem-solving approach with a background of ethical theory rather than through the imposition of any particular value system. However, we do not claim to have written a handbook which is value-free, as we espouse the rights of children (including those with disabilities) to high quality vision care – this assumes a rights-based ethic.

A distinction needs to made here between human rights and legal rights. The United Nations, in 1973, listed children's human rights, specifying that the best interests of the child (not the parents or other adults) should guide the formulation of legislation. Although this principle may be acceptable in many cultures it is not universally acceptable; this may be why the United Nations Convention on the Rights of the Child (1989) omitted any reference to the *priority* of children (Last, 1994), although the rights of children (including those with disabilities) to adequate health care are clearly expressed. Ideally, human and legal rights should correspond (Gelfand, Jenson and Drew, 1988, p. 441) but may not do so in reality. A 'bill of rights' for children in psychotherapy has been suggested (Koocher, 1976), and we propose that it may be considered equally applicable to the optometric context. It proposes, briefly, that a child has the right:

1. to be told the truth
2. to be treated as a person
3. to be taken seriously
4. to participate in decision-making.

Consent

The child's right to participate in decision-making has been assumed throughout this book but, from a legal standpoint, is it ultimately the child or the parent who consents to treatment? The topic of consent in paediatric contexts is fraught with difficulty. This is illustrated by the fact that a statement on consent and related issues was first presented to the American Academy of Pediatrics in 1985, but not published until 1995, after 10 years of amendments and re-presentations (AAP Committee on Bioethics, 1995). Consent is generally less of a burning issue in optometry than in fields such as paediatric medicine and psychological therapy given that optometric procedures are relatively innocuous. However, there is a trend towards the use of more procedures which are mildy invasive (Abplanalp, 1994), so issues of consent (and, more specifically, informed consent) may be increasingly of concern in optometry. In any event, it should be noted that any practitioner–client physical contact requires consent although in the case of relatively non-invasive procedures consent will invariably be implied rather than expressly given.

Age of consent may be established by law. For example, in England and Wales, the law presumes that 16 and 17 year olds, even though they have not reached the age of majority, can consent to surgical, medical or dental treatment without the need for reference to parents (*Family Law Reform Act,* 1969, section 8). Surgical, medical or dental treatment includes any diagnostic procedures and any procedures ancillary to treatment. Although optometric procedures are not expressly mentioned it will be noted that the definition is inclusive, which means that it is open to the interpretation that it does include optometric procedures.

Again in England and Wales, a person of 15 years or under may also give consent without reference to parents (or even in the face of express parental prohibition) if they are of 'sufficient understanding and intelligence to enable him or her to understand fully what is proposed' (*Gillick v West Norfolk and Wisbech Area Health Authority* [1986] AC 112). This has become known as 'Gillick competence'. This issue was clouded for a while by legal decisions which implied that a child whose competence was in doubt would be competent to consent to treatment but incompetent to refuse treatment (Devereux, Jones and Dickenson, 1993). It would now appear, however, that the right to consent includes the right to refuse. Recent legislation in Ontario, Canada, adopts similar principles.

In the Gillick case, Lord Scarman suggested a procedure for enabling a professional to comply with the law in the case of a child of 15 or under.

1. Persuade child to bring parents to consultation.
2. If child refuses to bring parents, only treat if 'Gillick competent' (if child is not so competent, parental consent must be sought).
3. Even if not so competent, can proceed in case of emergency, parental neglect, abandonment of child or other circumstances where reasonable to do so (see also Chapter 3 for discussion of child abuse and neglect).

In judging whether a child is capable of giving consent, a New Zealand author (Grant, 1991) has commented on the importance of an understanding of developmental psychology (especially cognitive development) and of communication skills. Good communication skills are also essential to ensure that *informed* consent is given, whether by child or parent. Even if the parent is the one who is legally giving consent, it is still desirable from an ethical point of view that the child understands and participates as much as possible, given the children's rights listed earlier and the fact that children are more likely to co-operate with procedures and interventions when they have been fully involved (Chapter 3).

Legal liability

By and large, the risks of facing litigation seem to be relatively low for optometrists given the nature of their work. Even the legalization of the use of therapeutic drugs by optometrists in some jurisdictions has resulted in few drug-related malpractice claims against optometrists in comparison with ophthalmologists (Classe, 1992a). However, several topics have received attention from a legal liability point of view and have the potential to be relevant in the case of children (they may also involve an ethical dimension). These topics include contact lens use, pupillary dilation, sports vision, traumatic eye injury, the need to advise, access to records and confidentiality.

Contact lenses are the major area for litigation in optometry in the USA. According to Classe (1994a), negligence is most often alleged, but informed consent and product liability may also be used as the basis for damages claims. For daily-wear clients, claims may be based on non-approved use of lenses or solutions, monovision contact lenses, negligence by a technician, failure to verify lenses before dispensing, mismanagement of corneal abrasions and inadequate monitoring of ocular health. For extended-wear clients, sources of claims include inappropriate client selection, inadequate client training, improper wearing schedules, improper management of corneal complications and inadequate monitoring of ocular health. Classe (1991), with particular reference to extended-wear lenses, advises adequate communication with the client and a systematic programme of examination and follow-up. Informed consent requirements obligate practitioners to document instructions, findings, warnings and recall examinations.

Pupillary dilation is a controversial issue, even in jurisdictions where optometrists are permitted to use it, because of the risk of angle-closure glaucoma, systemic side-effects and client inconvenience (Bartlett and Classe, 1992). Failure to warn of common and expected side-effects may create liability (Classe, 1992b). Premises liability may apply if a client is injured as a result of unclear vision after pupillary dilation (Gold and Classe, 1991). Also noteworthy is the fact that the US Court of Appeals found an optometrist to be negligent for failing to carry out a dilated fundus examination, which resulted in a 4-year-old girl being treated for accommodative esotropia while her retinoblastoma went undetected (Harris, 1995).

Sportspeople have brought claims after suffering ocular injury from lenses or frames, alleging that they were defective or that the practitioner was negligent. An adequate history of sports involvement should be taken and, when there is a reasonable risk of injury, polycarbonate lenses and frames meeting adequate standards should be prescribed (Classe, 1993a).

Occasionally, the optometrist is approached for care of a traumatic eye injury. Although he or she may be under no legal obligation to provide such care, an ethical obligation may be involved (Classe, 1993b). Timely referral, if needed, should be made, and the case details documented. As practitioners may be liable for employee acts or omissions, receptionists should be trained to determine the urgency of such cases.

Finally, the optometrist needs to consider whether a child has a problem which merits giving advice to return for follow-up evaluations or treatment if symptoms persist or become worse, in order to to avoid being sued for negligence, as has happened in the medical arena (Harris, 1991).

Records and confidentiality

Optometrists should be aware of any laws relating to client (and parental) access to information in records, trends being in the direction of open access. For example, in the USA, clients have access except under extraordinary circumstances, but the obligation to release contact lens prescriptions is limited to 17 states (Classe, 1994b).

Glossing over the fact that confidentiality is a confused and confusing concept (McMahon and Knowles, 1995), it is generally accepted that client records should be confidential. Cases where parents insist on being given information which a child does not want released are, we believe, unlikely to arise in optometry. Divorced parents who have joint custody are equally entitled to information about their child. In fact, in some jurisdictions, even a non-custodial parent may have an equal right in terms of information and decision-making. This became the case in Australia in 1996, with the old concepts of custody and access being replaced by notions of joint parenting; although this is a worthy ideal it has the potential to place professionals in some difficult situations when the parents cannot co-operate and have different views about their child's medical treatment.

Frequently, the optometrist may consider that the disclosure of clinical information to others, such as teachers, would benefit the child, and permission should be sought from parents for this. An exception is if the optometrist suspects that a child has been abused (for example, from ocular examination evidence), when there may be not just an ethical, but a legal, obligation to disclose the suspicion to the relevant authority (Chapter 3). In this case confidentiality is overruled.

Conclusions: guidelines for dealing with ethical and legal issues

1. Keep up with the literature on the ethical dimensions of optometric practice as these are becoming a matter of debate and concern.
2. When faced with an ethical dilemma, take a problem-solving approach. Consulting with colleagues may be helpful.
3. Be aware of any legal issues surrounding optometry in the jurisdiction where you practice, including informed consent and mandatory reporting of suspected child abuse. Local professional associations may be the best source of advice given the variations that exist between countries and states/provinces.
4. Be aware of any practice guidelines/codes of conduct laid down by your professional association. However, also be aware that in legal cases higher standards of care may be applied, so professional codes are not guaranteed to protect you in the case of claims. Entire professions can be found to be acting negligently.
5. Consider the 'bill of rights' for child clients.
6. Develop good communication with child and parents.
7. Warn of possible drawbacks of proposed courses of action and advise clients to return if symptoms persist or worsen.
8. Maintain thorough documentation of care, including information and warnings given.
9. Retain records for at least several years after child clients reach the age of majority so they have the opportunity to access their own records (Koocher, 1995). Also take into account any express

legal requirements for retaining documents and limitation periods for negligence/assault cases to be brought.
10. Maintain insurance cover and seek legal advice as necessary.

CONCLUSION

We have devoted most of this book to outlining the development of various visual functions, based on recent research evidence, and to describing ways in which eye care practitioners (optometrists in particular) can assess these functions and check the ocular health of infants and children, using a clinical problem-solving approach. We have seen that a certain amount of creativity and flexibility is needed in order to work effectively with children. In this final chapter we have addressed the question of clinical decision-making on the basis of assessment information. Topics covered have included: prescribing spectacles; managing ocular deviations and low vision; and communicating findings effectively, both in a face-to-face clinical situation and through report-writing. We have also sought to create an awareness of some of the ethical and legal issues which impinge upon children's vision care as these seem to have been given little attention elsewhere.

Overall in this handbook we have sought to create an understanding, amongst those new to child vision care, of the vital role of

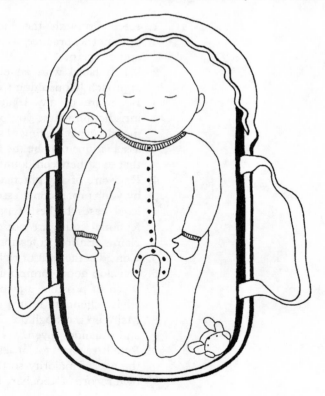

eye professionals in the early months and years of children's lives. The sensitive provision of high quality services to children and families is crucial in order to give all children the best chance of maintaining their visual potential and of using vision effectively in the fulfilment of their developmental tasks in childhood and throughout life.

REFERENCES

Abplanalp, P. (1994). Informed consent as an ethical issue in modern optometry. *Journal of the American Optometric Association,* **65** (5), 347–354.

American Academy of Ophthalmology (1994). Basic and clinical science course in *Pediatric Ophthalmology and Strabismus,* 1994–1995.

American Academy of Pediatrics, Committee on Bioethics (1995). Informed consent, parental permission, and assent in pediatric practice. *Pediatrics,* **95** (2), 314–317.

Atkinson, J. (1993). Infant vision screening: prediction and prevention of strabismus and amblyopia from refractive screening in the Cambridge photorefraction programme. In K. Simons (ed.), *Early Visual Development, Normal and Abnormal.* Oxford, Oxford University Press. pp. 335–348.

Atkinson, J. Braddick, O., Bobier, B. et al. (1996). Two infant vision screening programmes: prediction and prevention of strabismus and amblyopia from photo- and videorefractive screening. *Eye,* **10,** 189–198.

Bailey, I. (1980). Combining accommodation with spectacle additions. *Optometry Today,* **71,** 93–95.

Baldwin, W.R., West, D., Jolly, J., and Reid, W. (1969). Effects of contact lenses on refractive corneal and axial length changes in young myopes. *American Journal of Optometry and Archives of American Academy of Optometry,* **46,** 903–911.

Barraga, N. (1964). *Increased Visual Behavior in Low Vision Children.* New York, American Foundation for the Blind.

Barraga, N.C. (1970). *Teachers' Guide for Development of Visual Learning Abilities and Utilization of Low Vision.* Louisville, Kentucky, American Printing House for the Blind.

Barraga, N.C. and Collins, M.E. (1979). Development of efficiency in visual functioning: Rationale for a comprehensive program. *Journal of Visual Impairment and Blindness,* **73,** 121–126.

Barraga, N.C., Collins, M. and Hollis, J. (1977). Development of efficiency in visual functioning: A literature analysis. *Journal of Visual Impairment and Blindness,* **71,** 387–391.

Bartlett, J.D. and Classe, J.G. (1992). Dapripazole: will it affect the standard of care for pupillary dilation? *Optom. Clin.,* **2** (4), 113–120.

Bier and Lowther, G.E. (1986). Myopia control study: Effect of different contact lens refractive corrections on the progression of myopia. *AOA Proceedings,* December.

Brent, H. (1983). Contact lenses. In J.S. Crawford and D.J. Morin (eds), *The Eye in Childhood.* New York, Grune & Stratton.

Ciuffreda, K.J. (1991). Accommodation and its anomalies. In N. Charman (ed.), *Vision and Visual Dysfunction, Vol.1. Visual Optics and Instrumentation.* Ann Arbor: CRC Press.

Clarke, K.L., Sainato, D.M. and Ward, M.E. (1994). Travel performance of preschoolers: The effects of mobility training with a long cane versus a precane. *Journal of Visual Impairment and Blindness,* **88,** 19–30.

Classe, J.G. (1991). Liability for extended-wear contact lenses. *Optom. Clin.,* **1** (3), 51–62.

Classe, J.G. (1992a). Liability and ophthalmic drug use. *Optom. Clin.,* **2** (4), 121–134.

Classe, J.G. (1992b) Pupillary dilation: an eye-opening problem. *Journal of the American Optometric Association,* **63** (10), 733–741.

Classe, J.G. (1993a). Legal aspects of sports vision. *Optom. Clin.,* **3** (1), 27–32.

Classe, J.G. (1993b). Legal aspects of management of ocular trauma. *Optom. Clin.,* **3** (2), 103–113.

Classe, J.G. (1994a). Avoiding liability in contact lens practice. *Optom. Clin.,* **4** (1), 1–12.

Classe, J.G. (1994b). Management of contact lens prescriptions. *Optom. Clin.,* **4** (1), 93–102.

Davidson, G. (1995). The ethics of confidentiality. *Australian Psychologist,* **30,** 153–157.

Davis, H.D. (1993). *Counselling Parents of Children with Chronic Illness or Disability*. Leicester, The British Psychological Society.

Deller, M. (1988). Why should surgery for early-onset strabismus be postponed? *British Journal of Ophthalmology*, **72**, 110–115.

Devereux, J.A., Jones, D.P. and Dickenson, D.L. (1993). Can children withhold consent to treatment? *British Medical Journal*, **306**(6890), 1459–1461.

Duckman, R.H. (1984). Accommodation in cerebral palsy: Function and remediation. *Journal of the American Optometric Association*, **55**, 281–283.

Evans, B.J.W. (1997). Coloured filters and reading difficulties: a continuing controversy. *Optometry and Vision Science*, **74**, 239–240.

Evans, B.J.W., Wilkins, A.J., Brown, J., Busby, A. and Wingfield, A. (1996). A preliminary investigation into the aetiology of the Meares–Irlen syndrome. *Ophthalmic and Physiological Optics*, **16**, 286–296.

Family Law Reform Act, 1969, s.8. UK.

Faye, E.E. (1984). *Clinical Low Vision*. 2nd edn. Boston, Little, Brown.

Faye, E., Padula, W., Padula, J. et al. (1984). The low vision child. In E.E. Faye (ed.), *Clinical Low Vision*. Boston, Little, Brown.

Gasson and Morris (1997). *Contact Lens Manual*, 2nd edn. Oxford, Butterworth-Heinemann.

Gelfand, D.M., Jenson, W.R. and Drew, C.J. (1988). *Understanding Child Behavior Disorders*. New York, Holt, Rinehart and Winston.

Gillick v West Norfolk and Wisbech Area Health Authority, AC 112 (House of Lords, 1986).

Gold, A.R. and Classe, J.G. (1991). Premises liability. *Journal of the American Optometric Association*, **62** (10), 772–775.

Grant, V.J. (1991). Consent in paediatrics: a complex teaching assignment. *Journal of Medical Ethics*, **17** (4), 199–204.

Groenendaal, F. and van Hof-van Duin, J. (1992). Visual deficits and improvements in children after perinatal hypoxia. *Journal of Visual Impairment and Blindness*, **86**, 215–218.

Gwiazda, J., Thorn, F., Bauer, J. and Held, R. (1993). Emmetropization and the progression of manifest refraction in children followed from infancy to puberty. *Clinical Vision Science*, **8**, 337–344.

Haegerstrom-Portnoy, G., Schneck, M.E., Verdon, W.A. and Hewlett, S.E. (1996). Clinical vision characteristics of the congenital achromatopsias. 1. Visual acuity, refractive error and binocular status. *Optometry and Vision Science*, **73**, 446–456.

Harris, M.G. (1991). Failure to advise. *Journal of the American Optometric Association*, **62** (11), 867–869.

Harris, M.G. (1995). The five legal doctrines for dilating your patients. *Review of Optometry*, **132** (9), 90–93.

Hill, J.L. (1987). Rights of low vision children and their parents. *Canadian Journal of Optometry*, **49**, 78–83.

Hokada, S.C. and Ciuffreda, K.J. (1982). Measurement of accommodation amplitude in amblyopia. *Ophthalmic and Physiological Optics*, **2**, 205–212.

Ing, M.R. (1983). Early surgical alignment for congenital esotropia. *Journal of Pediatric Ophthalmology and Strabismus*, **20**, 11–18.

Ingram, R.M., Arnold, P.E., Dally, S. and Lucas, J. (1990). Results of a randomised trial of treating abnormal hypermetropia from age of 6 months. *British Journal of Ophthalmology*, **74**, 158–159.

Ingram, R.M., Arnold, P.E., Dally, S. and Lucas, J. (1991). Emmetropisation, squint, and reduced acuity after treatment. *British Journal of Ophthalmology*, **75**, 414–416.

Jan, J.E. and Groenveld, M. (1993). Visual behaviours and adaptations associated with cortical and ocular impairment in children. *Journal of Visual Impairment and Blindness*, **87**, 101–105.

Kalloniatis, M. and Johnston, A.W. (1990). Color vision characteristics of visually impaired children. *Optometry and Vision Science*, **67**, 166–168.

Karnes, M.B. and Teskla, J.A. (1980). Toward successful parent involvement in programs for handicapped children. *New Directions for Exceptional Children*, **4**, 85–111.

Klein, R. (1979). Public opinion and the National Health Service. *British Medical Journal*, **1**, 1296–1297.

Knoblauch, K. and Arditi, A. (1994). Choosing color contrasts in low vision: Practical recommendations. In A.C. Kooijiman et al. (eds), *Low Vision Research and New Developments in Rehabilitation*. Amsterdam, IOS Press, pp. 199–203.

Koocher, G.P (1976). A bill of rights for children in psychotherapy. In G.P. Koocher (ed.), *Children's Rights and the Mental Health Professions*. New York, Wiley.

Koocher, G.P. (1995). Confidentiality in psychological practice. *Australian Psychologist*, **30** (3), 158–163.

Last, M. (1994). Putting children first. *Disasters*, **18**, 192–202.

Leat, S.J., North, R.V. & Bryson, H. (1990). Do long wavelength pass filters improve low vision performance? *Ophthalmic & Physiological Optics*, **10**, 219–224.

Leguire, L.E., Fellows, R.R., Rogers, G.L. et al. (1992). The CCH vision stimulation program for infants with low vision: Preliminary results. *Journal of Visual Impairment and Blindness*, **86**, 33–37.

Lewis, T.L., Maurer, D. and Brent, H. (1995). Development of grating acuity in children treated for unilateral and bilateral congenital cataract. *Investigative Ophthalmology & Visual Science*, **36**, 2080–2095.

Ley, P. (1988). *Communicating with Patients*. London, Croom Helm.

Linstedt, E. (1986). Early vision assessment in visually impaired children at TRC, Sweden. *Br. J. Vis. Imp.*, **IV**, 49–51.

Mayer, D.L., Fulton, A.B. and Rodier, D. (1984). Grating and recognition acuities of pediatric patients. *Ophthalmology*, **91**, 947–953.

McConkey, K. (1995). Hypnosis, ethics and the ethics of uncertainty. *Australian Psychologist*, **30**, 1–10.

Mc Mahon, M. and Knowles, A. (1995). Confidentiality in professional practice: A decrepit concept? *Australian Psychologist*, **30**, 164–168.

Miles, T.R. (1988). Counselling in dyslexia. *Counselling Psychology* Quarterly, **1**, 97–107.

Millodot, M. and Millodot, S. (1989). Presbyopia correction and the accommodation in reserve. *Ophthalmic and Physiological Optics*, **9**, 126–132.

Nathan, J., Kiely, P.M., Crewther, S.G. and Crewther, D.P. (1985). Disease-associated visual image degradation and spherical refractive errors in children. *American Journal of Optometry and Physiological Optics*, **62**, 680–688.

von Noorden, G.K. (1996). *Binocular Vision and Ocular Motility. Theory and Management of Strabismus*. St. Louis/Baltimore/Toronto, Mosby.

Overbury, O., Goodrich, G.L., Quillman, R.D. and Faubert, J. (1989). Perceptual assessment in low vision: Evidence for a hierarchy of skills. *Journal of Visual Impairment and Blindness*, **83**, 109–113.

Pantell, R.H., Stewart, T.J., Dias, J.K. et al. (1982). 'Physician communication with children and parents', *Pediatrics*, **70**, 396–401.

Prior, M. (1996). *Understanding Specific Learning Difficulties*. Hove, Psychology Press.

Project IVEY: Increasing Visual Efficiency (1983). *A Resource Manual for the Development and Evaluation of Special Programs for Exceptional Students*. Volume V-E, Tallahassee, Florida, Florida Department of Education.

Ravault, A.P., Bongrand, M. and Bonamour, G. (1972). The utilization of prisms in the treatment of divergent strabismus. In *Orthoptics. Proceedings of the Second International Orthoptics Congress*, Amsterdam, Excerpta Medica Foundation, p.77.

Rest, J.R. (1983). Morality. In P. Mussen (ed.), *Carmichael's Manual of Child Psychology*. New York, Wiley.

Ritchie, J.P., Sonksen, P.M. and Gould, E. (1989). Low vision aids for preschool children. *Developmental Medicine and Child Neurology*, **31**, 509–519.

Rosner, J. and Gruber, J. (1985). Differences in the perceptual skills of young myopes and hyperopes. *Clinical and Experimental Optometry*, **69**, 166–168.

Rosner, J. and Rosner, J. (1987). Comparison of visual characteristics in children with and without learning difficulties. *American Journal of Optometry and Physiological Optics*, **64**, 531–533.

Rosner, J. and Rosner, J. (1990). *Pediatric Optometry*. 2nd edn. Boston, Butterworths.

Shute, R.H. (1991a). *Psychology in Vision Care*. Oxford, Butterworth-Heinemann.

Shute, R.H. (1991b). Treating dyslexia with tinted lenses: A review of the evidence. *Research in Education*, **46**, 39–48.

Shute, R.H. and Woodhouse, J.M. (1990). Visual fitness to drive after stroke or head injury. *Ophthalmic & Physiological Optics*, **10**, 327–332.

Sloan, L. and Habel, A. (1973). Problems in prescribing reading additions for partially-sighted children. *American Journal of Ophthalmology*, **75**, 1023–1035.

Spafford, M.M. and Strong, G. (1995). Design elements of professional ethics courses. *Optometry and Vision Science*, **72**, 10, 1–12.

Stein, J.F. and Fowler, M.S. (1985). Effects of monocular occlusion on visuomotor perception and reading in dyslexic children. *Lancet*, **ii**, 69–73.

Stone, J. (1976). The possible influence of contact lenses on myopia. *British Journal of Physiological Optics*, **31**, 89–114.

Tavernier, G.G.F. (1993). The improvement of vision by vision stimulation and training: A review of the literature. *Journal of Visual Impairment and Blindness*, **87**, 143–148.

United Nations General Assembly (1973). United Nations declaration of the rights of children. In: A. Wilkerson (ed.), *The Rights of Children: Emergent Concepts in Law and Society*. Philadelphia, Temple University Press.

United Nations (1989). *Convention on the Rights of the Child*. UN secretariat, Centre for Human Rights.

Whittaker, S.G. and Lovie-Kitchin, J. (1993). Visual requirements for reading. *Optometry and Vision Science*, **70**, 54–65.

Wilkins, A. (1994). Overlays for classroom and optometric use. *Ophthalmic & Physiological Optics*, **14**, 97–99.

Wilkins, A.J., Evans, B.J.E., Brown, J.A. et al. (1994). Double-masked placebo-controlled trial with precision spectral filters in children who use coloured overlays. *Ophthalmic & Physiological Optics*, **14**, 365.

Woo, G.C. and Wilson, M.A. (1990). Current methods of treating and preventing myopia. *Optometry and Vision Science*, **67**, 719–727.

Youngson-Reilly, S., Tobin, M.J. and Fielder, A.R. (1995). Multidisciplinary teams and childhood visual impairment: A study of two teams. *Child: Care, Health and Development*, **21** (1), 3–15.

Appendix 14.1

Reporting form used for children with visual impairments based on that developed by the Center for Sight Enhancement, School of Optometry, University of Waterloo, Waterloo, Ontario, Canada, N2L 3G1, and reproduced with their consent (N.B. slightly different forms are used for adults with low vision and for children with additional impairments). The form is carbonized paper, with the explanation of visual acuity terms on the reverse. The conversion from Imperial to metric is given as Imperial measures are still commonly known due to the proximity of the USA where the Imperial system is still in use. In many countries this conversion would not be necessary.

REPORT OF LOW VISION ASSESSMENT

Date of examination:

Child's Name: _____ Date of Birth: /   /

Ocular Diagnosis:

Issues Identified

☐ Reading   ☐ Functional assessment   ☐ Glare
☐ Writing   ☐ Hobbies/recreation   ☐ Boardwalk
☐ Mobility   ☐ Computer access   ☐ Other _____

Examination Results

Distance visual acuity: Right eye: _____ Left eye: _____
                              Both eyes: _____

☐ With present glasses   ☐ Without glasses

Detects lines of _____ cm. Pictures/letters should consist of lines at least three times this width.

Near visual acuity: Right eye: _____ Left eye: _____ Both eyes: _____

☐ With present glasses   ☐ Without glasses

Refraction: ☐ Myopia   ☐ Hyperopia
             ☐ Astigmatism   ☐ No significant refractive error

☐ No improvement in VA. Visual acuity improves to: R. eye: _____
                                                    L. eye: _____

Binocularity: ☐ No strabismus   ☐ Strabismus

Fixational status: ☐ Roving eye movements   ☐ Steady
                    ☐ Nystagmus: position of null point _____

Colour vision: ☐ Normal ☐ Abnormal _____

Visual fields: ☐ Full Constricted to _____ ☐ Central Defect

Additional information: _____
_____
_____

Recommendations

☐ New distance spectacles to be worn: ☐ Constantly
                                       ☐ As necessary   ☐ For distance only

☐ Reading spectacles/bifocals

☐ Magnifier

☐ Telescope

☐ Tinted spectacles for glare control to be worn: ☐ Outdoors
                                                   ☐ Indoors ☐ Constantly

☐ Place visual material to (position) _____

☐ Train in preferential looking before next assessment in _____
   months time

☐ Vision resource teacher recommended

☐ High contrast materials

☐ Vision stimulation programme

☐ Uncluttered visual material

☐ Closed circuit TV/Assesment for computer access

☐ Electro-diagnostic testing

☐ Other _____

Additional comments _____

(The following explanations of visual acuity should accompany the above form.)

Visual Acuity is a measure of the smallest detail that the eye can distinguish. Normally, visual acuity is tested using letters, numbers, or pictures of different sizes that are shown from a certain distance. The result is written as a fraction; for example 6/12, 6/6, etc. The upper number is the test distance, usually 6 metres (20 feet), and the lower number is the distance from which the normally sighted eye could see the same sized letter. Clinical low vision specialists regularly use a 3 metre distance, but these results can easily be converted to the more conventional format by multiplying both parts of the fraction by two; for example, 3/30 is the same as 6/60. Metric results can be converted to the older Imperial system using the table below.

Distance visual acuity equivalents

Imperial	Metric	Imperial	Metric
20/700	6/210	20/80	6/24
20/600	6/180	20/63	6/19
20/400	6/120	20/60	6/18
20/350	6/105	20/50	6/15
20/300	6/90	20/40	6/12
20/225	6/67.5	20/32	6/9.5
20/200	6/60	20/30	6/9
20/180	6/54	20/25	6/7.5
20/160	6/48	20/20	6/6
20/140	6/42	20/16	6/4.8
20/125	6/38	20/12.5	6/3.8
20/120	6/36	20/10	6/3
20/100	6/30		

Near visual acuity equivalents. Near visual acuity is usually recorded as the minimum size of print that could be read at a specified distance. In order to read at twice that distance, the print would have to be twice the size. Individuals are most comfortable reading print which is larger than this minimum size. We normally recommend that for fluent reading the print size should be at least twice this minimum size at any distance.

M Notation 40 cm	Reduced Snellen 40 cm	Point 40 cm	J Notation 40 cm (Jaeger)	N Notation[*] 40 cm	Common Usages
.4	40/40	3	—	3	Medicine bottle labels
.5	40/50	4	1	4	Stock market print
.6	40/60	5	2	5	Footnotes
.8	40/80	6	3	6	Telephone directories
1.0	40/100	8	5	8	Small column newsprint
1.2	40/120	9	7	10	Typing
1.6	40/160	12	10	13	Books ages 9 to 12
2.0	40/200	14	—	16	Computer display (80 column)
2.5	40/250	18	12	20	Books ages 7 to 8
3.0	40/300	—	14	24	Large print books
4.0	40/400	24	15	32	Subheadlines
8.0	40/800	—	16	65	Newspaper headlines

[*] Times Roman print.

Index